# The Wild Rainbow

*Journeying as Woman, Mother and Sage Femme*

**Sheree Stewart**

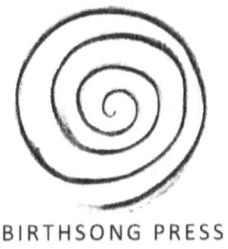

BIRTHSONG PRESS

2013 Birthsong Press, Melbourne

© Copyright Sheree Stewart 2013
© Copyright in individual pieces remains with the attributed authors

All rights reserved. No part of this book may be reproduced, stored or transmitted in any form, or by any means, electronic, mechanical, photocopying, recording or otherwise, without the written permission of the copyright owner.

Cover art © *Serpent Priestess* by Melissa Shemanna

The author gratefully acknowledges permission to reprint copyright material from the following:
*The spiritual practice of menstruation* by Jane Hardwicke Collings, Moonsong 2011, http://www.moonsong.com.au/spiritualmenstruation.html
*The Sacred Wound Exercise* by Jane Hardwicke Collings,
*Drumming During Pregnancy* by Jane Hardwicke Collings, Moonsong 2011, http://www.moonsong.com.au/drumming.html
*Meditation During Pregnancy* by Jane Hardwicke Collings, Moonsong 2011, http://www.moonsong.com.au/meditation.html
*Choosing Homebirth*, © Janet Fraser 2004 for Joyous Birth, joyousbirth.info
*Care of the Placenta*, by Shivam Rachana, Lotus Birth (2nd edition), Good Creation Publications, 2011
*The Placenta Garden*, by the author, first published in Lotus Birth (2nd edition) by Shivam Rachana, Good Creation Publications, 2011
*Medicinal Placenta Homeopathic Remedy* by Jane Hardwicke Collings, Moonsong 2011, http://www.moonsong.com.au/placental.html
*Breastfeeding, not special, just normal,* by Janet Fraser, Where Birth and Feminism Intersect, http://janetfraser.id.au/blog
*Alchemy of Midwifery and Women's Initiation,* a talk given by Shivam Rachana, Edited from International Homebirth Conference, Sydney University http://www.womenofspirit.asn.au/ArticlesAlchemyofMidwifery.htm
*Healing Birth, Healing the Earth* @ Dr Sarah J. Buckley MD 2005, published in *Gentle Birth, Gentle Mothering: A Doctor's Guide to Natural Childbirth and Gentle Early Parenting Choices* (Sarah J Buckley MD, Celestial Arts, 2009).

National Library of Australia Cataloguing-in-Publication :
    The wild rainbow : journeying as woman, mother and sage-femme
    / Sheree Stewart.

Dewey Number:   306.8743

    (1) Stewart, Sheree--Anecdotes. (2) Women--Anecdotes.
    (3) Mothers--Anecdotes. (4) Midwives--Anecdotes.

ISBN 978-0-646-90188-6 (paperback)

## *Dedication*

This book is dedicated to all of you

who dare to dream the impossible dream.

# Contents

| | |
|---|---|
| DEDICATION | i |
| CONTENTS | ii |
| ACKNOWLEDGEMENTS | v |
| FOREWORDS | |
|    Jane Hardwicke Collings | vi |
|    Shivam Rachana | viii |

## *Journeying as Woman*     1

| | |
|---|---|
| STAR BABIES | 2 |
| CHILDHOOD | 4 |
|    The Child of Light Who Lived In the Darkness. | 5 |
|    The Child of Magic. | 11 |
| RITUAL, LIFE, AWARENESS, WOMAN | 17 |
|    Ritual and celebration for our daughters reaching menarche | 22 |
|    Maiden Bleed Ceremony | 24 |
|    We welcomed a woman last night... | 30 |
| THE SPIRITUAL PRACTICE OF MENSTRUATION | 33 |
|    Some basic and stunning facts | 34 |
|    Ways to honour the menstrual cycle | 42 |
| WOMAN AND SELF LOVE | 48 |
|    Sisters | 52 |
|    Celebrating myself! | 53 |
|    Being a succulent wild woman | 56 |
| LOVER WOMAN | 57 |
|    Lilith | 57 |
|    Empowerment in sexuality as a mother | 64 |
|    Honouring my sexuality: this woman's story | 70 |
|    Living with an open heart | 75 |
|    Sheree and Steven: Real life love story | 78 |

| | |
|---|---|
| MOURNING WOMAN, WOUNDED WOMAN | 83 |
| The Descent of Inanna | 84 |
| My mourning | 90 |
| Eternal Love – a story of miscarriage | 100 |
| The One Who Steals the Innocent | 103 |
| WOMAN: HONOURING THE SACRED WOUND | 106 |
| The Wild Girl – A Sacred Wound Story | 107 |
| The Sacred Wound Exercise | 110 |

## *Journeying as Mother* — **115**

| | |
|---|---|
| MY WHIRLWIND, EXPLOSIVE, FAST RIDE INTO MOTHERHOOD | 116 |
| MY GENTLE BIRTHING & NEW WAYS OF BEING. | 121 |
| HONOURING THE MOTHER | 126 |
| Blessing Way Ceremonies | 127 |
| Monsterways and Letting go of fear | 136 |
| Overcoming Fear – the birth of Aaliyah | 140 |
| MAMATOTO CONNECTIONS | 144 |
| Dance | 145 |
| Journeying with the drum | 147 |
| Mandalas | 154 |
| Meditation During Pregnancy | 156 |
| PREGNANCY AND BIRTH | 161 |
| Birthing Rhiannon | 162 |
| Choosing Homebirth | 164 |
| Women Choosing Homebirth | 168 |
| Finding My Power -Bree's Home Birth After 2 Caesareans | 171 |
| Finding Your Birth Team – feeling safe and loved. | 176 |
| The Homebirth Of Lilith | 179 |
| For The Love Of Doulas | 183 |
| The Freebirth of Imogen | 185 |
| Siblings at Birth | 189 |
| PLACENTA | 193 |
| Lotus Birth | 194 |
| Ceremonies for the Placenta | 199 |
| Medicinal Placenta | 212 |

| | |
|---|---|
| **POST BIRTH** | **216** |
| The Early Daze. | 216 |
| Breastfeeding | 224 |
| Traversing the Underworld – my downward spiral with PND | 237 |
| Create Community | 244 |
| **JOURNEY OF THE WILD RAINBOW** | **248** |

## *Journeying as Sage Femme* — 265

| | |
|---|---|
| **FINDING THE MAGIC** | **266** |
| The Priestess | 266 |
| Alchemy of Midwifery and Women's Initiation | 271 |
| **MIDWIFE~MOTHER~WOMAN** | **275** |
| Rose Between Two Thorns | 279 |
| Big Dreamings | 282 |
| Ruby With A Red Bow – a story of adoption | 286 |
| Baby Lavender – the life and death of | 288 |
| Standing Together - a natural birth in a high risk ward | 291 |
| The Bright Eyed Baby and Me | 294 |
| **HEALING THE MOTHER WOUND** | **296** |
| Healing Birth, Healing the Earth | 299 |
| Myah's Birth – welcoming baby tiger | 308 |
| Taioma's Birth – welcoming baby bear | 312 |
| **TRAVELLING SAGE FEMME** | **319** |
| Ethiopia | 319 |
| Cambodia | 339 |
| Earth Midwife | 363 |
| **AFTERWORD** | **364** |
| **CONTRBUTORS** | **366** |
| **ABOUT THE AUTHOR** | **375** |

## *Acknowledgements*

I acknowledge my aboriginal ancestry – my tribes Wergaia and Wamba-Gourmanjanyuk. My totem animals – pelican, red crested black cockatoo, rainbow serpent and frog.

I acknowledge my Irish and English ancestry.

I acknowledge this planet I live on. She constantly keeps me alive, nourishing and inspiring me, encouraging me to always explore, learn and love.

I acknowledge 3 teachers who have been in my life and shifted my way of being in very big and real ways. Jane Hardwicke Collings, founder of The School Of Shamanic Midwifery, Denise Love a.k.a Mumma Doula, founder of LifeOptions, and Shivam Rachana, founder of The School of Spiritual Midwifery.

I acknowledge Melissa Shemanna, the incredible artist who has gifted me her sacred, powerful art to be the front cover of my book.

I acknowledge my Mother, Annie Joy, who carried me in her womb, birthed me and allowed me to grow into who I am today.

I acknowledge my brother Adam and my sister Kyana

I acknowledge my Rainbowtribe. My tribe of women whose hearts sing the same song as my own. They are the ones who will forever laugh, dance, cry, sing, rage and love with me.

I acknowledge my husband Steven. The one who continually encourages me to live my life to its fullest, who believes in me when I don't, who reminds me to dream the impossible dream.

I acknowledge my babies. My incredible 6 wild, fun, noisy, lovable babies. Caelan, Rhiannon, Aaliyah, Sage, Myah and Eli.

I acknowledge myself for being courageous and passionate enough to share my story.

## *Foreword*

This is a big story of a woman's brave journey through the dark and into the light and back again and again and again.

And this is the story of a woman who I know and love.

Sheree is a Rainbow Warrior.

She has travelled to the deepest places possible and returned with wisdom that she shares willingly, honestly and with love for us all, all her relations.

She bares everything, and her light shines and splinters into all the colours of the rainbow.

She invites us to answer for ourselves the questions she asked herself as she navigated the dark places, she helps us see our own rainbows.

Sheree's Australian Aboriginal ancestry brings another dimension to the story that needs to be told.

Sheree shares women's stories she has gathered of birth and death.

We hear about her own experiences of giving birth, her work in hospital, her work in the home, and her travels to third world countries.

Sheree is a woman of integrity and depth, she brings so much to her community and she is loved.

At the School of Shamanic Midwifery, a Women's Mystery School, we learn the art of midwifing the soul. Though various practices, processes and rituals and through bringing consciousness to menstruation, the cycles of the Earth, the Moon and our lives we can find a deeper understanding of the way of things. We bring back from the shadows the long lost story of the feminine, we reclaim feminine wisdom through reconnection with the Women's Mysteries. We re-member, put ourselves back together. For to be able to best serve others as a Shamanic Midwife, we must first do the 'work' on ourselves. We must uncover our fears, our predilections, our 'default' patterns and then we can bring choice to how we behave. Once we can do this, then we can serve others as the 'clear vessel', the 'hollow bone' and truly be of service to another's process rather than bring our personal agenda.

Sheree's story is an example of this. She takes us on her journey with deeply personal details through her wounds, her pain, her bliss and joy, and this, as it does, uncovers her passions and reveals her life purpose.

Sheree offers this pathway to the reader with her suggested questions for contemplation and through sharing her experiences of doing that.

I have sat in circle with Sheree in the Red Tent on many occasions and with her and her SiStars, we have co-created safe sacred spaces for each other and all our relations, "for healing, for insight, for happiness and for fun"….

When I light the Mother Candle on our central altar I give thanks that we all feel held and heard and healed, and then we share our stories.

Here, Dear Reader, is Sheree's story. May you too feel held and heard and healed.

Blessed Be

Jane Hardwicke Collings

March 2013

## *Foreword*

At time when many live with a sense of disconnection, where a population that is educated, well fed and well housed finds itself confronting epidemics like obesity, depression, diabetes, allergies and ever increasing mental illness and with pharmaceutical companies continuing to create more pills for a population that seems to be more and more in need of them, we need to look for cause rather than cure.

The primal time from conception to birth and into the first three years of life lays the foundations for our physical, mental, emotional and spiritual health. It is also the time when new families are established. The potency of this time of primal imprinting with its corresponding neurological development is largely unappreciated. We have strayed far from where nature requires us to be for optimal outcomes.

Few are born free of big phama's products coursing through their veins. Institutionalized rituals that impede the optimum situation for mothers and babies disrupt hormonal systems and deprive mothers of nature's tonic, those powerful hormones of birth, that ensure a happy transition to motherhood. Women are losing, nay have lost, the time-honoured knowledge of how to trust their bodies to give birth and fed their babies and instead are succumbing to the surgeon's knife and filling mother-baby clinics. Ever increasing numbers of little ones are away from their parents for ever increasing lengths of time in commercial 'care'.

We need conversations and examples about how it can be done differently.

This book is about Sheree Stewart's life as a mother and a midwife, as an adventurer and a devotee of living in the moment. It is a rollicking journey that is amusing, informative and generous in its sharing and unabashed honesty. This I find most refreshing and it makes you want to know what on earth she will be up to next.

There are many moving moments in this book and you will learn as you travel with Sheree and the other wise women who she has gathered together to share information and insights that will enrich your sense of yourself as a woman and encourage you to pay attention to aspects of your life that you may have overlooked.

This book abounds with the experience of living consciously. Savouring each moment whether it is a birth in Cambodia, Ethiopia, a Melbourne hospital or in the sanctuary of home. Death is here too and the challenges of a hard road childhood.

Sheree writes well and her conversational manner of inclusiveness brings you along with her as she embraces and discovers the depth of connection that is available at the time of birth and in being a mother and a midwife. This is most nourishing for the reader.

At 30 years of age Sheree is a well -practiced mother of six children this in itself is an amazing attainment. She is also a registered midwife. And now she has produced this book. She has established her own authority and this is where she comes from and at the same time she is ever the student of life learning from those around her.

Her aboriginal heritage enables her to bridge the divide between the oldest civilization with their esoteric connection to the earth and it's rhythms and today's contemporary society that seeks that reconnection. Whilst this is a truly women's business book it is so obviously held and supported within the partnership with the support of the masculine. It is a love story.

I think that you will enjoy this book and be a better person for having taken the journey.

Shivam Rachana

March 2013

# Journeying as Woman

When sleeping women wake, mountains move.
Chinese Proverb

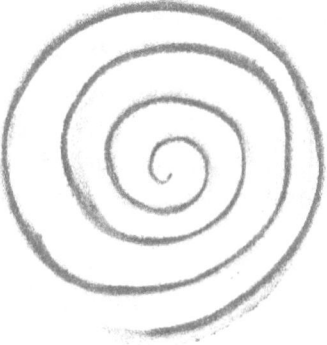

## *Star Babies*

When I was a Mother of 3, I overheard my 6 year old and my 4 year old have a conversation about when they lived in the stars and decided to incarnate to Earth.

> "I remember when we were Star Babies" said Caelan
>
> "Me too" said Rhiannon, "And we spun around like this"
>
> "Remember when we were deciding what was going to happen, Rhiannon?"
>
> "Yeah, you were coming first to be 'borned'"
>
> "Yeah and then you, Rhiannon, and then 3 more girls after you"
>
> "Yeah, and we take turns but I go first. I am the boy. I am strong. I always help"
>
> "Yeah, and we live with Mum and Dad. It was big in the stars wasn't it Caelan?"
>
> "Yeah, but that's because its space. It's where everything has to be before it can come here."
>
> "It's smaller here isn't it Caelan?"
>
> "Yeah"

Then their conversation ended and they were quiet for a short moment before they chatted about something else completely different. I felt my heart race in my chest. It was one of those moments where you know you are hearing a truth. In a single moment as I was walking passed their bedroom to put away some washing, my ears and heart just witnessed my 2 young children reveal a cosmic truth. We are all a part of something bigger than ourselves.

Journeying as Woman

*Nothing can stop us now, because we are all made of stars*

*-Moby*

I believe we all come from the stars. That we are all just stardust that has come together and formed this magnificent universe.

Even though we are completely our own entity, living our own lives, we are also connected to something else which is much bigger than ourselves.

It is all those fractals that make up that diamond. It is all those drops of water in the ocean that make an incredible world full of life, wonder and magic. It is all those individual leaves growing on the individual trees that make up a whole sustainable, life providing rainforest. If it wasn't for individual parts of these great things, then nothing would exist. Each of us matter. Each of us are so important, probably more than we would ever realise. We are all fractals in the diamond, and drops of water in the ocean. We are all the entire universe.

This book is my life. This is my contribution to that 'something bigger'. This is my fractal in the diamond.

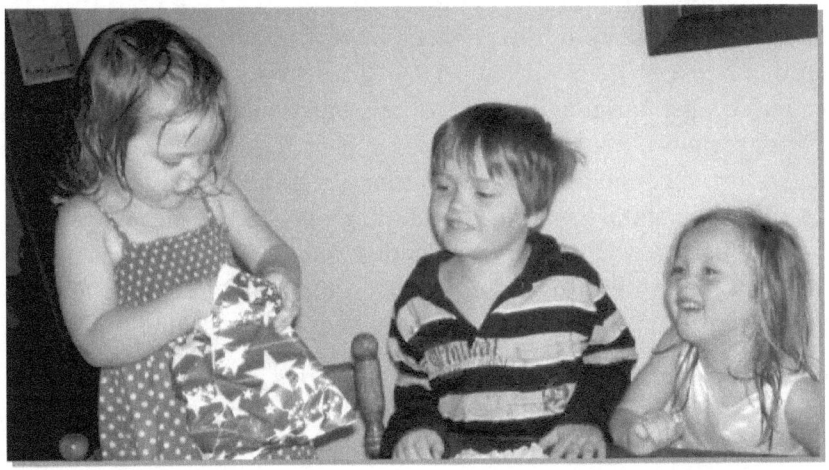

*"Star Babies"* - Photo: Steven Booth

## *Childhood*

When I think of my childhood, I feel as though I am living in 2 lives. Sometimes I remember the fun times: The times of sunshine, laughter and family. And sometimes I think of the times that make my heart sink: The times of violence, hatred and misunderstanding. When I try to explain my childhood to someone, I often feel as though I need to pick one story or the other, it's too hard to explain the love, laughter, violence, hatred, bliss and desperation to be part of one story, to make it a whole. So, here I have presented two stories. The first story is the story of my childhood as the wounded me. It is the story of my childhood where my heart was torn, where there were monsters lurking in the corners of my room, where you can't sleep at night because there are too many ghosts. The second story of my childhood is the one where I grow in sunlight, surrounded by beauty, love and adoration. I am the child that thrives, the child that sees her potential and is nurtured to pursue it.

None of my stories are better than the other. None of my stories are right or wrong. They are both my stories, and they are both true. This is the same for all of us. If we value our stories as a form of healing, as word medicine, then our hearts will be free and we will be less wounded, less burdened. We will feel validated, worthy and heard. Stories are word medicine in that it binds us together, even if we have never met. It connects us in a way that we feel deep inside more than we can understand or articulate. Telling our stories, no matter what they are unites us. It creates a collective, and we are woven as one in a grid of togetherness – we form understanding and compassion on a global level. Storytelling as medicine is its own special kind of magic.

Something beautiful I noticed about my stories is that with telling both sides of the same story, I ultimately end up on the right path, on the path of the heart, on the path where I win, and spiral, and become beautiful and whole. This is the path where I dream the impossible dream and ride with it.

## *The Child of Light Who Lived In the Darkness.*

There was so much violence. How could such a small town be full of so much hate? Why did everyone hurt each other? Why were everyone's eyes full of hate or sadness or bitterness or desperation?

How did I end up here? Was I in the wrong place? Was my incarnation faulty? Did something happen, a glitch in the matrix maybe, and I was stuck in the wrong place?

I was a small girl child with a heart full of compassion who felt every violent act that was laid upon another. My body constantly flinched as harsh words and drunken fists were thrown across the room. Most of the time, the hatred didn't make sense. It was alcohol and drugs. It was jealousy, rage, and self-loathing. These feelings were so all consuming to the perpetrator. It was vicious and poisonous and it gnawed the souls of many people who I loved.

One of the earliest memories I have of my life is of my father, bleary eyed and drunk with hate, trying to chop down the door to get to us in the bedroom with a small axe because he was angry of what Mum made for dinner.

He was a violent drunk and my Mum tried to keep us all safe by locking us in the bedroom together or driving us to our Nan and Pop's place. He once tried to set the house on fire with my Mother, brother and I inside. In a state of overwhelming rage, he tried to pull the water cooler out from the window to get

> *"Nature loves courage. You make the commitment and nature will respond to that commitment by removing impossible obstacles. Dream the impossible dream and the world will not grind you under, it will lift you up. This is the trick. This is what all these teachers and philosophers who really counted, who really touched the alchemical gold, this is what they understood. This is the shamanic dance in the waterfall. This is how magic is done. By hurling yourself into the abyss and discovering it's a feather bed."*
>
> — Terence McKenna

to where we were, but he lost his balance and he fell backwards with the water cooler on top of him, landing in the billabong. We just left him there moaning, muttering and swearing in the shallow water and drove to Nan's house. The next day when he was sober, he drove to Nan's with a bunch of flowers for Mum and said sorry. So we came back home.

My Dad once broke my Mum's nose by punching her in the face. I don't even know what the fight was about. As usual, it was probably about nothing. I just remember the blood and tears mixed together on her cheeks. I used to always tell Mum to move away. To just leave Dad. Even as a little girl around age 6 I remember telling her that we should just go away where we would all be happy. I remember thinking that it would be nice to not have to worry about violence when we were trying to sleep. I would dream of a little farm. A small white house, with a big verandah. We could set up for tea parties on the verandah and watch the sun go to bed every single night for the rest of our lives. We could live with some animals – chooks would be good, and some cats, a dog and twin lambs. We could live quietly and peacefully. I know she wanted to do this too. I know she wanted the courage to start a new life - One free from violence and disrespect, loneliness and alienation. I know she wanted to wake up in the morning and look into the eyes of a man that loved and respected her, that made her feel safe and supported. A man that valued her, and held her in his strong arms with admiration and deep love; a man that used his hands to love her, and not hurt her.

As a child I never knew why people stayed in situations that made them so sad. As an adult, I still don't fully understand but she tells me she did this because she loved him and she knew no other way to live. She loved the man he was when they first met. She loved the man who showed his gentle side in the moments he was sober. She loved the man who whisked her away from an unhealthy household and took her to what she thought was love and safety. In my heart I feel as though she put up with it because she felt like she deserved it and that this is the way that you live your life. She never knew deep love from any male figure in her life. She only ever knew subservience, powerlessness and lack of control. She was always controlled harshly by males and she had little self-worth or sense of self, so any male that showed at least some kindness was good enough for her for that is all she was taught she deserved.

It wasn't just my Dad that was violent. It seemed most of the males in my family were. We couldn't just get together as a family without the men fighting. And furthermore it wasn't even just my family, it was my community. My neighbours were violent and the people up the street were violent.

The men were violent to their wives and children and animals. The women were violent to their children and animals. The children were violent to the animals. It made the small growing heart in my chest weep. It was a deep wound witnessing cruelty being inflicted onto others. Why did they do that for? Why was there always blood spilled? Why did the men fight and the women cry? Why did everyone hurt each other? I hated it. Surely this isn't what life is about.

My life felt like I was always in fight or flight mode. Even now, I am able to wake up in heartbeat, ready for action in case I need to flee a dangerous situation. I can do it calmly, quickly, silently and easily.

When I was 10, we moved from our small Mallee town into the bigger town, 90kms away, for Dad's work. It was such a huge shift and one that changed my whole family forever. It was at this time in my life where I felt like my childhood had ended and I was beginning a new phase, with new challenges and new experiences unfolding in front of me. I was growing up, it was awkward, I had no friends, and I had no support. I feel as though that move was a big rip that tore our family apart even further, that left us all feeling stranded and separated in the middle of the big ocean, unable to swim, to reach the bottom or see any land from where we were thrown.

At 11 years old, my brother started seeing a counselor at school. He was awfully shy and such a gentle hearted kid. He had trouble making friends and he struggled with many aspects of his young life. At one point he mentioned to the counselor about Dad's behaviour. The next thing I knew, 2 adults came and took me out of my classroom to a police station and got me to make a statement against my Dad. I was so confused. This was so unexpected and I didn't know what to do. That day was the start of 18 months of my word against my brother's word against my mothers' word against my fathers' word. It was so stressful. I was so scared. I didn't want to be taken away from my mother or my brother. I wanted to stay with them.

* * *

When I hit puberty, I entered it alone. I felt full of embarrassment and awkwardness and I didn't know how to handle this 'growing up' part of me. As puberty came, I let my inner worlds shut down. I closed the gates to my magic kingdom. I started looking for friends, looking for others for answers. When I hit my teen years, I had no answers left inside me so I read the teenage magazines that tell you how to kiss boys and what shoes to wear. I barely had any friends and was often teased at school. Even when I tried to fit in, it didn't work. That part of me that was able to make light out of any situation was gone. The part of me that was able to easily escape the violence and heartache to an inner world of beauty and peace was gone. My magic was gone. I was so depressed. I had no control over anything. I developed an eating disorder that went on for years. I fell in love with someone who I thought loved me in return, but it turns out, they didn't even care. I had completely forgotten who I was. No matter what I did, I couldn't feel in control or sovereign of my own self. There was no spark, ritual or meaning to who I was as a person. I felt so blank, desolate and barren. I felt like I had nothing to offer – no spark in my eye, no dreams in my mind, no hope in my heart.

One day, after months of planning, I tried to kill myself. When I was on the edge of life and death, I called out to my Mum who somehow managed to hear me over the loud music that was playing in the sunroom of our home. In my faded, semi-conscious memory of it all, I thought that it was my Dad driving fast to the hospital with my head

> "It seems I am imaginary
>
> No one can see me
>
> You say that I have no meaning
>
> I've no insides to bare
>
> Am I just hollow space floating in the air?
>
> You say that I'm a liar
>
> I don't know what that means
>
> You say that I am nothing
>
> But nothing is what is seems"
>
> - - WRITTEN BY MY 15 YEAR OLD SELF.

was slumped on my mother's lap. I thought my uncle told me that I will be ok and that I'm a great kid. My brother wasn't there.

As it turned out, the story was slightly different to the story my mind had constructed and I didn't know this until 16 years later. My Mum had told me that it was indeed her that found me slumped in the land between life and death. She said she went screaming out to the sunroom to tell Dad but he was too pissed to care so my Uncle Shane and brother Adam helped carry me to the car. Shane sped into town whilst my Mother and brother sat with me in the back seat. She was keeping me awake, wiping my mouth as dribble and froth just kept coming. At the hospital it was my brother's strong arms that carried me to help. His heart was breaking, he was watching me die. The hospital wanted to know what I had taken so my Mum rang Dad to check in my room. He answered the phone but was so drunk, he told my Mum to get fucked and he hung up the phone on her. Shane drove back out there to do it whilst Mum waited in despair to see the fate of her only daughter.

Maybe it was that moment that my Mum decided she could no longer stay with this man. Was me trying to leave for the stars the catalyst she needed to decide 'no more'? It must have played some part in it, because the next thing I knew we were looking for a place to live. We found a little house in town, it was at the end of the street, by a creek and it was just what we needed. It seemed to happen so fast, but with the help of one of my Aunties, on a day Dad was at work, we packed up our things, and moved, just like that. It made me feel happy. It felt so right.

I can't remember the timing of things, but after maybe a week, my Dad found us. Of all the times Mum left Dad, this was the most drastic, the most real. It wasn't just going to Nan's for the night and waiting for him to apologise. This was a whole new phase. We had found a house and moved in and he was none the wiser until after the fact. When he found us, he wasn't full of rage. He wasn't there to apologise and he wasn't drunk. He was shy and sober and looked like he hadn't slept. There was something about him that had changed. A realisation of some sort perhaps? He said he hadn't had a drink since we left and whether it was true or not, I really wanted to believe him.

When I looked at his face, it was the first time I remember doing so in my life that wasn't in anger or sadness. It was the first time ever that I realised I had the same eyes as him. They were green and soft. For a single moment in time, I could see the gentleness in him that Mum often swore still resided there somewhere.

Mum decided she was going to stick to her plans. We were going to stay in the house until our lease was up. She was going to see what happened to my Dad, if anything, in the way changes.

Things were feeling nice. I had returned to my class in year 9 and settled my mind into what seemed like a new life, a fresh start when on a particularly hot summer's night I was woken in the middle of the night by two policemen knocking on our door.

What were they doing here? I wondered. My first thought was, 'is something wrong with my grandparents?' They came to tell us that my Dad had suddenly died. He was hit by a car in the middle of the night, on a dark, quiet country road. All of a sudden, my world had changed drastically. Again.

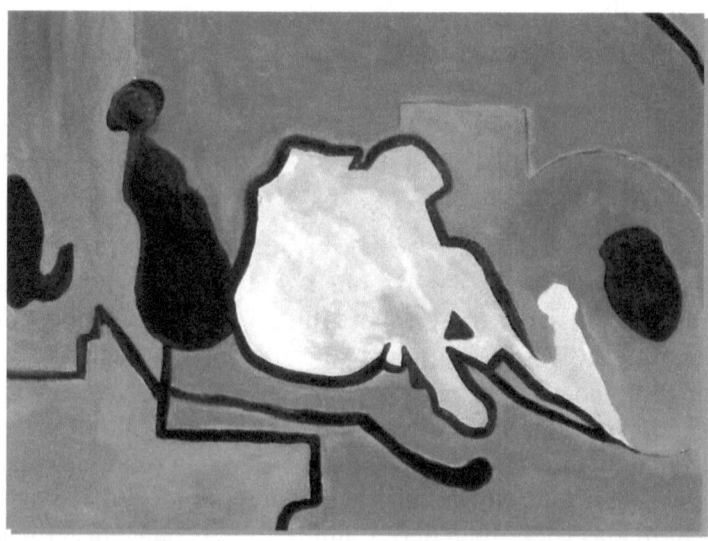

*"Grief"* - Artwork: Annie Joy

## *The Child of Magic.*

When I was a little girl, I used to play all day in the bush with my older brother. We used to play and climb trees, make cubby houses and call out to the faeries. We lived in the Mallee near an old unused railway station – a place that gave us years of adventures. We were pirates in ships looking for treasure and we used to search the empty paddocks for jewels. We collected ants and made cities for them out of broken glass and leaves and rocks. We used to take paint out to the bush and paint the trees in rainbow colours and we'd make bike tracks that weaved in and out of the dusty Mallee landscape. In our eyes, the horses were all unicorns, the roads were made of gold and rubies and the trees were the storytellers of the earth.

I often think of the Mallee and my heart remembers it fondly. I remember the smell of sunscreen and the hot Mallee dirt. The dirt would get so hot that it would burn our feet, and we would do a fast, scurrying dance to get to the shade of the peppercorn trees to cool them down. There were spitfires and bullants. Spiders and snakes. Kangaroos too. It was incredible. Every day was an adventure.

My Dad worked on the railway and my Mum stayed home and raised us. On my Dad's side they were farmers and on my Mum's side, my Pop worked over at the silo at harvest time, and would go carting sheep and petrol at other times of the year.

> *In my country I play with the morning star, sing the earths song, fly with the red desert dust, ride with the whispering wind, dance with the lightning clouds, slide down the river snakes rainbow, splash with the bush animals, chase the hiding sun, swim in the moonlight tide, sleep among the ghost gums, dream about my friends. I love my country.*
>
> — 'My Country' by Ezekiel Kwaymullina and Sally Morgan

## The Wild Rainbow

My Mum used to do baking with us as well as do crafts with us. She would make her own paint and clag and we would be busy for hours creating houses, people, cars and parks. On Sunday's our family would drive out to 'the farm', which belonged to my Margar - a strong willed woman who was widowed early in her life, and left with a farm and 9 children to raise. My Dad was the eldest of the 9. We would have a big roast: roast potatoes and roast pumpkin was one of my most favourite foods, but only if made by Margar. After lunch, my aunties and uncles would relax and me and my brother would turn on the sprinklers and take off our clothes and run through the water. Two of my aunties would always set up a little tea party when I came over. They would get out the good china and we would sit together and sip tea in the shade of the trees or on the covered verandah.

December to February was a busy time for the folk in the Mallee. It was harvest. During this time, my Mum would work at the silo in a tiny town where my Nan and Pop lived, with a population of 11, and my brother and I would catch the bus to my Nan's house after school. There were always cousins to play with at Nan's. My Mum was one of 7 children, and there were always lots of grandchildren around at her house. We were all similar ages so it was nothing but fun and noise! Nan had a pool set up for the kids under the row of plum trees. We would swim in the shade, and every now and then, ripe plums would fall into the pool and we would race each other to go and eat them. Fresh plums straight from the tree to our mouths - Yum!

Nan's chooks free-ranged in the day and went in the pen at night. It was always an adventure looking for eggs and we would find them in the most random places. I remember giggling once as my cousin and I found 3 chook eggs on the seat of Pop's tractor. We laughed all night and told Pop that he was clever and we didn't know he could lay eggs whilst plowing on his tractor!

My brother, cousins and I would often sleepover at Nan and Pop's. In the morning we would wake to hear the clanging of dishes, the smell of burnt toast and the sweet voice of my Nan humming and singing in the kitchen. She was always so busy, as you can imagine with so many kids and grandkids. Her toast would always burn, she would always forget to put the butter away and it would be a melted mess on the bench by the time she remembered. Gosh, she was beautiful. The middle of the day in summer was too hot to play outside, so my cousins and my Nan would sit in the lounge room by the fast blowing fan and watch looney tunes and other cartoons on the TV. The CB was on the dresser in case Pop needed to contact Nan, or when he would tell us he was almost home.

My favourite show as a child was Rainbow Brite. I remember watching it over and over again as a wide eyed little girl. Wisp was a humble girl, sent on a quest to find colour and restore it to the dreary world. I marvelled at how just your average girl could undertake such a dangerous yet important task for the good of humanity and I cried many times when she found her colour belt and was dubbed by the Spirit as Rainbow Brite. In Grade 2 I dressed up as Rainbow Brite at school for book week. It was one of the highlights of my life. My Mum made me the outfit, of course including the colour belt and I stood there in front of the school and said 'I am Rainbow Brite'. I had butterflies inside and felt like I was Wisp, who had succeeded at her task of bringing back colour to an ugly, unfair and evil world.

I used to love reading and writing. My Mum always told me that one day I would be a writer. I used to write about girls getting lost and finding castles full of crystals. There were always stories about horses in all its forms – the pegasus, the unicorn, the unises and there was often a middle point of chaos in which the girl/princess/shero would have to work out what to do in order to survive and then thrive, living happily ever after. The things about the stories I wrote was that there was never a prince or another character to come and save these girls. These girls would work the situation our on their own or with their sisters and then continue onwards in their journeys. I still have a lot of these stories I had written from those days. My Mum kept them in a cupboard, as she can't bear to give things away, and one day she handed me a bag that was full of the stories I had written as a child between the ages of 5 -8.

When I was 10, we moved from our small Mallee town into the bigger town, 90kms away, for Dad's work. It was such a huge shift and one that changed my whole family forever. It was at this time that I felt like my childhood had ended and I was beginning a new phase, with new challenges and new experiences unfolding in front of me. I was growing up, it was awkward, I had no friends, and I had no support.

My world of magic was left back in the Mallee bush amongst the trees, the snakes and the old railway station. My mind was changing, my body was changing, and the dynamics of my family were changing. It was a chaotic time in many aspects and when I think of it, I really feel as though that move was a big rip that tore our family apart, that left us all feeling stranded and separated in the middle of the big ocean, unable to swim, to reach the bottom or see any land from where we were thrown.

* * *

Hitting puberty was challenging. I felt so awkward and didn't have a great support network around me. I felt like my life was changing fast, right before my eyes. The magic moments of my childhood were fading, and I was entering a phase of looking to other places for answers instead of to myself. Looking to others ended up leaving me feel lost. Slowly, day by day, my heart was losing its fire.

I felt like I had nothing to offer – no spark in my eye, no dreams in my mind, no hope in my heart. One day, after months of planning, I tried to kill myself. It didn't work, I was still alive and I felt as numb as ever. Around this same time, my Mum had decided that it was time to finally leave Dad. Their relationship of jealously, violence and hatred was finally coming to an end. My Mum was so brave, I was so proud of her. Things moved fast, and before I knew it, my Mum, brother and I had a little home by a creek in town. This was a point in my life where I felt a positive shift. There was still depression, but I could feel something ignite deep inside of me. Was this the beginning of my new life?

Just as I was able to see something positive emerging in my life, a hot Mallee summers night bought two policemen to my door to bear the news that my Father had suddenly and unexpectedly died. He was only 40 years old.

The weeks after Dad's death passed in a blur. Things were so surreal, I wasn't well supported by my friends, my mother was deep in mourning and we had moved back into our old house.

It was a sudden change of turning my world upside down that I started to think about what life is. As a 15 year old who had herself almost went back to the stars too soon, to losing her father, I was confronted with death. Being confronted with death meant that I was also confronted with life. You can't have one without the other. So, this was my turning point of thinking about the point of life and what is life for. I could see death, I saw what that did. It took you away. So, what did life do? It made me think of my life and what I wanted. I wanted magic. And happiness. And a beautiful future, full of marvellous things.

In small and subtle ways, I started to think about how to reawaken my life to its magic. What things did I love? What gave me meaning? What is meaning? What makes me feel alive? What makes me feel worthy? What makes my heart sing? What do I need? As a then 15 year old girl who tried to enter the afterworld way before her time and who had just lost her father, I began to open my mind's eye to the possibilities of what could make my life worth living seeing as though I was still alive. As I type this, Mythologist and author, Joseph Campbell comes to mind when he succinctly puts it: It is by going down into the abyss that we recover the treasures of life. Where you stumble, there lies your treasure.

One of the things I felt strongly pulled to and connected to was the sense of support, community and ritual I once had when I thought of my times as a child living in 'my magic forest'. My fondest memories of childhood were at my grandmothers' homes, which were full of children, full of laughter, playing, noise and life. I wanted support. I wanted connection. I wanted community. I wanted my own tribe. A place of fullness where my needs were met and where I felt wanted and loved – always in the arms or heart of someone.

The other was ritual. My understanding of ritual was that it helped to form your life in a meaningful way. It gave you depth, sustenance, nourishment. I wanted my experience on this blue planet to be one that was fulfilling and meaningful to the core and one that could be felt through every cell in my being. Bringing ritual into my life meant that my whole mindset undertook a huge change. That 15 year old girl who was nothing but a crumbling shell, started to look for meaning in things, meaning in herself. I remember thinking back then that 'ritual is as simple as waking up every morning and saying 'today is going to be awesome'. Ritual to me was a way of bringing my inner being in harmony with the outer world – and then I felt connected and 'plugged in' to something bigger than myself, and something extraordinary. It made me feel alive and the thought of death no longer consumed me. I felt that by being alive, truly alive, was what magic actually was.

When I realised this, I started opening myself instead of closing down, and I allowed magic back into my life. When I did this, I slowly began to see magic everywhere. It was in everything. It was a bright, clear pulse. It radiated. It filled me and the person next to me and the birds in the sky and the flowers in the soil. I remember looking out the window at school one day and staring at a tree that was glowing with a violet aura. It was both subtle but radiant at the same time. And in the same week I sat near the side of the house while my cat birthed her kittens in the middle, darkest part under the house where it was deep and safe. I sat there for ages and at one point she came out, I gave her some milk and patted her. When she was ready to bring her babies out to the world, she first bought them to me.

Community. Support. Ritual. These were my keys to the door, the answers to my questions, and the music in my heart. My life began to open and unfold right before my eyes. I was making positive changes and magic was happening. And so I started to follow my bliss.

> *"Follow your bliss and the universe will open doors where there were only walls."*
>
> - JOSEPH CAMPBELL

## *Ritual, Life, Awareness, Woman*

I often imagine what life would be like if there was no violence. I would imagine what it would be like to start our life in pure love, deep trust, hope, and wholesome nourishment. Imagine if bliss was ours for the taking – with no conditions and no restrictions. Imagine how it would be if bliss and ecstasy was handed to us at birth. Imagine if all of us, as newborn babies, were born into the arms of our parents who were conscious, aware and present. Imagine how our psyche would be. Imagine how our foundations to our life would be if we were to be born in to a place of deep connection, magic and awareness. Imagine if our very life was considered sacred, if it was revered as holy, perfect and beautiful. Imagine how when we grow as children, we are acknowledged and validated as who we are as both unique individuals and who we are as a collective whole in our community. Imagine if when you reached puberty that it wasn't awkward or embarrassing, but it was embraced and honoured. The young men go out with the elders for a Sun's Journey and they engage in 'secret mens' business'. The young women who start their bleed are circled in the Red Tent by elder women who honour their bodies, who teach them how their bodies work in relation to the moon, how we work in a cyclical perfect harmony with nature, how we are always connected to this natural magic. Imagine feeling as though your menstrual cycle was a magic tool, something to be revered, not shamed. Imagine knowing this and then entering motherhood, where we had already spent our childhood and adolescence in tune and honouring of the sacred magic nature of who we really are – where there is no fear, no mistrust, no stigma around our bodies abilities and wisdom, but rather, there is a reverence.

As years have passed, I have come to learn that all of this is not a fantasy, but can be reality. We are actually designed to be born into bliss. The natural magic that lives within a woman's body, has the capacity and instinct to make the mother and baby fall in love and become chemically addicted to each other. This actually is our birth-rite. I have come to learn that women in many places in the world still understand and honour their body's natural timing and tuning with nature. Many women bleed in sync and in tune with the moon –

bleeding on the dark moon and ovulating on the full moon. Even in modern western culture where we seem to be so out of sync with nature, close women friends will naturally sync with their menstrual cycle.

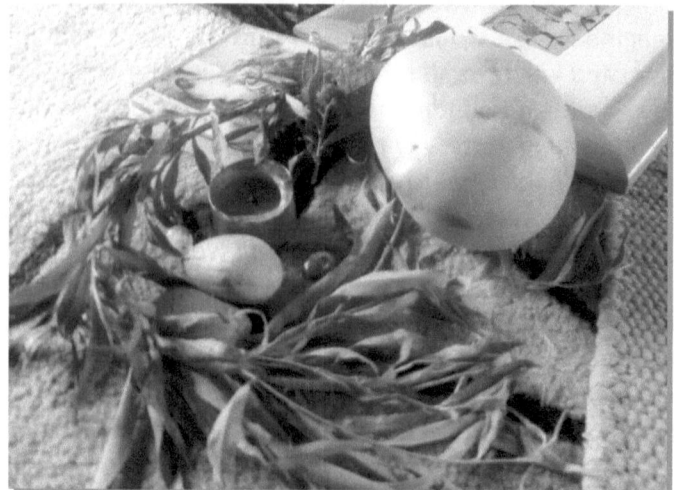

*"Summer Offerings"* – Photo: Sheree Stewart

As a teenager, I wished that things weren't so awkward. It was so hard to feel beautiful. It was so hard to feel worthy. I never had a body that was 'perfect' by the standards of the magazines and TV shows. I was too short, I was too shy, I didn't want to go to the back oval and smoke in the lunch break with the other girls, and I didn't like pop music. It all felt so shallow and lacked depths and substance. I wanted more. I wanted to feel beautiful from the inside out. I wanted my inner beauty to radiate outwards and be noticed. I wanted to be honoured for who I was. I didn't want to feel embarrassed and awkward. I wished I had strong female role models around who would love my gentleness, who would honour my creativity, who would allow me to be me. I wanted to feel empowered and I wanted to reach woman hood with a strong self of self and worth. I wished that normal parts of who we are as women were respected and not made into a joke.

I used to think about rituals that could be done for girls who reach menarche. How that would be a beautiful, empowering celebration - feeling that it would enable the young woman to feel confident in herself, and gain awareness of her body. It would give her insight, acknowledgement and validation. It would normalise something that

# Journeying as Woman

is indeed normal. It would give her a clear view of what it is like to be fully alive and connected to the world. I didn't realise that these thoughts of having these rituals are ones that have been around since the time began. Rituals such as the ones I used to dream of have been happening since women have graced the Earth.

I wish there was more openness and honesty around bleeding when I was growing up, but like most women I know in the western culture, menstruation in my family was 'something we don't talk about'.

One day in my late 20's, the ever so wise Jane Hardwicke Collings, founder of the School of Shamanic Midwifery, asked me a question around my menarche and what it taught me about being a woman. It seemed like such a huge question and my mind started ticking over as I thought of my menarche. What was my menarche like? What was my introduction to womanhood? What did this pivotal time teach me about being a woman?

As I was thinking about it in the quietness of my own room, with my other children asleep, I was munching on an apple, which bought me to the awareness of the cycle of nature and how it harmoniously works. The apple in my hand was so ripe. It gives me the awareness of how this apple had fallen from the tree, as the treemother had served its purpose. The treemother had nurtured and nourished this apple until it reached her full potential. When the apple was ripe and ready to leave the 'nest', it left for bigger and better things.

Who ever would have thought that eating an apple whilst thinking could lead my heart on a great journey of awareness and awakening! Thinking about this apple, and its journey from the seed, to the tree, to flower, to fruit to ripeness, made me think of my own journey through life. From birth through to menarche to motherhood and how this nurturing (or lack of) has created the woman I am today.

Thinking back to my menarche, I realised that I didn't even know about women's mysteries at all. I wasn't even aware that women bled every month until I was 10 years old and one my friends at school told me. No words were ever really spoken about menstruation by my mother or my grandmothers, except that it is private and we keep it to ourselves. Once I did start bleeding at age 12, I felt so shy that I didn't even tell my mother. She knew of course, but she didn't say anything to me either. She would just leave a packet of pads on my drawer every few months. It didn't really feel shameful. I guess I felt a bit embarrassed and felt awkward, not knowing what clothes to wear and I didn't want to play any sport or go swimming. I didn't know what was considered normal and I was too shy to ask. One of my friends mothers spoke about it more openly but it was always described it as a 'nuisance'. I never really thought of it to be a nuisance. My flow was always light, painless, predictable and easy. It was never 'in the way' of anything.

I guess for me, it was when I started my training in the art of midwifery did I start to learn of the potency and magic of a woman's body, of her blood, of her incredible womb space. The years learning all about a woman's body opened up so many locked doors in my heart and psyche that I began to marvel in the natural magic that exists within a woman. I had a lot of practice at being open, and not closed off, of speaking feelings and truths with other women. Sharing space with other women enabled me to slowly, slowly, slowly unravel, open and appreciate my own mysteries.

With each child that I birthed, I felt unravelled and opened more. Each baby bought new awareness, new magic, new openings. Each birth made me feel and appreciate the magic naturally within me.

I pondered on the original question that Jane had asked me and thought of what the experience of menarche taught me about being a woman. I felt disheartened when I actually realised what this experience taught me about who I was, and who we are as women.

I felt my menarche, and experience of becoming a woman, showed me that women:

- need to be quiet and keep things to themselves.
- have times when they are 'dirty' and 'messy' (and that those 2 things are not desirable qualities)
- are hormonal and 'all over the place', and are controlled by their hormones
- have parts of themselves that they aren't allowed to talk about
- have a shameful, embarrassing side that can't be expressed

Having this knowledge and reliving those feelings in my mind those feelings I was having, I had a deep sadness and felt as though I wasn't 'connected in'. I felt like I wasn't part of a whole. My dreams of women living in communities: where they support, share and nourish one another, where they are revered and honoured as the beautiful beings that they are. It seemed like this surely wasn't possible if I was unconsciously living in a space constructed of the beliefs around 'what women are' based on my my menache experience.

I think the main feeling I got from looking back at the time around my menarche, at the time of when I 'became a woman' was that I have learned a lot of lessons from it. Although it wasn't what I wished it was, it has given me insight into what it can be for my four daughters.

I do feel excited at this unravelling and feel as though it is enabling me to teach and live by example the natural woman/moon/earth magic that is alive in all women across the earth. I have daughters I can teach this to. I have 4 daughters and many nieces who I can honour and show them the respect. Hopefully by me doing my part in this, the next generation of young women will grow up with awareness, self-respect and confidence in who they are.

And that makes my journey worthwhile.

* * *

Since this dreaming has become more alive as I've grown more in to who I am as a woman, I decided to talk to women in my community who live with at least some parts of their life in accordance with nature and the natural cycle of life. It was incredibly exciting for me to see women choosing to live with this awareness and empowerment and passing this onto their own daughters. Where once a childhood of seeing women being controlled by men, I was starting to see generations of strong, knowledgeable and empowered women being shown to me, right before my eyes! It was wonderful and encouraged me to keep following my heart and to know all the thoughts and dreams I had as a child were not only possible, but were my right to have as a woman.

## *Creating ritual and celebration for our daughters reaching menarche*

*By Julie Bell*

You've been seeing the signs like a farmer notices the spring. And now the time is here - your daughter has begun her menses. Your graceful gazelle of a girl is emerging into a woman.

You sew her a wheaty-pack in soft crimson velvet. You trim it with purple ribbon and scent it with lavendar. You find your longest shawl for her to use as a rebozo. You buy her a set of cloth pads and a calendar. You talk to her about keeping an extra pad or two in a special pocket of her bag, just in case. You give her herbal tea and a herbal bath sachet of fragrant, nourishing herbs.

You think about perhaps a mother-daughter trip to somewhere special, for a night or two ... a place where you might bathe in the sea, soak in hot springs, or climb a fern-shrouded mountain and paddle in a shallow stream.

You wonder if you will talk a lot, or hardly at all. Either way, it is OK. Either way, you create a kind of Red Tent for your daughter to come to. You wonder if she would like you to draw henna on her hands, or make a daisy chain for her hair ... or is that too the top, will she feel bashful?

And then, the time is right to give her the little book. It is a slim, small volume, formed of re-cycled brown paper. The decorations and illustrations are hand-drawn. The prose is practical, truthful, honouring and lyrical. The writing swirls and curls as the vines entwining the pages do. The wisdom is brief, yet profound, easy for a girl to enjoy and absorb.

**The Little Brown Book**

- What is within this little brown book?
- What would you like to see on the pages?
- What wisdom do you wish to bequeath your daughter?
- What blessing would you bestow to honour your woman-child and help her embrace this new phase of her life-cycle with grace and dignity?
- What essential knowledge would you wish for her to have, about her body, her moon-cycles, her fertility, her birthing self, her soul-self, her spirit-self?

For more of Julie's wisdom, you can follow her on blogspot.

http://melbournedoula.blogspot.com.au/

## *Maiden Bleed Ceremony*

*By Simone Surgeoner*

For my eldest daughter, who started her period at 12yo, I thought long and hard about how to celebrate it. I learnt from personal experience (my second daughter is now going through the same stage) that in the year or two leading up them getting their period, their bodies start to change in many other ways, some of the more noticeable signs being their nipples swell, the breasts start to bud and they develop underarm and pubic hair. I find for the 1-2 years before the period arriving that my daughters become very self-conscious, all of a sudden my little girl, who happily and unconsciously undress in front of me, won't let me in the room when she's getting changed or in the bathroom when she's in the shower. And it can be quite a violent and angry reaction "GET OUT of my room!" - Something that wasn't a problem just a week ago!

I also found that they became much less affectionate and didn't welcome hugs or kisses. Or ANY mention of their changing bodies. I once tried to bring up the subject of periods with my daughter about six months before she got her period and it ended up with her shouting at me in tears to stop talking about it. She was very distressed at the time. But by the time her period came around she was open to talking about it and once she got her period she became open to affection once more and me seeing her body again (although never again with the same unconscious freedom and innocence of a young girl).

I realised later that it is a deeply emotional time as the girl grieves the loss of her childhood and it's a true awakening into a whole new phase of life. The girl begins to look outside herself to the world around her and starts becoming "self" conscious. She is aware on an unconscious body level that a huge responsibility is soon to be born in her (literally the ability to bring forth new life) but has no real mental awareness of what this truly means (beyond any simple mechanics taught about the female human body). It's a deeply emotional time which means the girl needs to spend much time inward and she naturally retreats, especially from her mother and father at this time.

Of course, I didn't know how long it would last. Now with my second daughter at the same stage I have been quite relaxed about it and know that my normally affectionate daughter will come back to me :)

So during that time I also stayed with my feelings, the grief I felt as my eldest daughter was leaving her childhood (it's always hardest with the first!) and my new real feelings of impotency as I noticed her for the first time going inward to find her own resources and rejecting my offers of wisdom and advice. Of course I knew all these things were good and as they were meant to be - I just didn't realise how hard it was to go from being the centre of your child's world to suddenly a sideline observer! I also felt excitement for her and this new stage of life. And I was present to the insights into myself that I lacked at that age - where the onset of menstruation was treated just matter of factly (not bad, not good - certainly not with any meaning).

One of the ways I dealt with the withdrawal was to give my daughter a diary for her to start writing in. I also gave her a lovely pen, some beautiful paper and a wooden carved cylinder that I had and we set up a system where she could write a letter or question to me, put it in the cylinder, place it in my room and if I saw it I could read it and then write a reply. She used it a couple of times to tell me things that I did that made her unhappy and I appreciated the chance to take it in and not react defensively in the moment. Sometimes she asked me questions she felt awkward about. There wasn't communication that often, but I found it was amazingly effective for my daughter to open up to me about her feelings in a way she felt safe and still keep the lines of communication open. Once she came out of that stage she started confiding in me verbally again (sometimes it takes a little prodding) and I was grateful that we had found a way to traverse the awkward stage.

Because my two eldest daughters spend every second week with their father, I wanted to make sure she was prepared for the onset of menstruation. I admit there was a part of me that hoped she would get it when she was with me (she didn't) but I certainly didn't want it to be an experience she shared with her father's then girlfriend. So I bought her a little pretty bag and filled it with disposable pads, cloth pads, tampons and a couple of small plastic bags as she was going away on holidays with her father for a couple of weeks. I explained to her how they all worked. I encouraged her to use cloth pads at night (good for her body, good for the environment) but also said I understood if she didn't feel comfortable using them at school etc. She didn't get it when away on holidays, but a couple of months later she got her first period when at home at her dad's. I found it interesting how intuitively I could feel the event coming closer and closer.

As she was in Grade 6 and all the girls in the class were, one by one, starting to get their period, as well as it being their last year together before all going off to different High Schools, I organised an afternoon ceremony facilitated by Tanishka (www.starofishtar.com) for all the girls and their mothers to attend together. In the end only five mother daughter pairs attended and we had a wonderful afternoon. Tanishka is funny, real and very down to earth and speaks 'teenager' very well. She talked to us in a group about cycles and mother/daughter relationships changing (us mothers got a lot of out of that part!). Tanishka had also arranged for us mothers, prior to the afternoon, to write a letter to our daughters and at one point in the afternoon we all went off for a private walk in the bush with our daughters, found a quiet spot and read out our letters to them. Another part of the circle the mothers gifted to our daughters something personal to us. I gave my daughter my gold ring that I bought when I was about 18 years old - it was my first independent purchase of valuable jewellery (ie: I bought it on my own, with no consultation from family or friends, with money from my job) and I wore that ring most of my twenties.

That was a beautiful afternoon and all of the mothers and daughters enjoyed it much more than we expected!

Then I wanted to do something with all the family women in my daughter's life (women on my side and her father's side). Given that most of them belong to a strict Christian religion I had to come up with something that was honouring to my daughter in the way I wished but also did not come across as hippy trippy, pagan, or too 'out there' for the women - as it would just end up being met with resistance and spoil it for my daughter.

I had read lots of things on the internet about maiden ceremonies and had explored the topic quite a bit in mini workshops I had done with the likes of Jane Hardwicke-Collings. In the end though I just sat and meditated and then came up with something that suited our families. Initially I thought we could all put in for a beautiful, expensive piece of jewellery for my daughter and I shared a picture of a stunning crystal necklace with my sister. She came up with the idea that we all buy her a charm for a charm bracelet (we ended up getting her a necklace instead) and I extrapolated on the idea and asked everyone to buy a charm that held meaning to them in some way and think of what they wanted to say to my daughter when they gave it to her.

I booked a dinner at a Moroccan restaurant in South Yarra - the red, exotic, lavish interior of the restaurant lent itself beautifully to the evening - without me having to go all 'red tent' on my family. There were 10 of us in total - me (I also had my 6mth old third daughter with me), my daughter, on the maternal side: her grandmother (my mother), her great grandmother, her aunt and her great aunt. On her paternal side: her grandmother, her aunt and her two adult female cousins.

We had all dressed up for the occasion and it felt so wonderful all of us women being together. It was especially amazing because my husband and I had been separated for over a year and it was the first time we had all come together (our families were relatively close) and it felt very poignant and emotional for me and all of us on many levels. We enjoyed a banquet dinner and then after dinner, before the dessert, we all focused on my daughter and one by one we gave her the charm we had chosen for her. As each woman gave it to her we expressed why we had chosen that particular charm, along with some words of advice or wisdom they could pass on to her as a woman.

I went first and I gave her a snake charm. I spoke of how a snake symbolised the shedding of skin, which literally represented what happened to her monthly with the shedding of the uterine lining. I also told her that there would be many times in her life when she would "shed her skin" and find herself letting go of old things and embarking on new adventures in her life, that she could choose whoever she wanted to be at any time in her life. I also told her I love snakes (my name even begins with one) and that it was my personal symbol.

My sister gave her a pig with wings and spoke of how she should always believe in herself, in her dreams - even in the face of people who might say it was not possible.

My aunt gave her a seahorse. My aunt is known for her love of the beach so it was a fitting symbol. But she also spoke eloquently of the ocean, how sometimes it was calm and tranquil and other times stormy and how life was like that. There was also mention of how the ocean tides are governed by the moon, just like her menstrual cycle.

Everyone spoke so richly and at length and I was quite overwhelmed by how much I had underestimated these women to be present to my daughter in this way, because they did not normally appear to explore life with such purpose and depth as I do (they certainly don't live very in tune with nature and they belong to a very patriarchal religion). I know that sounds judgmental, it is just my observation, and their own expressions at the end of the night, thanking me for organising such a beautiful evening for my daughter and how unusual it was but how much they valued it, made me aware that they had no reference for this kind of thing. Even though it felt slightly peculiar to them at first, they ended up completely seeing it as gift for my daughter and some even expressed that this should be a given for all young women. I realise, given the right circumstances (such as what was created that evening) the wisdom in all women comes forth. How much we live in alignment with that wisdom in day to day life is another matter, but it is there for all of us to access.

As everyone went around the table we all became more and more emotional and there was many a teary eye. My daughter started crying at one point when my mother spoke. My daughter was completely overwhelmed by the experience, in the most beautiful way. She's a child who tends towards being passive and quiet, so she was unused to that level of attention and focus on her. She loved it, she told me in the car on the way home that she was crying because of all the love she felt for her.

One other thing I did become mindful of was to ask a few women to become mentors in her life. One is her piano teacher, a friend of mine. I spoke to my daughter how I understood she may not always want to come and talk to me about events in her life (as much as I would like her to) and I felt it important that she had other women she could talk to, so we discussed who these women could be. I realised it was also important she had other healthy female reference points in her life so that she could draw on many aspects of the feminine, I don't want her just to take my words unquestionably and I want her to experience the broad range of the feminine.

## *We welcomed a woman last night...*

By Jessica Pritchard

I am so exceptionally blessed to have some of the most amazing women in my life. Last night my daughter (who is 7) and I were invited to join in blessing the way for a young girl who has just entered womanhood. What an experience! I have never been to a "red party" before and as a woman who has a less than perfect experience of the first bleed, I found it unexpectedly emotional.

Tiana and I received the invite in the mail. As usual the timing was bang on. I had been a bit taken aback by a friends' daughter who had just begun bleeding at the tender age of 9. This is just 2 years older than my baby girl. I knew that I needed to talk to my wee one about it all but with very little to framework to go off I found myself floundering somewhat.

Periods were never talked about in my house. Kind of strange seeing as there were 3 girls. I learnt about women's business through the matter-of-fact Singaporean school system. So when it came to being open and honest with my own daughter, I really didn't know where to start and felt really very uncomfortable.

Working as I do I have had to face my issues of embarrassment around all things women. I ask women about their menstrual history; talk to them about sex after birth, about stretching vagina's, secretions, abnormal bleeding and all things breasts. It has taken me a while but I am very comfortable and confident now. So my dilemma was then transferring this to my relationship with my daughter.

So those were the sort of things that were going through my head around the time we got this beautiful invite. And after all the angst and thinking and talking (to other people), I simply explained what the invite was for. I was met with a very matter-of-fact response followed by quite a show of excitement. Problem solved.

We attended such a beautiful ceremony and I got quite teary through the ceremony. Especially the part where the young woman's mother took hold of both of her hands, look deep into her eyes and told her about how wonderful it was to be a woman and about how all of these women were here just for her and always would be.

The ceremony started with only those that had bled. The younger girls were somewhere else with the guest of honour and it was their job to make her beautiful for the occasion. They talked about their experiences of being girls. We older women formed a circle and sung as the younger girls entered:

> **We all come from the Goddess and to her we shall return,**
>
> **Like a drop,**
>
> **Of rain,**
>
> **Flowing to the ocean.**

The girls formed their own circle within the larger one and after a few words, were invited to join with their elders.

We went around the circle and talked about the women who have inspired us the most and how we knew the young woman. We then shared with her a stone or a pebble. The point of the pebble was explained by her older sister.

She explained that all the women at her red party had given her a rock that they had picked specifically. Whenever she felt alone, afraid, scared or upset she would go to the bowl in her room that contained all the stones that the women in her life had collected for her. She would hold each rock and know that there were many, many women out there who loved her and who would always love her. She told us how she would draw energy from all the rocks and the intentions with which they were given.

We then closed the circle and shared in a wonderful meal that was provided by everyone who came (the theme was red food). We ate and then sat in a circle around the young woman and told her stories of our menarche.

It was an amazing feeling for me, being surrounded by women who were honouring the cycles of the woman, who were acknowledging the wonder of a woman's body and who were openly and passionately passing their wisdom on to the younger generation.

It was liberating and fulfilling and I am so blessed that the circle of silence, in my family at least, has been broken. My daughter will grow up with a solid sense of what it is to be a woman, without the shame and secrecy that has surrounded my own growth.

To the young woman who invited Tiana and I into your sacred space, thank you. I have learnt so much from you.

To all the women who shared last night with me, I love you, I honour you and I am in awe of you. Thank you for sharing such an intimate part of your life with me and making women normal and beautiful for myself and my daughter.

## *The spiritual practice of menstruation*

By Jane Hardwicke Collings

There is so much more to the menstrual cycle than the biology lesson given to explain it, in the same way that there is so much more to sex and childbirth than the mechanics. The menstrual cycle is a cycle to base your life around, in fact your life is based around your menstrual cycle whether you realise it or not, whether you pay attention to it or not. And everyone who lives under the same roof is under the influence of the menstrual cycles of the women who live there.

So, why not pay attention?

So much more will make sense and you will make more sense to yourself!

With the introduction of drugs to suppress menstruation completely - "Feel the same every day", is their catch cry, with the wide spread, almost epidemic use of The Pill by our young women, with the Earth, the feminine, in crisis, now more than ever we must seize our birth-rite and know our bodies and reclaim the 'women's blood mysteries'.

There is magic inherent in the menstrual cycle. Each cycle provides a woman with the opportunity to understand and read the messages her body gives her for any specific healing she needs. Each cycle creates the opportunity for as much spiritual growth and personal development that she could want. All a woman has to do to connect with that potential is simply to be with what is, her cycle, happening over and over.

The distressing symptoms that so commonly surround a woman's menstrual cycle in our day are often due to women simply not being connected with their cycle and ignoring their body's messages or symptoms, messages there to indicate specific emotional or physical needs or imbalances. Our menstrual symptoms are usually 'wake up calls' about the amount of toxins in our lives, whether that be in the food we eat, the company we keep or the stress levels we create from our lifestyle.

## *Some basic and stunning facts*

### *Women's cycles are effected by the moon.*

A women's cycle and the lunation cycle (moon phases) are the same cycle. Before electricity, women ovulated when the moon was full, and bled when the moon was dark. The pineal gland in our brain sends messages to our ovary, by hormones, to release an egg based on the amount of light our brain senses in the night when we are asleep. At the point of most light in the night, the full moon, we are programmed to ovulate.

Women who live in the country are more likely to be in synch' with the moon, as are women living in primitive cultures.

Ovulating at the full moon means we bleed at the dark of the moon, the time when the energy is more inwardly focused anyway. The average menstrual cycle is the same as the lunation cycle 28 days.

Modern life with the artificial light and constantly bright nights has disrupted our natural inclination to be in synchrony with the moon. The biological blueprint for our fertility cycle is very different to how it happens now. Imagine the disruption this creates. Not only are we meant to be synchronised with the moon phases, we are also meant to be synchronised with each other. Like we are sometimes.

Many women have no connection with the moon and no idea what particular phase it is in. When they begin the practice of regularly observing the moon, tracking its path across the sky, noticing its waxing and waning, most often their cycle begins to synchronise with the moon phases. They ovulate with the full moon and bleed at the dark of the moon or the opposite, depending on their phase in life. And sometimes they change again, depending on external influences.

### *You can ovulate twice a month.*

Each woman has the potential to ovulate a second time in her cycle when the phase of the moon is the same as it was when she was born - her lunar return. This is called the Lunar Ovulation and explains all those pregnancies that happen when women think they are not fertile.

This second ovulation happens unless the lunar return occurs at the same time as your normal cycle's ovulation, or you are fully breast feeding (although that's not the case for everyone), pregnant or on The Pill. It's easy to find out your lunar return and so when you ovulate the second time each month. You just need to find out the phase of the moon on the day you were born. Many books have that info, such as an ephemeris, and you can find out online by visiting menstruation.com.au.

## *The World's first Shamans were women.*

Shamans are medicine men and women. In ancient cultures they were the healers who used their special talents to access the hidden realms to receive information to facilitate the healing process.
They used trance and drumming to communicate and connect with nature to receive information. It has been supposed that the Shaman was a man's role but in fact anthropologists and archeologists have discovered that the first shamans were women.
This is obvious when the tendencies of women at different times of their cycles for prophetic dreams and other worldly communications are considered.
The Sanskit word for ritual and menstruation is the same - *r'ku.* The word root for menstruation *mens-*, is the same for moon, month and measurement.

## *So, the cycle:-*

The first measurement of time, the first calendar was based on the menstrual cycle. The menstrual cycle is a cycle within a cycle. The bigger cycle is the woman's life cycle, her life seasons, which are just like the Earth's seasons.

Spring – Maiden, Summer - Mother, Autumn - Maga, Winter - Crone.

Every cycle is the same as very other cycle, just different lengths.
The cycle goes - birth, growth, full bloom, harvest, decay, death, rebirth. The menstrual cycle is the same cycle. It is also divided into four quarters like the Earth's seasons. Weeks 1, 2, 3 and 4.

If you have a cycle that is consistently longer or shorter than 28/29 days it's the first half of the cycle that is shortened or lengthened.

Provided that you are ovulating, the second half of the cycle is fixed and is always the same either 13, 14 or 15 days.

Each week of the fertility cycle is as different to the other weeks as the Earth's seasons are different to each other. It's the characteristics of each of these weeks that are the opportunities for the spiritual practice that I speak of. Week one resembles spring energy. Week two summer. Week three autumn, and week 4 winter.

Each week our inclinations, energy levels, and the messages from our body are different. They speak of the physical situation of that point in the menstrual cycle and the related emotional situation.

So if you know where you are in your cycle you can much more easily 'go with the flow' so to speak. You could even manage your life around it. Start new projects in the first and second week of your cycle. Express you creative urges when you have them.

Have parties when you're ovulating, finish off things in your third week. Stay home, and be on retreat when you're bleeding.

You'll have a lot less strife in your third and fourth week if you know you will be retreating when your blood comes, you'll actually be looking forward to your blood coming, and be ready 'to let go'.

Here's an outline of the emotional and psychological energies of the cycle, week by week that you are dealing with, or if you aren't consciously, give it a go. If you are aware of the specifics of the lunation cycle you will see the direct connection.

**Week One** (day 1 - first day of bleeding - day 7): Death Rebirth Phase
Inwardly focused, quiet. On retreat or wishing you were or creating situations in your life so people will leave you alone (for example fights).
Life review.
Visions of how it might be this new cycle.
Letting go of ways or beliefs and attitudes that no longer serve - both metaphorically with your prayers and intentions and literally with your blood.
Spring energy, building as your blood stops flowing.
A time for metaphorically planting seeds for the new cycle.
During bleeding: "I feel quiet, inward", "I don't want to be disturbed".

After bleeding: "I feel soft, a bit vulnerable", "I feel as if I'm peeking back out at the world " "Here I come again".

*Week Two* (day 8-14): High Energy Creative Phase.
Summer energy
Increasing physical, sexual and creative energy building to a peak at ovulation.
Urgent creative feelings.
Heightened awareness of self and others.
More interested in physical appearance.
"I feel happy, excited, full of energy", "I can do anything!"

*Week Three* (day 15-21): Coming Down and Harvest Phase. Autumn energy.
Post ovulatory descent - can be positive or negative, a sense of pride or failure.
May experience feelings of failure or elation depending on what you achieved from your creative peak in the few days after your egg has died unfertilised.
"I lost my chance", "I feel useless".
"I am so awesome, look what I did!"
May feel relief or regret (at not being pregnant, literally and metaphorically).
Feelings of wanting to get rid of unnecessary things around you or in your life. Wanting change.
Things or ways of being that are no longer working for you show up. This may be confronting or a relief or both.
Depending on how long you've been ignoring these promptings will depend on how you react to them showing up again. This happens to get your attention so you can let go of them in this and the next phase.
"Everything seems to be hard", "Nothing feels like its working".
"I've been so busy, I'm so glad I can rest now".

*Week Four* (day 22-28):Distillation and Clarity Phase.
Winter energy.
Lessons from this cycle are available to be seen and felt.
Either glad of the where you're at with your life or fed up (again).

Feeling ready to let go and surrender or feeling frustrated and annoyed.
Less interested in everyone else, less available emotionally to others. Inwardly focused.
"Don't ask me to do anything, leave me alone"
"I get it now, I'm letting go of this and not taking into my next cycle."

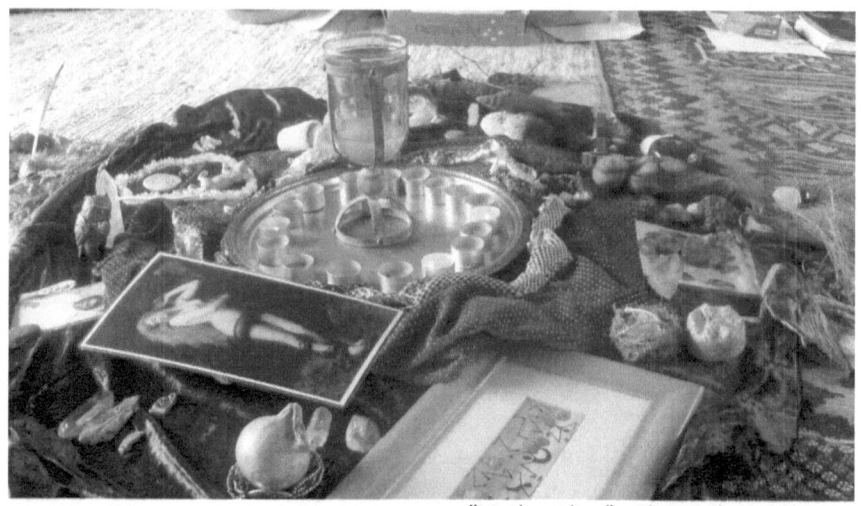

*"Mother Altar"* – Photo: Sheree Stewart

And of course this all goes for the corresponding moon phases and the seasons as well. Understanding the way of cycles brings with it an awareness of the flow of energy, the wisdom in that flow and the opportunity to be in synchrony with that flow.

I believe, honouring her fertility cycle is a woman's responsibility. It is in fact one way she can participate, in helping to correct the imbalances that have been created through not honouring the feminine.

An issue that we must address so that we can live harmoniously on our planet. Through honouring your menstrual cycle, you help heal the "wounded feminine" the symptoms of which ravage the Earth and most of her people. By honouring her cycle a woman honours the feminine, the dark, the juicy, the mysterious, the feminine power of creativity, sexuality and our Mother Earth.

## Symptoms of the Menstrual Cycle or rather messages from your body.

I was talking to a young woman about her cycle, starting to lead into the flow of the energy in our cycles and how she could be with that to best suit her life and I asked her 'Are you on the pill?' 'Yes', she was 21 and had been on it for seven years because she had bad period pain at 14. I suggested the concept that her body was giving her a message that she wasn't heeding, that maybe she needed to rest in bed with a hot water bottle. She said nothing had worked, her mother even needed to take the day off work to look after her. I didn't feel I had the license, so to speak, to take the conversation deeper, but if I did I would have asked her about what she needed to do at 14 to get her mother's attention, to get her needs met? And I would suspect that her whole story would unravel and she would 'see' that what had been going on in her life regarding her needs being met or not, was manifesting through her cycle, her period pain. Instead of taking the opportunity to 'hear' her body speak to her of her needs - physical, emotional and spiritual needs, and any imbalances, she was subjected to the enforced regulation of The Pill. The fake version of a cycle, in fact when you're on The Pill, you're body 'thinks' it's pregnant. I've heard also that when you're on The Pill your inbuilt pheromone radar system that checks out likely mates for their suitability ceases to work.

The different physical and associated emotion symptoms that you experience through your cycle, are your body, your Self alerting you to a particular need you have that requires meeting. If you chart your cycle you will see that the symptoms happen at different times that have different needs.

The crankiness, impatience or annoyance so infamously called Premenstrual Syndrome, that we may experience in the last two weeks of our cycle, is really more about the feelings you have because you are not flowing with what your body really wants you to do - that is slow down, withdraw from the busyness of the outside world and look after yourself, not everybody else.

In your premenstrual week you feel less interested in the outside world and desire quiet time to yourself. If this doesn't happen or isn't possible because of your living arrangements, you may become very edgy, easily upset and in a 'bad mood', this serves its purpose and usually drives others away from you anyway.

There's one sure way to get some space to yourself and that's have fights, so no one wants to be around you!

Often times, the bad moods, so to speak, associated with the end of the cycle are due to the woman knowing that even though she'll be bleeding next week, and would really rather be having sometime to herself to do that, she will have to carry on regardless, looking after everybody else and not herself. If she knew at this time, that next week she was going to have 3 days to herself, to rest, read, write, draw, whatever, her moonlodge, red tent time she wouldn't be cranky, she'd be looking forward to it.

The other thing that happens in the third and fourth week of the cycle is that everything that's not working in your life shows up.

Like, ways you've been behaving in relationships, ways you've been meeting your needs, or not, old patterns, anything, everything. Its Nature's design that at this time, you notice outmoded ways of being so you can let them go with your blood and replace them with their evolution next cycle.

Each month when you bleed you can consciously let go of old ways, patterns and beliefs that no longer serve you. You can do this for yourself and also "for all your relations", the collective feminine.

It's the contemplative and reflective energy of this phase of the cycle that facilitates this great opportunity, your inner autumn pruning, as it were.

Cramps at bleeding time are to get you to apply some heat to your belly or back, and to get you to withdraw, from the outside world, so you notice what you're feeling and thinking. You will hear your inner wisdom and have new ideas about how to do things differently for those outmoded ways you let it go of with your blood.

When we bleed we are more tired and when we sleep, when we bleed we may dream more than usual and it is common to have prophetic dreams at that time. So that's why your body sends you messages of tiredness, so you will sleep more, and have those dreams.

When you emerge from your raw bleeding state, hopefully you will bring with you what you have learned from listening to her inner wisdom. In the tradition of the Native American's Moonlodge, the community waited for the wisdom that the women returned with from their moontime retreat. They would come back with information about when and where to move camp, about where the buffalo were etc. The community valued this highly and made their plans around it, they honoured the wisdom of the feminine.

Watch the cyclical nature of your libido, your sexual desire and your body awareness.

Women usually experience increased libido around ovulation for the obvious reason that there's a chance they will conceive, and that's the case even if that's not their plan.

They pay more attention to the clothes they wear and how they look, leading up to and during ovulation.

Sometimes women feel more sexual just before they bleed too.

This is because their vulva and vagina is more filled with blood in that fullness we feel around our pelvic area, just before our blood flows. And because relative to the lower levels of oestrogen and progesterone at this time of the cycle, our testosterone level, responsible for many things including libido, is high.

The severity of symptoms you experience throughout your cycle will be a direct result of all the things that influence your state of health. What you eat, what you think and what you do with your body. Eating a good diet, and a regular yoga and meditation practice are the best things you can do to regulate your system and ensure it functions from a harmonious space rather than out of balance.

## *Ways to honour the menstrual cycle*

The flow of the energy through the cycle gives us the clues for how to honour it. It's a good idea to let the people you live with know if you are going to change the way you do things at your bleeding time. Their support will be important to the success of you implementing these life changes.

### *Week one*

Retreat from the busyness of the world, even just for an evening.

Have a relaxing bath by candle light with essential oils. Try geranium and rose.

Create your moonlodge or red tent, this is as much a state of mind as a physical space.

Wear particular clothes or jewellery when bleeding, red stones or appropriate crystals. This can also serve the purpose of notifying the people you live with that you're bleeding.

Suggestions from Cassarne, my crystal advisor:

> Two crystals resonate with the bleeding time and the choice can be made depending on which the wearer is more drawn to.
>
> <u>Carnelian</u>: this relates specific to the sacral chakra and our creative centre, it brings balance to the female sacred organs and empowers the feminine in its process.
>
> <u>Moonstone</u>: provides a balancing healing energy, especially of the emotions which may be in a vulnerable and fragile space. It assists in the balance and awareness of our hormones in their "dance" through our cycle. It is also a lovely stone to wear when it's one's bloodtime as it reminds us of our connection with the moon and all her & our rhythms. Moonstone reassures us when we are in retreat at this time.

Garnet could also be worn purely because of its deep blood red hue and its resonance to our physical experience at this time. Plus it keeps one grounded and strengthens the healing energy of the Earth with our heart.

Experiment with dreaming by asking particular questions of your dreams.

Invoke a particular Goddess archetype to be with you during your bloodtime, perhaps Maeve or Kali.

Draw or paint.

Meditate - with or without questions and perhaps focused on what it is you will let go of with your blood this cycle.

Do gentle exercise such as walking in nature and consciously connecting with it.

Feed yourself well.

Use special linen at bloodtime, like red coloured!

Use red towels.

Be kind to yourself - go with your flow!

The bleeding phase of the cycle is as if a monthly enactment of a vision quest. On day 3 of your cycle, just like in a vision quest, do a meditation and ask for a vision. You will be gifted with a vision to inspire and fuel you for your next cycle, write about it, draw it and refer back to it.

Make Blood Prayers - collect your blood by soaking your pads, and return the blood to the Earth, in a ritual with your prayers and intentions for your next cycle and beyond. With your blood that you give, return to the earth, metaphorically attach the unwanted ways you want to let go of. The Earth transmutes everything that returns to her, your prayers for your new cycle are made new from that. Pour the blood on the garden, many women have a special blood rose to pour their blood around, and they grow so beautifully!

The red dot that the Hindu women put between their eyes, on their third eye, used to be menstrual blood and was done so to invoke the potential visionary aspect inherent in the bloodtime. Your blood carries with it all your genetic information and your ancestors' genetic information, so this practice could open your third eye to specific personal information and ancient knowledge. The third eye area is also the place of the pineal gland, referred to in ancient knowledge as the "seat of the soul", so this practice could well increase connection and communication with one's 'higher self'. This practice could be done at bed time with a special invocation to remember your dreams in the morning.

Once you've stopped bleeding, when you are ready, gently reintroduce yourself back into the world.

## Week Two

Use your creative energy, make something (make your own pads).

Express your sexuality, beautify yourself, be indulgent.

Celebrate the energy of your ovulation (just like you would the full moon).

Dedicate your egg to something you wish to give the creative life force to.

## Week Three

Celebrate what you have achieved, created, succeeded in this cycle and let go of what you haven't. Don't be hard on yourself.

Start to notice the things that aren't working in your life in readiness to let them go with your blood.

Don't start any new projects, rather finish things off.

## Week Four

Be ready for your approaching bloodtime, adjust your plans around it.

Cook in preparation for your retreat time.

Make a pot of hearty soup that you can easily feed yourself and everyone else from during your bleeding time.

Slow down.

Start to imagine how you want your next cycle to go.

*"The whole menstrual cycle is an alchemical process in itself, during which every woman who bleeds goes through a transformation inside herself.*

*To menstruate means to live through a cyclical transmutation in which the past is shed and the new in embraced.*

*Experiencing this transformation through conscious ritual awakens us to our connection with the cycles taking place all around us and to our relationship with all life."*

Lara Owen - "Her Blood is Gold"

## *Honour the Rites of Passage*

Welcome your daughters to womanhood with an honouring ceremony, as little or as much as she will allow you! What happens around a rite of passage teaches you about what's expected of you in your new role.

Think about what happened around your menarche - What did it teach you about being a woman? Maybe you want to re-enact your menarche.

Honour and understand peri-menopause and menopause - it is a time of transformation, a labour of sorts with a birth of a new you.

Create a Women's circle and share together your experience of your cycle.

So, there you have it - the menstrual cycle is such a gift if you bring your awareness to it. It's that extra special thing about being a woman, not only can we create new life but we can re-create ourselves anew each cycle. And it's so important to get this, because this happens whatever the energy is, whatever thoughts and feelings you start your cycle with will be what sees you through that cycle, it will be the theme (just like at a new moon).

So if that's negative, like yuk, here I am bleeding again, I'm so tired, what about me, I'm in pain etc etc, then those thoughts are the metaphoric seeds you've planted at the start of the cycle that will grow, full bloom, harvest, decay, die and then be reborn again. So make sure you spend time at the start of your cycle, and on the new moon, setting your intentions for the new cycle, planting the metaphoric seeds that will nurture and feed you as they grow to their fullness during your current menstrual cycle or as the lunation cycle takes its course.

So in closing I shall say again, there is so much transformational magic available to women through their cycles. Such opportunity!

And I'll leave you with a thought...

You know, if we, all the women, got it together with our prayers and intentions maybe even resynchronise our cycles with the moon and with each other - we could use this energy to heal the planet.

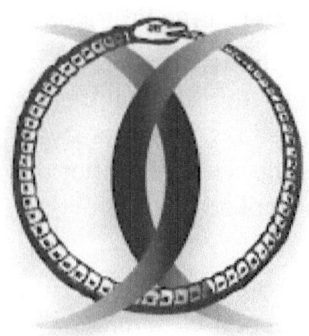

Logo: *The School of Shamanic Midwifery*

There are many references on the effects of the moon on our cycles.

For further information read *"The Wise Wound"* by Penelope Shuttle and Peter Redgrove (particularly chapter 4) and *"Lunaception"* by Louise Lacey (chapter 6), and "The Woman in the Shaman's Body" by Barbara Tedlock

## *Woman and Self Love*

After many of my teenage years spent with eating disorders and a life time of low self-esteem, self-worth and confidence, I can now look at my body and marvel at the wonder that it is.

My body has grown 6 babies. Each pregnancy has been changing its shape a little bit more.

When I was pregnant with my first born, I got no stretchmarks. I was in the 'normal weight range' and was healthy enough. Pregnancy fit easily into my skin. People would say that my belly looked so neat, it looked like I shoved a basketball up my shirt.

My 2nd pregnancy changed the shape of my body dramatically. The body of a first time mother was no longer and I struggled with these changes. My muscles were not so taut and my belly stretched and stretched as the babe grew. It wasn't a neat little package like it was with my first baby. It didn't look like I had a basketball under my shirt. People asked me if I was having twins when I was only 20 weeks pregnant. My body felt lumpy and bumpy. I didn't feel pretty or like a sexual or sensual being at all. Stretchmarks made roadmaps all over my belly and it made me feel so self-conscious. It didn't help that when I went into the labour, the first thing the midwife said when she saw my belly was 'wow, what a lot of stretchies. You must have put on so much weight.' I don't have very thick skin and I took her comment to heart. I didn't feel that I had any qualities of a woman that was considered 'desirable'.

When I had my 3rd pregnancy, I just made sure that my belly was always totally covered so no one could ever look at it. Although I enjoyed my pregnancy and loved growing my little spring baby within, I couldn't help but feel jealous of the Mumma's with the beautiful tight, glowing, golden bumps. I felt like I was 'just a mother', no longer a woman. My self-esteem was so low.

> *"Imperfection is beauty, madness is genius and it's better to be absolutely ridiculous than absolutely boring."*
>
> ~Marilyn Monroe

My pregnancy with my 4th baby was one of self-discovery. It was while pregnant with this baby that I learned so much about my Self and much of life began to make sense in where I had been, where I was and where I was going. It was during this pregnancy that I started to unravel those old beliefs and attitudes I had about myself and my body and started looking at how amazing my body actually was. A slow opening and experiencing allowed me to gently feel a deep love and appreciation for my body. I was understanding it, and paying attention to how it worked.

With this baby, I was planning a freebirth, which means that I was planning on birthing her without any medical staff in attendance. Because of this, I began to tune in to and rely on a deep trust and intuition to my Self and body. I HAD to have the trust and knowledge in my body if I was going to birth this baby with no other assistance. I had overcome some deep seated fears and beliefs with this pregnancy. The little sage I was growing was teaching me a lot. After her birth, I had overcome a lot of issues around my body's abilities. I could see the magic in it.

It wasn't until the pregnancy with my little tiger, my 5th baby, I realised I still had poor self-image. I did love my-self, I did honour myself, I did feel good about who I was as a person. However, I was not able to share this with others. I still didn't love my body. I would shut off and not let anyone in this space. No one could see my growing belly babe underneath my shirt. On the warm sunlight filled days, I refrained from putting my belly in the sunshine in case people were grossed out about the many accumulated stretchmarks I now had. I had an obvious 'muffin top'. Oh, how I loathed that word. Didn't even know it was a word to describe a certain body shape until I saw it in a pregnancy and birth magazine. I felt self-conscious if people touched my belly and I was afraid of the intimate connection that could be shared if I allowed people that closely in my life that I allowed them to touch me, even if it was to connect to the baby growing in my womb. But why!? It was beautiful! I knew deep down somewhere that my belly was beautiful.

I began to tell myself everyday how beautiful and normal my body was. As a midwife, I had seen many, many bellies of all shapes, sizes and colours. And this was fine. It didn't bother me in the slightest. I didn't even have to think 'that is a normal body'. It was just an understanding. We all have bodies that are made of the same stuff. And in reality, up close and personal, none of these bodies are airbrushed and painted and perfect! I had seen so many stretchmarks, so I actually knew that stretchmarks were so common, yet still I felt so ugly that I had them. It also seemed illogical to me, when I thought about it, was that the women who I have been attracted to in my life have all had stretchmarks and a little belly that shows that they have had a baby. I, personally, find it incredibly attractive.

Thinking about that fact that so many women have 'imperfect bodies' made me realise that all of our bodies are actually perfect. Furthermore, I started to realise just how we must be so conditioned in our culture to what is beautiful and desirable that we are trying to rid ourselves of characteristics of our bodies that are actually normal. I thought about all the 'get rid of your unsightly stretchmarks' messages that are out there in our culture and understood that my self-loathing of my body wasn't even that I didn't like my body, it was a fear that others wouldn't like it, and I hated that idea that people wouldn't find me desirable. There are so many different creams, tablets, oil, surgery, injections, etc to get rid of our stretchmarks that it made me understand how common they actually are.

With this in mind, it didn't make me feel better, but it gave me some perspective of where my-self-loathing came from. My body didn't look like other bodies I see plastered on billboards and in magazines, which is silly as they are all airbrushed and photo shopped anyway – they are actually impossible bodies to attain.

So, I decided to pretend for a few days that I actually loved my stretch marks and that all the parts of me I was unsure or uncomfortable about where actually the parts of me that were desired and preferred in our culture. I pretended that my breasts that are big and milky were the 'standard of beauty'. My belly that was round and full of baby, with a bit that hangs down that millions of sit ups couldn't fix, was beautiful. It was an honourable mark of being a mother. I would look at my stretchmarks and think 'how beautiful' and at my not so pert boobs and think 'how great, it shows that you have grown and nourished so many babies'. All these affirmations and changes in my thoughts around my body image didn't make a massive difference to how I felt, but it certainly shifted something in me. I did notice something stirring within me. It, at least, was a start.

Then a few times, a close friend asked if she could touch my belly, with her hand under my shirt. She was so close to me in my life and thought of it made my heart race, but I said yes. And when she did, I felt wonderful! I felt beautiful and loved. My body quivered with acceptance.

I started taking photos of my belly and made a pregnancy blog, which was a huge step for me. I had my photos there, of my belly, for people to see! And guess what! No one said that they were yuck or gross or unattractive or that I need to hide it under a shirt. In fact, people just said wonderful things. And they opened up to me and told me stories. They told me that they too have stretchmarks. They told me their nick names for stretchmark's. They called them life lines, love lines, marks of honour, stripes of honour, special maps, baby maps, knowledge lines, courage marks, tigress stripes.

And they said that my stretchmarks look wonderful, normal and real. Their validation of me reinforced my sense of self-worth as a woman.

Some days I still feel as though I need to remind myself, but I think that is normal and just an aspect of being human. Love the skin you're in. Celebrate yourself. You only have one physical body. Love it.

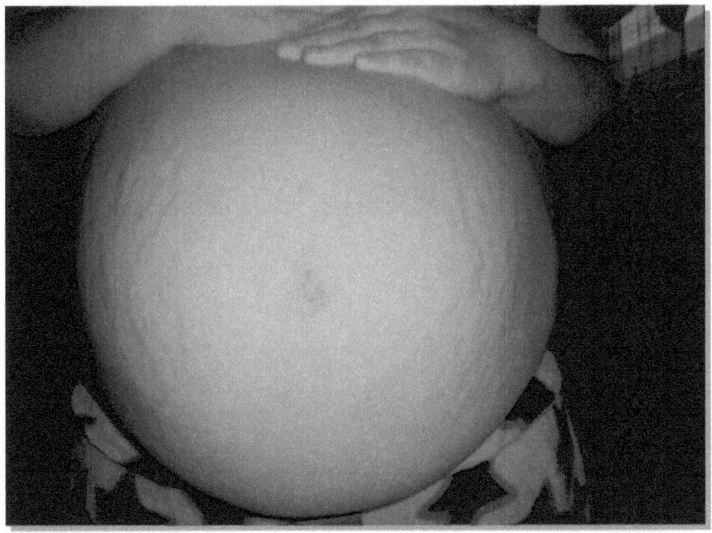

*'Full Moon Belly'* – Photo: Rhiannon Stewart

## *Sisters*

*I am dreaming back my sisters
Whisper-worn footfalls on the Temple steps
Skywalkers
Storm dwellers
Heavy-breasted cauldron keepers
Songweavers
Snake sisters
Darkmoon dancers*

*Labyrinth builders
Star bridgers
Fiery-eyed dragon-ryders
Wind seekers
Shape shifters
Corn daughters*

*Wolf women
Earth stewards
Gentle-handed womb sounders
Dream spinners
Flame keepers
Moon birthers*

*Come home sisters, come home*

~ Marie Elena Gaspar

http://moonflowercreations.org/

## *Celebrating myself!*

### *30 amazing things before I turned 30*

1. Having 6 wild, outrageous children. They have taken me on this path to where i am now. And have taught me all I know.

2. Getting my bachelor of midwifery. Pretty shitty climate for midwives in Oz at the moment, but my heart sings that I have learnt this knowledge.

3. Travelling to the remote highlands of Ethiopia to work in the hospital and villages supporting mums and babies. Although it was extremely sad as there were 4 baby deaths and one maternal death whilst I was there, it fuelled my passion even further for women's rights and empowerment

4. Working in villages in Cambodia, promoting safe women centred care. Providing support for women and their babies post birth. Travelling to remote villages for postpartum care.

5. Finding my tribe! I never knew it was possible to find a group of people who you love so much that you just want to live with forever! I've found mine and I love them so much!

6. Finally marrying the man I love after 13 years of being together. We got married in our backyard, with our children present and our best friends in Feb, 2012

7. I got interviewed on MTV with musician Kate Miller-Heidke at a charity event, talking about my time volunteering with birthing women in Cambodia

8. Been published in 3 separate books, the first when I was 16 for a poem I wrote.

9. I have given my breastmilk to 10 babies, only 6 of those babies my own.

# The Wild Rainbow

10. Rode my bike 350kms from the capital of Ethiopia to the remote highlands. I raised $7000 for a maternity hospital from doing this.

11. Have painted with my menstrual blood, breastmilk and my childs' placenta

12. I made a shamanic drum out of deer hide

13. Danced naked under the full moon with sisters

14. Have fallen in love

15. Have supported women from all walks of life, from white upper class women, Sudanese refugees, women in jail, homeless women, heroin and other drug addicted women, young mums, older mums, celebrities and everything in between. Each has their own story to tell, and each inspiring in their own way.

16. Wrote a book! This book!

17. Have had more than 20 pet cats in my lifetime! Lots of those were from my childhood. I only have 2 cats at the moment. I may or may not be a crazy cat lady.

18. Had a baby named after me, on my first day in birth suite as a graduate midwife.

19. Had 3 unassisted births.

20. Got to hang out with 80 year old traditional birth attendants in Cambodia.

21. Spoken to the last surviving survivor from S21 prison during Pol Pot's atrocious genocide in Cambodia

22. I had rainbow coloured hair for my wedding. Colours make me happy. There were 8 different colours.

23. I used to play bass in a band with my now husband called 'Moonfire Angels'.

24. I have been given an Aboriginal name by my Mother.

25. I caught my friends' baby into my own hands.

26. I've been witness to some of the closest people to me as they birth their babies. Thankyou sweet babies - Seven, Raven, Taioma, Blake, Imogen, Archie, Maisie, Woodley and Ethan for honouring me with your earthside journeys

27. I had 2 photos of myself – (one pregnant with my 5th baby and another breastfeeding my 5th baby while she was still attached to her placenta) inspire one of my favorite artists and these images were painted by the incredible Daisy Mabel.

28. I used to be in a corroboree group when I was in primary school. We used to travel to schools around Victoria doing aboriginal dance

29. I was dressed as a mutant bug, modeling nipple piercings at Melbourne's Fringe Festival when I was 17

30. I had the first 19 years of my life with the best brother on the planet. He is the reason I want to create a marvelous life for myself. Thank you, Adam.


**Now, write your own list!**


**Remember just how perfect and unique you are.**

# The Wild Rainbow

## *Being a succulent wild woman*

SARK is one of my most favourite authors, and she encourages us to all live as succulent wild women. This is her advice!

Bathe Naked in the Moonlight
Marry Yourself First, promise to never leave you
Buy yourself gorgeous flowers
Practice extravagant lounging
Paint your soul
Investigate your dark places with a flash-light
Make more mistakes
Weave your life into a net of love
Invent your life over if it doesn't feel juicy
Cradle your wounded places like precious babies
Be delicious
Eat mangoes naked. Lick the juice off your arms
Discover your own goodness
You are enough, you have enough, you do enough
Celebrate your gorgeous friendships with women
Tell the truth faster
End blaming
Smile when you feel like it
Shout: I'm here! I'm succulent and I'm loud!
Be rare, eccentric and original
Describe yourself as marvellous
Dress to please yourself
Let your creative spirit rush flow tumble leak spring bubble stream
dribble out of you
Be inwardly outrageous
Seek out other succulent wild women.
Encourage the sharing of mutual treasures

By Sark

## Lover Woman

Lilith reawakens us as women to honour and share our sexuality and sensuality with ourselves and those we love. Lilith tells us to express ourselves as lover.

## Lilith

Story retold by Mikailah Rachael Gooda

*The earliest origins of the story of Lilith were in ancient Sumeria. Lilith was a Goddess who resided in the bottom of the garden, under the tree of life with the great serpent. The great serpent represented the great blood mysteries of women. It was our ability as woman to be revered in this matriarchal society for our psychic gifts, for our ability to be the Creatrix so that we could give birth and our children would be considered gifts of the Goddess. We were honoured for our sensuality. Our sexuality was also revered as part of another gift – it was the same as honouring the harvest and seasons and cycles of change.*

*A role of Liliths was that as the handmaiden of the Goddess Inanna (who is known as the goddess of the harvest, fertility, sexuality, love). Lilith would call the people in from the fields to come back and worship in Inanna's holy temple for the sacred sexual rites. She represented feminine sexuality as free, instinctive, sacred, healing.*

*The next time that Lilith is mentioned in history is in the Old Testament, in patriarchal times, where she is the 1st wife of Adam. Lilith did love Adam but she wanted a partner of equality, respect and fairness. She wanted him to love her as an equal partner, so she confronted him and said 'I love you, but you need to treat me as your equal to stay'. Adam wanted a subservient wife and one who would lie beneath him so Lilith voluntarily chose to leave her family and her tribe and go and live in the desert. Lilith does not forsake her own ethical truths and values to bolster another person's self-worth or esteem. She always honours her own integrity and truth. The ancient patriarchal leaders of the tribe vilified and demonised her for this. An exiled outcast from her own tribe because she did not obey her husband and the patriarchal ruling of marriage. So, over the ages, the folklore of Lilith became one of fear, that she was a demon (when really, she was not a demon, she was demonised). A wild woman is to be feared, not embraced or honoured. A wild woman is vilified as a harlot, a bloodsucker, a witch, a hag. And so with this, women began to separate and disown themselves from their menstrual sacred potential, their birth-rites, their psychic ability, their magic as prophetesses and enchantresses, because in the feminine psyche of collective unconsciousness, there was a fear of embracing this. Because if you embraced it, you lost your life.*

*Thankfully because of suffragettes and 3rd wave feminism, we can liberate her energy and resurrect her potency as she cuts away all the false pretensions of who we are. It's the negative energy of Lilith that needs to be cut away so that she can come to embody not only the many aspects of the feminine shadow but to integrate these aspects within ourselves. When we can meet and own these, we can truly aspire to the illumination, magic, healing and rejuvenation that is our gift as magical wise sacred woman, as shamanic woman.*

*As the handmaidens to Inanna, we bring the people in from the fields to the holy temple where our expression of sexuality and love is a holy, sacred act of the Goddess.*

> "You were once wild here.
>
> Don't let them tame you."
>
> - ISADORA DUNCAN

## *Your own Lilith*

Lilith asks us to explore who we are as woman and lover. She encourages us to ask ourselves some these questions and see how you react to them. You may not know the answers but you may get a feeling - it may be a knot in the stomach, a pain in the heart, a love buzz, an excitement. It is those feelings you get when you first ask yourself the questions are the real answers to what is happening, rather the answer you 'think' of.

- How do you feel about your own sexuality?
- How do you feel about sex?
- Are you able to express what you want in a sexual relationship?
- What are the power dynamics in your sexual relationships?
- Do you allow your sexual nature to be its free, wild, instinctual form?
- Do you embrace your 'wild woman'?
- Do you both 'give' and 'receive' when making love or is it more one way? If so, how?
- Do you restrict what you want/need/desire?
- Do you feel repressed in your sensual and sexual nature?
- Is there shame or negativity around your sexuality?

# The Wild Rainbow

## *My own Lilith*

When I first heard the story of Lilith through the voice of Mikailah, something stirred so deep within me that it felt like a bubbling of water deep from within the Earth was coming up to the surface. A once desolate piece of desert land was about to be watered for the first time in a very long, long time.

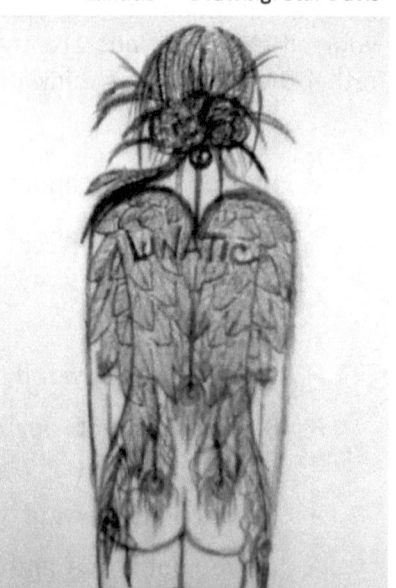

*"Lunatic"* – Drawing: Star Davis

I understood my own journey as Lilith Woman, and saw with my heart what our society has done to suppress women. Sensuality and sexuality in women is not often revered. It is taken from us, we are shown by the media what we are supposed to look like, what is and isn't desirable, how it is appropriate to behave, what the 'rules' are. Menstruation and childbirth are now medicalised to such an extent that we no longer look to ourselves for answers, directions or wisdom. We rely on machines, medication and men to do this for us. We have a whole part of ourselves that is in the 'things we don't talk about' category. Menstruation is taboo, natural birth is taboo, breastfeeding is taboo. I feel that women are not revered as sacred, holy beings, powerful and autonomous in their own right.

Lilith resonated with me because I felt as though I could see parts of myself that is repressed and exiled, just like metaphor of her story. I have my own wounding where I feel as though I can't push myself out into new territory because I have had very little sense of self-worth. A lot of the time I don't allow myself to trust my instincts of flashes of inspiration that come to me. Because of this, I sometimes hide away. I sometimes feel like a bear in the winter time, hibernating in the cave. Not wanting to come out because I don't feel safe. Not revealing who I really am in case it is too outrageous, too disgusting, and too politically incorrect. I don't want to be seen for who I really am. I don't want to be in the public eye, I don't want people to look at me, in case they hate what they see when I reveal myself. So my protective mechanism is to hide away.

I often shut myself off. My husband always recognizes this in me and lovingly reminds me that I am doing it. Shutting myself off, turning myself down is how I survived through my childhood. As a child I was sometimes sworn into secrecy, where I was threatened of terrible things if I told anyone. If I was too loud and expressive, I faced the wrath of my Father who didn't like me making noise. As a teenager, if I wore shorts that were too short, my Aunty would call me a slut. I was always taught by my mother to just be nice to my Dad and my Aunty, even though they were the people that hurt me. "Sometimes people just act silly when they are drunk" she would tell me. "But they are nice to you when they are sober". So, instead, I just shut off. Closed down. If I had to be nice to people in my life who abused me, then I could only do that by changing who I was, by just shutting down and becoming something else that was safe to be.

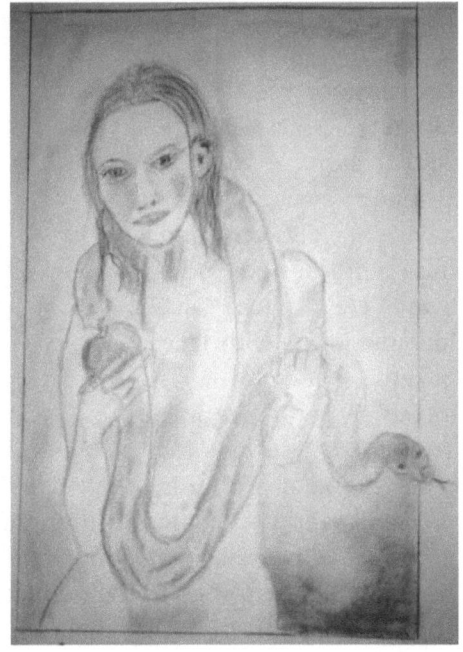

*"Lillith and Sammael"* – Drawing: Steven Booth

Lilith's story also deeply reflects my own journey as woman as a sexual being. I have often felt so shy and nervous, not wanting to express what I wanted in lovemaking in case it turned my partner off or s/he was disgusted with me. I have been sexually attracted to only a handful of people, and with that I haven't even slept with them all, but when I have been, it has to be a full package deal. I have never been able to just have a fling, a one-nighter or have casual sex with someone. My sexual nature

# The Wild Rainbow

has also been about deep, long lasting connection that is emotional as well as physical. My Lilith wounding has shown me that a lot of my sexuality has to do with feeling safe, loved and equal. I don't want to be laughed at, shamed, ridiculed or abused for expressing my self. My deep fear and wounding is that I don't want to be vilified and exiled for feeling and acting on what I do so I share that part of me only with a very close few. I want to be gently held, supported and encouraged by my sexual partners. For the wound to heal, I need to feel safe. When I feel the Lilith wounding in me, especially around my sexuality, I become bitter, resentful, angry, suppressed and not valued for who I am as woman. It was a sad realisation for me when I realised that I push parts of myself down that I actually don't to, because I am scared of being vulnerable and of not being held. I'm scared of 'getting into trouble' for what I want in relationships of a sexual nature. I want to be able to fully embrace and celebrate my free and wild side.

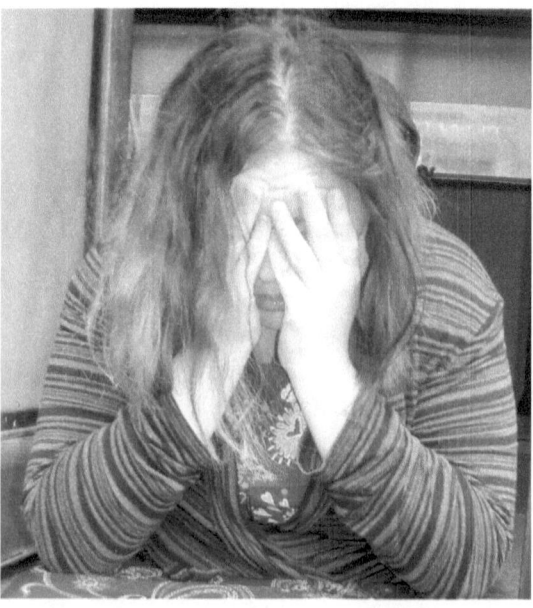

*"Anxious Anticipation"* – Photo: Steven Booth

In reclaiming Lilith, reclaiming my sexuality as my own, I am able to see the healing that takes place. Being able to be free in my own sexuality, to me, is the ultimate truth of the Lilith story. To be stripped away and to have our illusions and false pretensions cut away, and to look and love ourselves with true naked honesty is incredibly empowering. This is the journey for me. This is my journey that I feel I am really just beginning to recognise and understand. I suppressed my sexual nature for so long, in fear of being ridiculed or of upsetting and causing disturbance that I just didn't let myself go to the depths as much as I honestly wanted to. For the most part of having children, I felt as though my sexual nature was suppressed even further, which to me sometimes seems silly, as it is course our sexual nature that gets us pregnant in the first place! But just the whole culture around mother and lover being separate, where you can either be one or the other, not both, left me abandoning my feelings as lover and sexual being for a long time. As the years passed this obviously left me feeling dissatisfied with my life as woman and lover. Staring at it now with fresh eyes has forced me to take all the layers off and 'start again' in a sense. There has been the recognition that I can't live my life as woman and lover if I hide away my true individuality and life path. It just doesn't work and ends causing disturbances anyway, just in a different way to my original fears around it.

As Demetra George so succinctly states in her book Finding our Way Through the Dark, *"Lilith enables us to penetrate the delusion of our false needs which have forced us into roles that are not in accordance with our true selves. She makes us dissatisfied with the part of ourselves that pressure us to deny our needs and beliefs. She makes us reject sexual partners who do not honour or allow us to express our full erotic passion and abandon."*

After a lot of unraveling, I have come to learn more and more about myself as lover. Having a great sense of self and acknowledging that even though I am in the midst of 'mother', that I am still a sexual being, with sexual desires and needs has been one of the biggest shifts I have had to make. Also, getting rid of fear and shame around what my needs are has been probably the biggest challenge so. At least I am aware of it and I know that if I am open, and willing, that with the right people I can be slowly encouraged to be acknowledged and honoured for who I am as woman and lover.

## *Empowerment in sexuality as a mother*

Avalon Darnesh

The journey of pregnancy and birth gives us the opportunity to transform more deeply into the woman we came here to be, with each child bringing new gifts and insights. During pregnancy we become more open, vulnerable and raw. During this time many women feel emotional and out of control, and the smallest things may trigger powerful reactions. These moments are potential gifts if we look beneath the surface and delve more deeply into ourselves. What are we really needing in that moment? Do we need more quietness, are we craving peace and wanting to withdraw from the world? Do we need to be more gentle with ourselves, to slow down, to nurture ourself more? People often blame these mood swings and irrational behaviours on hormones, when in fact those hormones are simply allowing us to feel more deeply, so that we can connect with our intuition, our body and our unborn baby. We become more sensitive, more aware, more perceptive. We find it harder to witness aggression, injustice and disrespect. We are less able to overlook things about ourselves, our partner, our family, our friends, our children or our society. All things that are not in alignment with our deepest truth become glaringly obvious and harder to ignore, and these situations can trigger emotions in us. Assisted by the new life growing within us, we can access our personal power like never before, speaking our truth clearly and loudly. We become the archetypal feminine in all her fluidity and changeability, we become unpredictable and wild. This is the gift of pregnancy. When we honour these hormonal changes, we gain access to a deeper wisdom within us. This prepares us to go into the spiral of birth, and emerge transformed into motherhood.

As we access our intuition and become more tuned into our body, we become more receptive to heart connection and embracing the sensual aspects of ourself if, we really honour our body's yearning to soften into our feminine energy. As mentioned above, anything not in alignment with our heart is harder to tolerate during pregnancy, and sexuality is no exception. If our sex life has been less than fulfilling, it can become outright repulsive during pregnancy. On the other hand, we are able to drop into a deeper, loving space, we can open into more pleasure and bliss than we have ever experienced before. Our hormonal changes support this opening. Oxytocin, or the love hormone, is a beautiful energy to have flowing through our bodies as much as possible during pregnancy and birth, bathing our baby in this bliss. Whether we are with a loving partner, or on our own, this is a magical time to open gateways into more fulfilling sexual pleasure, assisted also by the increase in blood supply to the reproductive area, making it much easier to be aroused. Combined with this personal power to speak our truth and ask for what we want, the potential is there to blossom into new realms of sexual pleasure and fulfillment we have never known before.

This is contrary to our cultural conditioning, where the mother and the sexual being are seen as separate entities. It is rare for us to have grown up with, or seen examples of a mother with an integrated sense of self, including her sexuality. Culturally, the young maiden is considered the essence of sexiness, and many people, both men and women alike, buy into the fallacy that it's all downhill from there. There is a stigma attached to the mother as sexual being, which is ironic as sex got her there in the first place! To embrace our sexuality as mothers, we need to let go of limiting beliefs, and surrender into the true beauty of our blossoming self. This might mean transforming our ideas about what sexuality means. From the extremes of religious suppression, to pornographic objectification, sexuality comes frought with a complex history, both personally and culturally, of wounding and disempowerment. If we consider sexuality as our life force energy, both women and men have been kept from experiencing our full potential in this area. For many women, sexual fulfillment has become a source of frustration, which may be exacerbated during pregnancy, birth and mothering. Old sexual wounds may arise, and this is the perfect time to allow this pain to be seen and healed, assisted by the pregnancy hormones that allow us to feel deeper, so we can move into birth without these energetic and emotional blockages. It may be wise to seek specialised support in this area if things are coming up for you, to be guided in a loving and safe space to heal from the past. Do not be afraid to face these things during pregnancy, because unresolved issues can surface during birth, so it is much easier to address these things prior to birth. It is also wise to have supportive and understanding support at your birth itself, so if unresolved things arise, you can be held with love so these things can be shifted and your birth flow freely.

On a practical level, how do we make the most of this opportunity to embrace our sexual power during this time? One way is to focus on more heart connection and expand beyond the conventional approach to friction-based sex, which may be less appealing now. Explore ways to connect with your sensual nature, which goes beyond the bedroom. Sensuality is a much broader way of appreciating our senses and surrendering into our feminine softness. Anything that brings a sense of warmth and connection, from seeing a beautiful flower blossoming, to tasting a juicy mango, or cuddling a snuggly child, or immersing in a relaxing bath, all of these things connect us with our sensual nature and help us to relax into our bodies. All of these delicious experiences connect us more with our sensuality and are wonderful preparation for relaxing and opening for birth.

Sexually, pregnancy is a beautiful time to learn to relax and slow down with lovemaking. Take the focus off orgasm and expand your sexual experience to involve much more of your body. Take time to allow yourself to receive sensual touch from your lover, really breathing deeply into your body and feeling the warm, sensual energy flowing through you. Without any goal in mind, shift the focus toward pleasure for pleasure's sake, and indulge in the sensations of being touched affectionately. Indulging in sensual touch and the oxytocin that flows through your whole body is a gift to yourself and your unborn baby, who is immersed in whatever you are feeling. This might be a drastic change of pace for some couples, or may be an expansion of what you already enjoy. Enjoy the softness of your femininity, blossoming with fullness and new curves to explore. Practise connecting in your heart, bring your attention to your breasts and breathe deeply as you allow yourself to feel the love radiating from your heart. Look deeply into your partner's eyes and feel that loving connection, sharing this precious time of your baby growing within you. If you are single, gift yourself time and space to surrender into your love, to feel your softness, celebrate your opening and experience your pleasure. As you move toward birth, this softening and opening expands. Allow yourself to feel any emotions that arise in this sensual space. You may grieve the past, times when you weren't as connected in your heart. You may feel an overwhelming sense of gratitude for this beautiful baby growing within you. You may feel fear, anger, sadness, joy, celebration, or a mixture of things. Honour whatever arises and does not judge yourself. Be gentle and allow yourself to feel what flows through you. As mentioned above, seek support if you need to. Pregnancy is the perfect opportunity to clear old stuff, release old emotions and release tension that you may have subconsciously been holding onto. Celebrate this emotional cleansing, as it allows more love to flow through you as you blossom into your feminine power in preparation to welcome your baby into the world.

Birth is the ultimate sexual opening, so by clearing any blockages or resistance prior to birth, it will be much easier to surrender to the flow of birthing energy. A woman's reproductive area is very receptive, and can hold years of emotion and tension, resulting in varying degrees of blocked energy which affects our sexuality and our birth. We can consciously choose to release this tension and prepare ourselves for a more expansive and blissful birth experience, by setting our intention to do so, and allowing ourselves to feel what arises in each moment. Either alone, or with an intimate partner, there are simple yet very effective practical exercises we can do to release some of this energy so that we can open more easily for birth. One way is to create a sacred space in your home and set an intention to clear any blocked energy held in your vagina. In this safe space, have your partner or yourself gently insert a finger into the vagina feeling for any areas of tension, numbness or pain. Once found, hold the finger on that spot, no firmer than you would place pressure on your eye ball, and simply breathe into this sensation and be open to what arises. You may feel sadness, pain, grief, or not much at all. This process is different for everyone, and the key is to keep breathing into the sensation and trust that you are helping clear any tension held in your vagina. Continue doing this gently in other areas of the vagina, until you feel complete, or make another time to do some more. This is a very simple yet powerful way to prepare for opening for birth. There are other exercises I share with women in my sessions that are beyond the scope of this book, feel free to contact me for more information (www.blossomingwoman.com.au).

Anything that helps you relax, and surrender into your body is wonderful preparation for birth, and connects you more deeply with your sexual energy. During birth itself, support the natural process by doing things that increase your feelings of love and get your oxytocin flowing, which helps your body soften and open for birth. Kissing, hugging, massage, touch...anything that brings you out of your mind and into your body, with feelings of warm sensual energy, allows you to surrender into birth. In fact, the conditions that help you relax into orgasm are the same as relaxing into birth. These include warmth, privacy, safety and love. Consider this when making your choice of birth place and support people who will be present. Do you feel safe to open intimately in this environment?

After birth, most women put all their energy into the new baby and get into a pattern of exhaustion, neglecting other aspects of self, which is a common experience. Men can feel left out of this mamatoto (mama & baby) bubble, and this can be a challenging time for intimacy within a family. I challenge you to make intimacy a priority, to keep the love in your family alive. Even just share a loving embrace, or relax while your partner touches you softly, or if you are single treat yourself to a relaxing massage. It is very helpful to soften into your sensuality after birthing your baby, not as a luxury but as a necessity to experience more love, warmth and connection. I imagine the rates of PND would plummet if women were pampered, nurtured and showered with love after birth!

After birthing my third baby I was riding high with oxytocin for days. Then my milk came in, and sleep deprivation started to kick in, and I started feeling a bit sore and uncomfortable in my body. All my energy was going into my newborn baby, and I was still ecstatic from the birth, but I didn't stop to think about my sensual needs. Sure, there is a sensual connection that comes from breastfeeding a new baby skin to skin which is totally delicious, but I am talking about a different kind of sensuality and energetic flow. When my man hugged me, I melted into his arms and cried that I just needed to be touched. After the baby was asleep, he laid me down and very gently caressed my whole body, bringing delicious waves of pleasure through me. I surrendered to this bliss, and my sore, engorged breasts started leaking milk, relieving the pressure and softening, making big milk puddles by my sides. It was the most delicious relief, I cried with gratitude and joy, only a few days after birthing my baby to feel such pleasure in my body again. There was no pressure about sex, simply the joy of intimate touch and receiving pleasure.

It is understandable that after birth, women are not wanting conventional orgasm focused or friction based sex, but to avoid intimacy altogether they are missing out on the much broader connection with their sexual energy flow, which deepens with pregnancy and birth. If birth has been traumatic, this is even more reason to be open to nurturing touch, to reconnect with that pleasurable energy flow that is within every one of us. This energy overflows into every other area of our life, bringing more love and joy into our family. In this way we truly morph into the mother as sexual being, and we re-write the cultural beliefs that have limited us in the past. Each woman is different, and the important thing is to listen to our bodies and take all the time we need to honour our re-emergence into sexuality after birth. Explore new and more expansive ways of intimacy, including tantra and sensual massage, and learn how to give and receive pleasurable touch without any expectations, pressure or goals in mind. Step out of the past and feel more of yourself!

Reborn fresh with each baby, into a deeper expression of womanhood, we have a chance to reclaim our sexual power and embrace a richer experience of love and intimacy in our lives. Communication is the key, being authentic, connecting with our body, being open to what arises, moving into more expansive and pleasurable ways of relating. We need to use our voice, ask for what we need, slow down into more gentle and expansive ways of receiving and sharing pleasure. Imagine the gift we offer our children as we step into a more whole and integrated sense of self as a woman and mother, teaching our daughters how to be fully expressed and teaching our sons how to relate respectfully with an empowered woman. Let's embrace these gifts and reclaim the power of women's sexuality.

## *Honouring my sexuality: this woman's story*

At one point I was going through a difficult stage in my life, where I felt very vulnerable and open. I had fallen in love with a woman and she loved me back in return. This might sound okay, except that I am married to a man, and we have a family together. It was strange territory for my husband and I, as we navigated our feelings as to how this would work. At the time, I really didn't have any knowledge of polyamory, or any friends that lived in this way and I had no idea what was 'allowed' and what was 'forbidden', or what was even possible.

I remember going through a huge amount of inner turmoil. Thinking I was a terrible person, thinking that I was not worthy, that there was something wrong with me, thinking that I was faulty. I didn't know who to talk to. I didn't want to see a counsellor, I couldn't talk to my friends. What would they think of me? What if they stopped talking to me? How do I even start to explain it? What about my children? The woman who I loved didn't want to share it with the world, or with our children, although she was like a mother to them when she was around, so I felt stuck in a strange place of feeling like an alien, all alone, who had come from another planet where upon arriving here, nothing made sense.

> *A heart filled with love is like a phoenix that no cage can imprison.*
>
> *- - RUMI*

It also wasn't just a 'thing', it wasn't a crush, it wasn't a passing moment of lust. I liked her for more than a year before I admitted anything to myself, let alone my husband, or this woman. I had no idea what to think or what to do with these feelings. He wasn't interested in her, in the same way I was. He wanted me to be happy. Gosh, it was difficult. It was so incredibly fucking difficult. I felt so terrible for having these feelings. I knew I would never ever cheat on him. I didn't know what to do. It was so confusing and I felt so faulty.

\* \* \*

The woman's name was Phoenix and she was gorgeous. Her eyes were gorgeous, her lips were gorgeous, her cheekbones, her chin, her long dark red hair was all gorgeous. Her body was small but firm and strong. Her arms were muscled and tattooed and she was just divine.

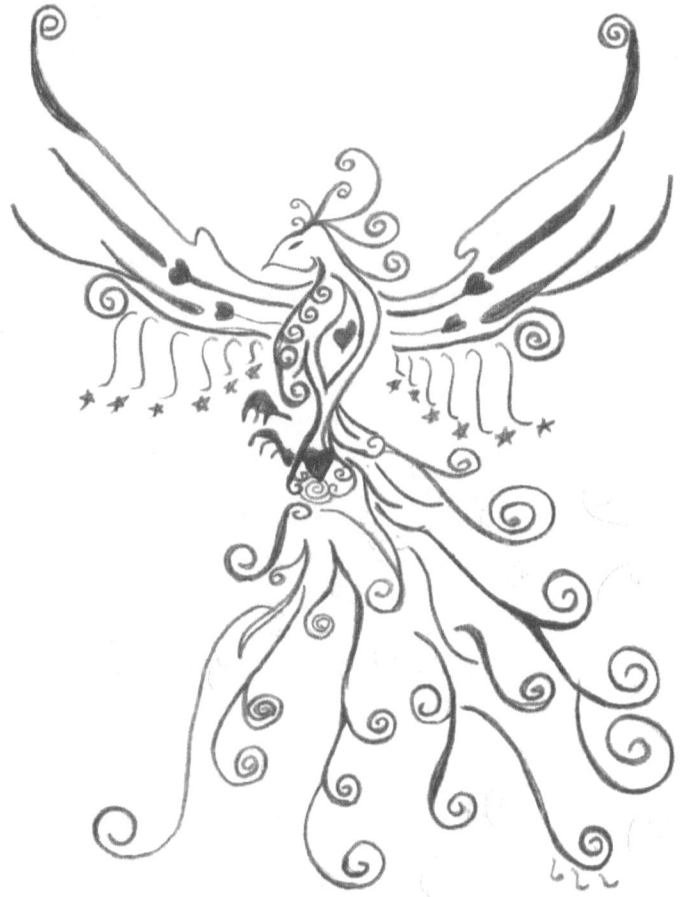

*"Phoenix"* – Drawing: Sheree Stewart

She came into my life one day by accident when I was sitting with my younger sister in a cafe. She had come and joined us for a coffee as she was friends with my sister. I was having a conversation about doctors' attitudes to vaginal births after caesareans. I made some comment about the fact that the uterus doesn't normally burst and explode during labour as much as doctors think and Phoenix burst out laughing. It wasn't just a small giggle, it was a big full belly laugh. It was big and loud and echoed through the whole cafe. It was so marvellous. It made me laugh big too. She made me smile.

We started spending a lot of time together and it felt as though we had so much in common. It was like we were aiming for the same dream. I could see her potential, who her heart truly was and who she going to become. She was just beautiful. We would spend time together drinking wine, looking at the moon whilst sitting in the backyard. We would pull out our junk food stash once the kids were in bed and watch shows that made us laugh out loud and big. We always had lots of fun together and she made me feel as though I was special. One day when I was over at her house, I asked her why she hadn't kissed me yet when we had spent the whole day with each other. She said she wanted to but she didn't want to fuck things up. I thought that was sweet.

One thing that happened in this time was that at some point I realised that that I was actually not faulty with what I was feeling. I learned about polyamory and I started opening up to my husband. What was imperative to the marital relationship was that I needed to communicate to him (seems simple, but excruciatingly difficult at the time). My husband and I had to put each other first and be clear, truthful and authentic in who we were as people. By keeping the lines of communication open, we were slowly able to work out and understand one another and see what the other of us needs. It has been a slow, cautious journey of working out what we are and are not comfortable with and what would and wouldn't work. We talked so much. I don't think we have ever talked so much in our whole relationship. It was so difficult, but in some sense, I actually was starting to feel free. I felt more open, more respected. I felt like the chrysalis undergoing the transformation and emerging as the butterfly. It was as though I had unblocked a part of me that was repressed for a long time. It was a part of me that I felt ashamed and embarrassed about. I didn't want to express this part of me in case I lost my husband and with fear of being hated or persecuted by my friends.

It turned out that this woman wasn't the one for me after all. She began on a different journey to the one that my heart first saw her going on. She has her reasons why she has chosen that path and I can't argue with that. It's not my place to, it's her life. I was childish in the process as well; it was not just her doing why we are not together. It is mine too. She was making herself more distant to me. The more closer I would try and get, the further away she would go from me. It must have been intense for her, for me to come into her life with huge ideas of what we could do together, what we could accomplish, what dreams we had that we could manifest into reality. I loved her so much. I wanted us to live happily ever after.

We ended up having a huge fight and left on sour terms. I often found myself wondering if she even loved me. She is a woman who likes to be with lots of people, whereas I have only been with a few people. I can't just have casual sex or one-nighters with people. When I am with someone, I am completely with them and I have to love them deeply. I have relationships that last for years, she doesn't, and she probably never will, it's just not in her nature. I did know this about her, and I was fine with it. I think I expected too much of her, put too much pressure on her. I was so all consumed by her and a part of me knows that she would never feel that loving and passionate towards me. I am sure that she didn't love me as much I loved her.

A year later we realised that we missed each other and we both apologised for our behavior and intensity. Seeing each other again made me wonder if I still loved her, which even though I realised I still did and she thought that maybe she felt the same way, we decided to just stay friends. This realisation made me sad, and I cried for a long time, but with respect and grace, we said goodbye as lovers. We are still apart of each other's lives, as friends, and I am thankful for that.

I am incredibly grateful for Phoenix and what she did bring to my life. She reminded me of my true nature and to live from the heart. She was the catalyst of me living in fulfillment and following my hearts journey. She reminded me of who I am, and if it wasn't for her, it is quite possible that that part of me would have been hidden and buried forever, which is sad, as it means that I would never feel free to grow to my full potential of who I am. If I hadn't experienced my love and commitment to her, I probably never would have known what that deep, lonely feeling that had been lingering in my heart was.

## The Wild Rainbow

It was such a trying, exhausting time as I was in the midst of this transition and chaos. It was a time where pieces of my true self were emerging, and possibilities of love, magic, chaos, bliss, destruction, rebirth arose around the idea of following and honouring my heart. Sometimes I just wanted to give in to the internal fighting and thought 'what happens if you just open your heart, feel what is there, and let it embrace you, take you away, sweep you off your feet and carry you on your life journey without you even fighting, complaining, resisting or feeling lost?'

When I allow my self to be in this, to feel this, to live with an open heart, it is not that it made things easier. But it made them more fulfilling. It made me more open, because I had to say things I wanted, what I didn't want, what did and did not work for me. I had to stand on my own 2 feet and say 'this is what I'm feeling, I've no idea what it means, but I feel it in my heart, and it feels right'. I've had to speak the truth, even when my voice shakes and I've had to say my thoughts out loud, even if I didn't want others to hear them. At times I felt like I had nothing left to give or say. I felt like a skeleton that had bared all, I had nothing left in side. But in doing so, I have set my self free. I have allowed myself at times when I needed to be, be stripped bare, to show I have nothing to hide, so that others could see right through me and see who I am. I have lived by the rule of non-violence, and that what I do is not violent or hurtful to myself or another, and I make decisions that I think and feel on before I react to them. I feel more free as a result. I feel as though I have climbed a mountain and I can see the view and I am not afraid to try and fly. It feels right for me.

Thank you, Phoenix.

## *Living with an open heart*

- What happens if I live with an open heart?
- What happens if I take away all the embarrassment, all the shame?
- What happens if I take down all the barriers that tell me I am wrong, I am ugly, I am disgusting, I am gross?
- What happens if I open my heart and let what is in there, free?
- What happens if the judgements of others no longer concern me?
- What happens if I let myself cry?
- What happens if I let myself feel?
- What happens if I say 'Yes!'?
- What happens if I let myself be vulnerable?
- What happens if I let myself be open to being hurt?
- My pericardium is the heart protector, it defends it.
- So how do I let love in?

How do I feel about my heart being exposed and open and there for someone to touch it and connect with it, without its protective casing surrounding it? It puts me in such a vulnerable position. Perhaps I could even die!

Perhaps living with your heart is just that - being willing to be vulnerable - confronting the parts of ourselves that we once used to protect and help us survive and letting them go, again and again and again so that we can be soft and full with each new experience the heart wants us to have. It's not easy. It's hard. It is really, really hard, but something that I strive for and am determined to achieve.

*I will always aim to live with my heart.*

### Her Wild Dragon, Her Wild Phoenix

Dragon & Phoenix,
         My wild lovers
            Who take me far from Eden
            to the borders of the world
            where nothing exists,
                  but them
Whoever thought that chaos could be
                    so beautiful?

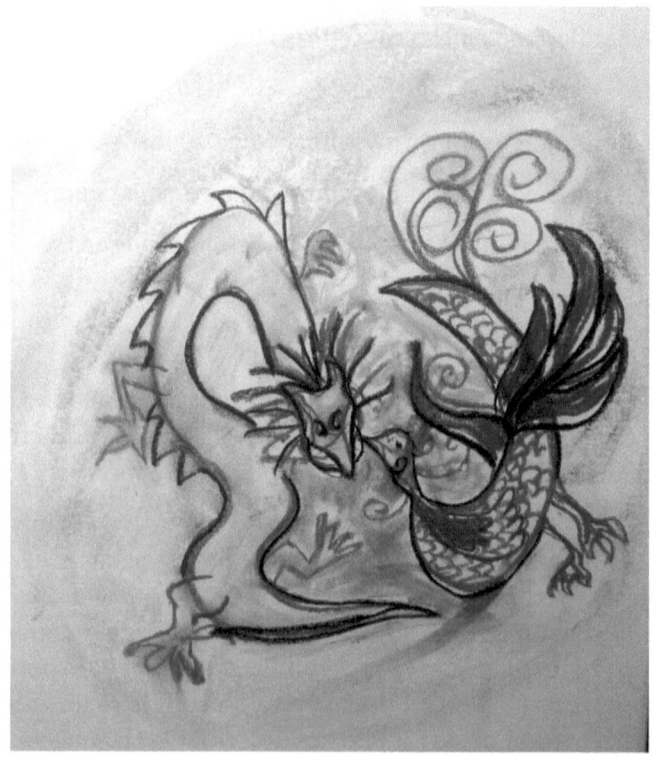

*"Dragon and Phoenix"* – Artist: Sheree Stewart

## Take Me Somewhere

Can you take me on a ride somewhere
On mountaintops and on the plains?
Can you hold me in sweet longing
Until the sun comes up
And the day begins?
Can you sing me a song
About love at first sight
And being swept away in a land of dreams
And kisses where everything is right
And peaceful and beautiful?
Can you take me on a ride somewhere
Where there is only sweet loving bliss?

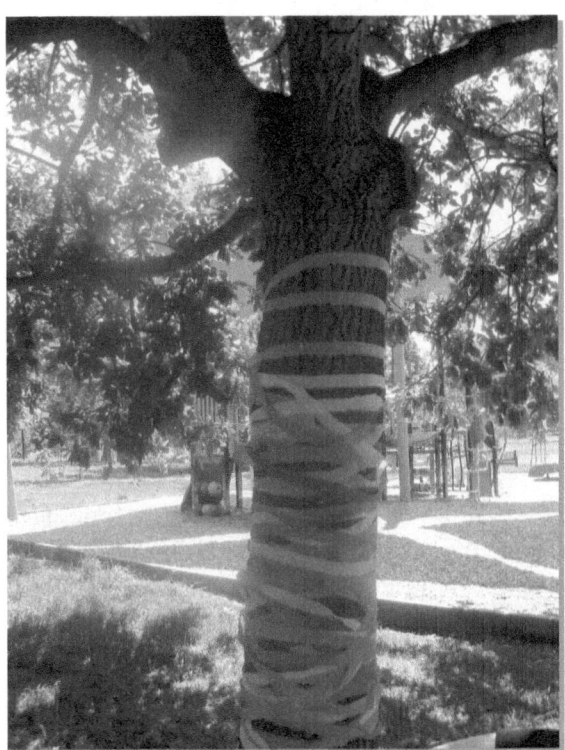

*"Tree Weaver"* -Photo: Sheree Stewart

## Sunday Dreaming With Her

She creates the world
With her magic hands
The clay, the wood, the leaves, the rocks
'It all belongs to her' she said
She sculpts and dreams
And kisses the sky
Love is in the universe
Love is in the stars

## *Sheree and Steven: Real life love story*

*Close your eyes, fall in love, stay there. - Rumi*

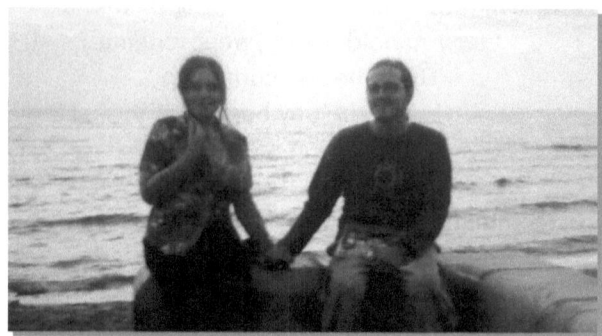

*"Forever and ever" – Photo: Star Davis*

I met Steven when I was 16. He had wild curly black hair and even wilder blue eyes. He played music and was incredibly intelligent. Growing up in a town full of rednecks, who would drive around in utes with bumper stickers blurting out 'no fat chicks' and 'rum injected ute', I thought that I would have to fly across the ocean before I found a soul mate who danced to the same music as my own.

As soon as I saw him, it was love at first sight. I looked at him and knew that he was mine. I knew that he was going to be the father of my children, the man in my life, my dream buddy. I knew that he was the one who I was going to wake up to every single morning of my life, and he was the one who would be able to understand and accept who I was in my entirety. He was my soulmate and I loved him straight away.

It didn't take long for the sparks to fly or for our dreams to merge and match each other. It was a fast, whirlwind, passionate love. It took us by storm and we were all encompassed with each other. After 6 weeks, we moved in together. By the end of the year, he was moving to the city for uni, and I couldn't let him go alone, so along I went with him.

We played music together. His hands were strong and melodic as he played the guitar, it was magic to listen to. When he would be playing the guitar, it stirred up my mind and lyrics would bubble and form within, then my voice would sing them out loud. We wrote many songs together.

Our lives were difficult at this time of our young love. It was wild. It was chaotic. It was full of teenage angst. At times we felt we were left with nothing, but in all of this, we had each other. And that kept us sane. As the years rolled past, we softened each other's hardness, we calmed the others fears and we chased away each other's demons.

When I was 18, the unexpected and sudden death of my brother left me in the throes of misery. It seemed to me that life couldn't get any worse and I was hanging by a thread. My Mum was in her own world of grieving and I felt so far away from everything. Steven held me in those darks hours. We tried to find solutions that kept us alive. At that point, being alive was the only thing I could manage. I couldn't expect much more of myself than that, I couldn't imagine a future, I couldn't imagine what my life could be. I couldn't see any possibilities of what life could become. I simply had to 'just live' and hope that life got better.

A few months passed of my brother, Adam's death while I was still clinging to the edge of life and death, I found out that I was pregnant. A little baby seemed to arrive from the depths of nowhere and awaken my heart in a way I had never dreamed. Although very unexpected, Steven and I smiled. It was a love child, a child of hope, a gift from the stars. It seemed that after so many of my close family members were so suddenly taken from me in the few years previous, I was now bringing a family member to us, into the world. Steven and I were making a family. It was the start of something new. It was a new beginning. I felt bliss inside, that things were going to be ok. Steven stayed beside me through both love and despair. Gosh, I love him. That mysterious man with the wild hair, my Steven, was now the King of a family. Of his family. Of our family. Of our future.

Years have passed, and with it, more babies were born. Each child took us on an exciting new journey of self-discovery. Each child gave us a new perspective, a new love, a wider heart, a more fulfilled life. Steven traversed the worlds of each birth with me and held me tight with whatever was going on, whatever I was feeling, he was there. Through the first birth which was fraught with fear and medical interventions that led to medical emergencies and a long time for my

## The Wild Rainbow

body to heal, to blissful, quiet births at home, where I laboured in water with his sweet company by my side.

I like to think that we allow each other to follow our dreams. To accept the other for who we are, to allow the growth of ourselves, of our potentials to climb to its heights. It is not always easy, and it takes a lot of team work, love and dedication to each other to raise ourselves, our children, our families and follow our passions and dreams. Steven and I have never been people that could just live an ordinary life – a 9-5 job, 2.5 kids, working for the machine, losing our hearts in the process.

So, it's been wild. And fun. And I am looking forward many more years of this ride with him.

After 13 years of being together, once we thought we had finished having all our children, we decided to finally get married. We did it true to our style and had a small backyard wedding, that was impossibly beautiful and Alice in Wonderland inspired. When Steven and I were first together, people told us it would never work out, that we were too young, that we were foolish, not thinking clearly and most other negative things you could think of. "It would never work out" said many people, "Teenage sweethearts don't last" they would say. Yet, here we were. Just like Alice who went on a journey that was seemingly impossible, where things were not always what they seem but here they were anyway. Our journey together was the one of Wonderland that was impossible. It was mad. It was bonkers. It didn't make sense to most. But it worked for us. And it continues to do so.

So, in front of 30 of our closest friends (and around 30 children!), we married the backyard of our home – a home that was built by Steven's grandparents, a home that that has their ashes scattered within the garden, a home where 3 of our babies were born, a home where we have children's placentas and pets now passed buried in the garden. Our sacred family land. It was so beautiful and the ceremony of marriage tied our hearts together even more and upon our ring fingers we have tattooed infinity symbols that permanently show our everlasting commitment to each other – from this life time to the next, to the next, to the next.

And we lived happily ever after.

### *My wedding vow to Steven:*

*Steven, Lets live like Dragonling, in our garden on our time on Earth, to look after the Baby Dragons that have been put into our care.*

*It's been an amazing, wild ride this last 13 years.*

*I feel like this spiraling path has led us here, to this cleared, opened space.*

*From this space we have the view of where we came from, where we are now, and what we can do next.*

*Let's be free together and live in bliss, ecstasy, contentment and love.*

*Let's create Heaven together and live it every single day with our Baby Dragons.*

*I am honoured to share this journey with you as your wife.*

*I love you with all parts of myself, through all lifetimes, through the cosmos, spiraling together forever.*

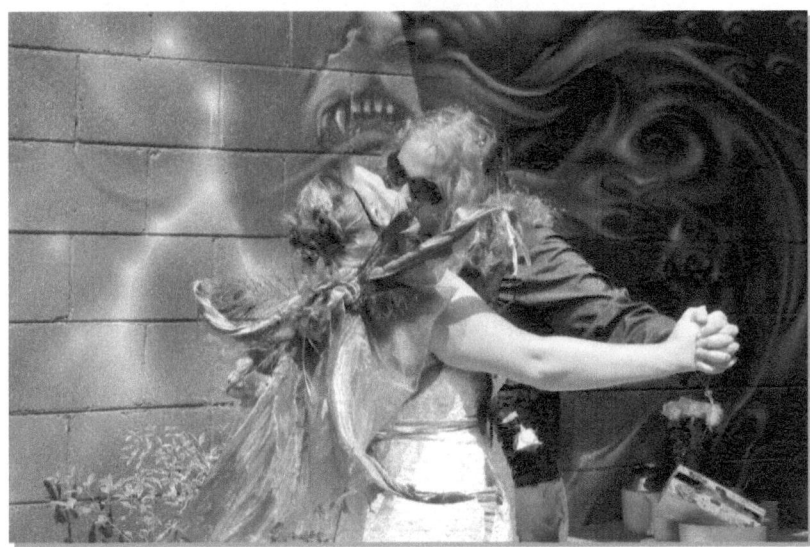

Photo: Paula Booth

### *And Stevens vows to Sheree:*

*My beautiful girl, Sheree,*

*As the galaxies infinitely wheel and turn, it is a privilege and honour to be journeying with you together through space and time.*

*Together we have courageously overcome challenges that we have faced, and welcomed the blessings and good fortune we have received.*

*Through the birthing and raising of our amazing Star Children, we are creating a new world and future together.*

*Today we celebrate our journey, and our joining together as one*

*As we continue to swing on the spiral of our divinity, I offer you security, support, my attention, loyalty, and love*

*I offer to meet your needs as you require, and embrace the totality of who you are, and to assist you in the fulfillment of your potential.*

*Most of all I offer you my heart, for all time*

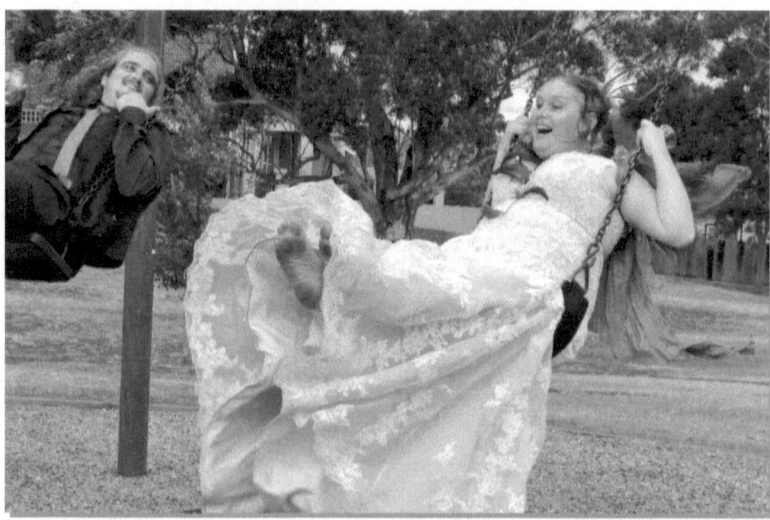

Photo: Paula Booth

## *Mourning Woman, Wounded Woman*

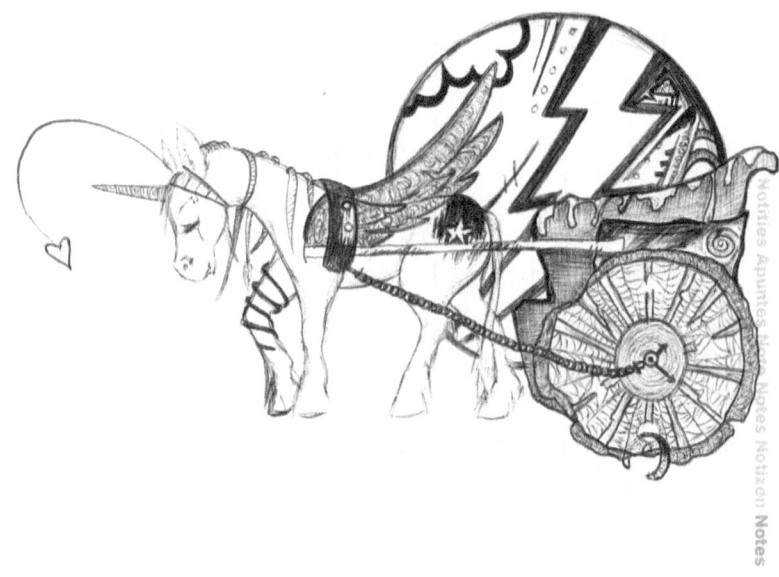

"Beast of Burden" – Sketch: Star Davis

Even if we lived where everything was handed to us, there will always be a time in our lives were we travel to our own hell. There is always a time in our lives when all is stripped of us, where we feel we sit on the edge of despair, staring into the abyss where there is nothing in front of us and nothing behind us. We sit in mourning until a time where something will remind us and reawaken us, and we can start our journey out of the centre of the labyrinth, out of the depths of hell, to our new found place. A place where we first came that is still the same in one regard, but different in another. We come out changed, transformed. We come out in a beauty that says to the world 'we survived it, we made it, we are still here'.

## *The Descent of Inanna*

> Re-told and re-imagined by Charlie Young.

From the great above, she opened her ear to the great below.

The goddess from the great above opened her ear to the great below.

Inanna from the great above...she opened her ear to the great below.

A long, long time ago in ancient Sumeria lived Inanna, Queen of Heaven and Earth—she of light, glory and movement. When she heard the call, Inanna knew she had to go.

Inanna also knew her loved ones would try to stop her so she told only her faithful servant Ninshubur of her plan. As expected, Ninshubur pleaded with her beloved mistress,

"Please, dear Queen, do not to go to that place. You will have to give up all your heavenly and earthly powers to descend to the Underworld. You will face a certain and horrible death. Oh PLEASE, do not go!"

Inanna smiled gently yet paid her no heed, saying, "Ninshubur, I have heard the call and I must go. Of that I am certain. But listen..."

Ninshubur was obedient and swallowed her wails.

"...You must wait for me here and be my witness. If I do not return in three days' time, beat your drum and run to the temples of my fathers. Seek help from those who dwell there."

Ninshubur swallowed again, nodded and then could contain her wails no longer.

Inanna set about preparing for her journey. She would need as much protection as she could muster. She chose seven aspects that represented her power and with magic she transformed them into feminine allure. Inanna stole away in the night and descended. She approached the dark temple slowly. Its walls glittered with lapis lazuli, and she stood before the great black gate; courage seeping out of her, foreboding creeping into her.

Slowly the gate opened. Inanna peered in; it was so dark inside. A face with small eyes and yellow teeth suddenly thrust up close to hers.

"Inanna! What brings you here?" The pungent breath of Neti, the chief gatekeeper, hung between them.

Inanna wiped his fleck of saliva off her cheek and pulled herself up straighter, remembering who she was.

"I am the Queen of Heaven and Earth, the place where the sun rises. I have come to visit my sister, Ereshkigal and to attend the funeral rites of her husband, Gugalanna; I have heard he is dead and I wish to grieve with my sister."

With that, Neti slammed the gate in Inanna's face and rushed down to report to his mistress. Ereshkigal was enraged to hear her heavenly sister had asked for the rite of passage to enter the land of no return.

After she had considered the situation for some time, Ereshkigal said, "Bolt all of the seven gates of this Underworld, Neti. Then let Inanna enter one by one—open each gate just a crack and before she passes through, make her take off her things, one at a time. The holy priestess of Heaven will enter my kingdom bowed, low and naked."

Neti ran back up, rubbing his hands with glee. He was going to have some fun at last. He opened the huge gate with laborious ceremony and ran a dirty fingernail over Inanna's arm, "You may enter," he said and let her step through the entrance to the Underworld.

At the first gate Neti instructed Inanna to stop.

"Take off your golden crown, Priestess".

Inanna was indignant.

"What is this?" She asked.

"Shush Inanna! Do not question the ways of the Underworld for they are perfect." And with that he snatched her crown. Inanna instantly felt bereft and alone; the link to her divine origins had been severed.

They walked slowly along the gloomy passageway. At the second gate Neti took the jewels from Inanna's third eye and ears.

"What is this?" she asked.

"Hush Inanna! Do not question the ways of the Underworld for they are perfect."

Now Inanna felt fearful; she could no longer see or hear her inner voice.

The Queen of Heaven put her hand out and felt the jagged damp walls as she trailed Neti deeper into the Underworld. At the third gate, Neti pulled at the necklace around Inanna's throat. Before he broke it, she reached up to unclasp it. She went to say something but found she could not speak. She had been silenced. Neti smiled.

"You are learning quickly Inanna. The ways of the Underworld are perfect."

At the fourth gate, Neti tugged at Inanna's breastplate. As he pulled it off, she was consumed with self-pity, her heart closing in the darkness. The servant sniggered.

The fifth gate creaked as Neti opened it just a crack and before he let the priestess pass he snatched the measuring line and rod from where she always held it, just above her navel. Inanna froze; her power was gone. She felt blocked. Empty.

Neti shoved her and she stumbled along, bowing lower as she went. Before he let her pass through the sixth gate, he yanked at her golden hip girdle and it fell to the ground with a dull clang. Inanna gasped as hatred and shame were borne inside her.

At the seventh and final gate, Neti took his time opening the bolts, going slowly, enjoying the sight of Inanna bowed low and nearly naked.

"Your royal breechcloth if you please!" He said, reaching out, leering and snatching at the last of Inanna's feminine allure. Inanna felt her connection to the earth vanish completely. She no longer knew who she was or where she was.

Ereshkigal waited on her throne, exuding power and anticipation. Although she knew that the naked and bowed figure who stumbled into her royal chamber was indeed her sister, the Queen of the Underworld did not recognise her. She stood up, eyes aflame, as Inanna started towards her.

All of a sudden the many judges of the Underworld, the Annunaki, flocked around Inanna and passed judgment upon her. Ereshkigal then fastened the eye of death upon her sister and uttered against her terrible words that tortured her spirit. Although she cowered, Inanna looked up at Ereshkigal and their eyes met briefly. Then the Queen of Darkness struck and Inanna fell. Her body morphed into a mass of rotting flesh.

The Anunnaki withdrew silently into the shadows and all that could be heard was Neti dragging the corpse over to the wall where a huge meat hook hung. The dead weight almost defied him as he struggled to get the body wedged upon the spike.

When it was done, Ereshkigal swayed and gave way to the ground; this loss suddenly biting into her bones. All her life, she had suffered deep wounds of rejection; hatred, rage, shame, abandonment and more. These had been hers to face in solitude, in the darkness. And all the while her sister had moved freely in the light. But now Inanna was gone, Ereshkigal felt completely and utterly alone. The dark goddess imploded with grief.

On the surface of the Earth, Ninshubur beat her drum. Her mistress had not returned and three days and three nights had passed. Ninshubur went to the temples of Inanna's father, and her father's father with the news. They were both furious and sent the maidservant packing, shouting as she went; Inanna had transgressed their law. She had sought a different path from theirs and for that she must pay. Inanna had known the Underworld was a place of no return and they would not help her.

Ninshubur beat her drum once more and made her way to the temple of Enki, Inanna's mother's father. The servant was, by now, beside herself and made barely any sense as Enki, the God of Wisdom, listened to her tale. Enki knew of the ways and the anguish of the Underworld and he understood what it was to heed the call. He agreed to help.

Using his powers of creation, Enki took the dirt from under his fingernails and fashioned the Kurgurra and the Galatur, ego-less, sex-less creatures who could trust the life force even when it sounded in misery. They entered the Underworld like flies. Their instinct took

# The Wild Rainbow

them to the Dark Queen who still wailed and moaned, contorted with grief. She had lost the other side of herself. The Kurgurra and the Galatur moaned with Ereshkigal, mirroring the desolate queen's emotions and for the first time ever she felt what it was to be witnessed; she was no longer alone!

Ereshkigal was immediately awash with gratitude and generosity. She offered the Kurgarra and the Galatur bountiful gifts of fertility and growth but they needed neither. The Queen of the Underworld asked them what it was that they wanted and they looked upon the corpse, hanging from the wall. Feeling less alone now, Ereshkigal was able to grant them their wish and feeling lighter still released her dead sister to them.

The Kurgarra and the Galatur flew about the corpse, sprinkling their magic—the food of water and life—upon the rotting meat that began to transform instantly, before all of their eyes.

Inanna was reborn in the Underworld and the sisters were re-united, each now with a little of the other in their hearts.

The Anunnaki reminded the sisters of the Underworld's law; passage out of the Underworld was prohibited. They would not allow Inanna to leave the Underworld.

Finally a deal was struck; for Inanna to return she would have to provide someone in her place. The demons of the Underworld, the Galla were summoned and instructed to cling to Inanna's side until she chose someone to take her place.

Ninshubur, dear faithful servant had not stopped the steady beat of her drum. When her mistress reappeared on the surface of the Earth she went wild. Bang, bang, bang went her beater and drum as fast as she could manage. Then she flung her sacred tools high in abandon and the big-hearted Ninshubur raced to greet her Queen.

The Galla started to leave Inanna's side but she stopped them, "No!" She shouted. They would not take Ninshubur.

Inanna enjoyed the hearty, surprised welcomes she received from her loved ones who had mourned her absence and dressed in their mourning cloths. All that is, save Dumuzi, her beloved. He had barely noticed his queen was gone. She came upon him lounging languidly on his throne, dressed in his finest. When the Queen of Heaven and Earth saw him thus, she nodded to the Galla and they left her side to claim their prize.

Dumuzi fled, pleading with the God Utu to help him get away. First he was transformed into a snake and then into a gazelle. But each time the Galla caught up with him and eventually he was captured.

Dumuzi's sister, Geshtinanna and his mother wept and wailed over his fate. Inanna saw them and was moved; she knew now what it was to suffer. Geshtinanna cried out suddenly that she would share her brother's fate and so Inanna, who knew what it was to suffer, softened. She decreed that brother and sister would take it turns, each spending half the year in the Underworld. Thus they became immortal.

And so it was that Dumuzi came to know and love both queens, She of light and dark. The Queen of Heaven and Earth and the Queen of the Underworld; each now, with a little of the other, in their hearts.

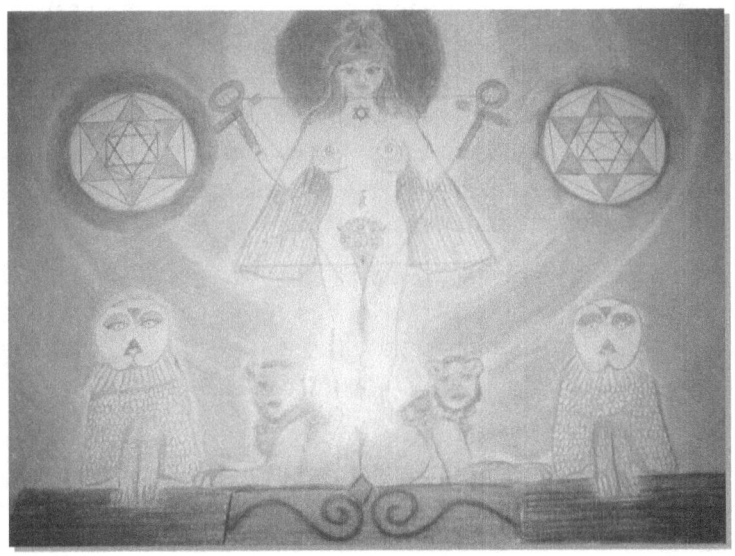

"Innanas return" –Drawing: Steven Booth

## *My mourning*

> *You flash like lightning over the highlands, you throw your firebrands across the Earth, your deafening command whistling like the south wind, splits apart great mountains.*
>
> *Holy Priestess, who can soothe your troubled heart?*
>
> —Wokstain and Kramer

### Father Of Mine

When I was 15, my Dad died suddenly. He was the first person who was close in my life that had died. I wasn't really sure what I was supposed to do. When the police came knocking on our door bearing the heavy news, I felt sad. I had a sinking feeling in my heart. I think that sinking feeling was my heart feeling heavy for my mother. I started crying. I think I was crying for my mother. I was sad that the man who she loved deep inside would never be around again. Even through those dark and hard years, I know she still stayed by his side, in case he changed, in case his gentle side emerged more fully than his hard side. I understand that because I do that too.

I went to wake my brother who was sleeping. I was meaning to just wake him and bring him to the lounge room so that someone else could tell him what had happened. But as he stirred and opened his eyes, I blurted out in one shaky, uncontrollable sentence "Dad's dead, Adam, Dad's dead".

We all sat in the lounge room together. I can't remember much else. The week of his death went by and I have memories of sitting in the blazing hot sun in the backyard of my grandmothers' house seeing my aunties and uncles cry.

My Mum's eyes turned blank, her heart was the heaviest I had ever seen it in my 15 years of being with her. On the day of Dad's funeral, she turned to me and said "I'm a widow and I'm 36 years old. What am I supposed to do now?" I didn't have the answers. I didn't even know what I felt, what my own feelings were about my father dying. I knew my brother was devastated, I knew my mother was lost. My grandmother cried at the thought of burying another child. "No mother should ever have to do this" she said to me. Some people told me 'about time he was in the ground'; others mourned 'the loss of a great hard working man'. I don't know what I felt. I only felt as though I was an observer. I didn't even feel as though any feelings I had were my own. Instead, it felt that my feelings around my father's death were merely a reaction to what other people were feeling about it. I went back to school the day after he died, I think because I wanted some normalcy. I wanted things to be 'normal' and 'right'. But of course it wasn't. And living in a small town meant that everyone knew everything. I was walking to my locker when I heard 2 boys chatting; One said 'Did you hear about that man who got ran over by a car on a quiet road in the middle of the night?' and the other said 'Yeah, what an idiot'. "Fuck off!" I yelled at them. Then they laughed at me and I heard one mutter to the other "what's her problem? She must have her period!"

Life went on and I adjusted to life without my Dad. We lived on a one acre block, just out of town. We had lots of animals and fruit trees. We used to listen to music and sing. We no longer went to bed worrying around drunks in the night. I was sleeping better and my dreams weren't always haunting me. In a way, I felt better. Life seemed easier. I did miss him, but I wasn't mourning him. I think the hardest part for me was I felt as though I lost my Mum and brother. My Mum and brother spiraled into a different direction to me. Their eyes were red from so many tears, their dreams taunted them and their hearts couldn't handle the loss. My mother didn't know how to handle her grief so she painted the inside of our home. Colours made us feel happy so the brighter the room the better. By the end of a year, the walls were purple and greens, blues and pinks, oranges and black. Some walls had painted faeries, some with pixies. It was a way to cope. A way to put some colour and hope into her life of mourning. My heart couldn't bear staying in that place, so a little over a year after Dad died, I left the dry, harsh Mallee and the burdened people with chained souls and moved to the city in hope to find myself a life.

## *Marlie The Lionheart*

So, moving to the city was a culture shock, especially at 16 years old and with no family or friends with me. All I had was my boyfriend. I was glad to be away from the small town of red necks driving around in their ute's with bumper stickers plastered over their windscreen with slogans like 'no fat chicks', 'rum injected' and 'looking for your daughter? She's in my trunk'. I was overwhelmed with delight when I saw 'people like me' walking down the streets without being abused. I remember the first time I walked down Smith St and I saw a girl wearing a tutu and mismatched knee high socks. Her hair was green and purple, just like mine, and she had so many piercings in her face. No one was shouting abuse at her, no one looked at her or made remarks about the way she looked. She was accepted for who she was in that part of the city. It was a shock to me, as I had never been in a place where differences were not only tolerated, but accepted.

When I moved to the city with my then boyfriend, the only connection I had with anyone was with an ex-girlfriend. She was the only other person I knew in this city of millions. We had a kind of awkward break up and I thought it would be strange to reconnect with her, but I did it anyway. It was nice to see her. Her face still looked the same, but I remembered she looked a 'little weathered'. She was such a resilient young woman. It seemed her life was a constant battle of surviving against the odds. Her whole life was a story of unimaginable abuse and neglect. I fell in love with her because despite everything that had happened to her in her life, she still had a spark in her eye. She dreamed big that I believed in her. Once she told me that I was the only one who told her that she was amazing and could do what she wanted with her life.

A few months after we reconnected I got news that she had died suddenly. She committed suicide. She had intentionally overdosed herself.

All of a sudden, between one moment to the next, she became a memory. Her shoulder length hair that was always violet I would no longer admire. Her eyes with the spark and the lashes that were always so thick with mascara I would no longer see. I would never have the chance again to lay my head against her chest and listen to the sound of what a courageous heart beats like. I don't even know what happened, as she seemed ok. Well, really, I guess I do…. Years of trying to be light whilst living in the dark must have eventually taken its toll. I understand that world of trying to be your best, to strive for something more than what you have been given but being shot down every time is like. It's like a beautiful flower kept in the dark with no sunshine or moist soil. The spark in her eye must have faded. The darkness in her world must have been too much to bear. I grieve for her. I grieve for the life that she missed out on. I mourn for the life that she deserved but never got. A part of me felt relieved that she could finally rest but another part of me was full of rage that she died alone and never got to see the full beauty and potential of what actually is possible in our world. And so she became a memory. I don't even have a photo of her. All I have is an anger that sits in my throat, wanting to scream out, to call out to the universe and ask it why was this life so cruel to her? I wrote a lot after she died. A lot of poetry flowed onto paper. It was the way I could cope as I didn't have anyone to talk to that was compassionate and understanding.

Some people I tried to share my sadness with told me it's her own fault. They called her a junkie and they called her weak. But to me, she was a shero. She was a woman of strength. A woman of resilience. A woman who protected those younger than her who needed to be protected, at any cost. She was a guardian of children, of girls. She was the watcher and the gatekeeper. She was the monster – hunter and she protected the innocence of children.

Her death was my beginning. After she died, I felt it imperative that I live in beauty for her. I would experience beauty and what is beautiful, so that her death wouldn't feel like 'the end'. I went and got a piercing on my face on my 'beauty spot'. My fascination for collecting beautiful things grew stronger and I would soon have an altar of feathers and rocks – gifts of beauty from the Earth to remind me, and her, that life can be beautiful.

# The Wild Rainbow

### *Savage, Wild*

Savage, wild
There she was born
From the eruption of a volcano
Like lava she came
Straight into the claws
of a crooked teeth monster
And though they tried
She never faulted
Her heart was made of gold
And her spirit of violet fire
She would never be broken
And now she flies with wings
Being watcher of the innocent
In her home in the sky
Where she is safe and free

### *Beautiful Things*

Though she was raised in fire and ice
She was made of beautiful things
She could dance like she was made of light
And her laughter made the faeries appear
The ones who called her worthless
Did not see her magic wings
They were tucked away, the beautiful things

## *Nan The Gentle*

When I was 17, my Nan was diagnosed with bone marrow cancer and she began her year long journey to death. She was in her early 60's and it wasn't fair. She was too kind to have to die so soon. The world needed her. I couldn't believe this was happening. Nan was the one who made me feel safe. In fact, she was the one who made me feel safe. Nothing was better than being with Nan, enveloped in her arms, listening to her laughter. Her place was my safe place where I went to in my childhood. She was the physical representation of my safety. She was the one who took my fears and my burdens for me and she returned them transmuted into love and kindness of the deepest kind. How was I supposed to feel safe if Nan wasn't around? How could I live in world that my Nan wasn't in? How would the world cope without someone so kind and compassionate living in it?

Over that long, dreadful year, each time I saw my Nan, my heart broke a little more. She was so sick. The cancer was killing her body. It was taking her spirit away. Her eyes were sunken, her big squashy soft body we loved to hug was gone. She lost half her body weight. She could no longer sing or tell us stories. All the medication made her blank and lifeless. My heart was breaking.

The last time I saw her, she was lying on her bed and she was so weak that she couldn't even talk. She opened her eyes, but it was as though the world was too bright for her. I kissed her hand and told her I loved her. Then I left the room before she could see my tears and I went to the dried up creek alongside her home and cried and cried and cried.

One night, when Mum called me at a strange hour, I knew what that she was going to say that Nan had died. I answered the phone and I said 'I know'. I felt so relieved that her journey was over. That the cruel suffering of a saint had ended.

Since Nan's passing, I've always felt her presence around. She is always with me in spirit. She comes in my dreams, she is guardian of her great grandchildren, and she comes and tells me stories or reminds me that she loves me. Her spirit is living in a soft place now. A gentle space of dreams and bliss and she is being nurtured by Angels as they sing her soul to sweetness. Gosh, I miss her and I wish she could be physically here to drink tea with me and play with her great grandchildren. But I smile at the thought of her being free, without pain and enveloped in love and bliss.

## *Adam The Brave*

Adam was soft. He was a gentle warrior. He was an Earthkeeper and a Starman. He was my brother and I loved him so much.

One night I awoke in tears. I sat up abruptly from my sleep and started crying. I don't think I had been dreaming. I was having no nightmares. I looked at the clock and it was 3:39am. Steven woke and asked me what was wrong. "I just can't do it anymore" I said over and over and over. I don't even know why I said that. And then I lay down and went back to sleep.

That morning my Aunty came to my doorstep. How strange, I thought. I didn't even realise that she knew my address.

"Sheree, I've got some bad news" she said slowly.

I readied myself. She was going to tell me that my grandmother had died. I was working out ways in my head how I would cope when she told me that news.

"It's Adam." she said.

~*~*~*~

I was 18 when Adam was ripped away from my life so suddenly and unexpectedly. The day he died was Friday the 13th. . Black Friday. It was also Good Friday.

My Aunty took Steven and I in the car and we travelled the 4 hours to my Mum. We stopped on the way at several service stations and milk bars. The roads were busy and people everywhere were smiling because it was Easter long weekend. "Good day for travelling" one old man with kind eyes said to me. "Happy Easter!" exclaimed a handful of others. I didn't respond. Instead, I retreated to the backseat of the car and shut the door, wishing I could disappear or become invisible to the whole world.

When I got to Mum's house, the curtains were drawn. It was dark inside. It smelled damp and the air tasted like tears.

"I knew when I opened the door to the police what they were going to say to me" my Mum told me. "I should have just got him when he rang me last night. You are all that I have left, bubs."

I was so numb. I hated this. I wanted Adam to be alive. I didn't want him to be dead. He was only 20.

Family didn't know what to do. A lot of my family on my Dads side were loving and helpful but on my Mums side; they just didn't know what to do or how to cope. Instead of staying around to support Mum and I through our grieving, they left us completely. Some even stopped talking to us. My Mum and I were just a harsh reminder of the realness and rawness of sorrow and grief. Most of my friends disappeared too. Slowly but surely I was being left out of parties, not receiving invitations to things. Friends stopped ringing me. Grief and mourning is hard enough to face when you are supported and loved by others. Grief and mourning when you have to do it alone is almost unbearable.

~*~*~*~

Adam's death was almost my own death. I lost hope. I started to think 'what is the point of living when we just all die?' Everyone around me was dying. In a space of 4 years, 4 people close to my heart had died. And they were so very young. My emotional descent into darkness and into the underworld was very real.

I felt as though I had met my shadow sister, Erishkagel, many, many times. As soon as I would start to feel the beginning of peace, hope or rebuilding, Erishkagel would drag me back down the seven gates until I was a groveling, naked mess at the feet of the shadow sister. My life felt as though I was being stripped bare, again and again and again. I didn't know how many times I could keep being dragged through the depths of the underworld. After my brother died, I told my shadow, my Erishkagel, that I don't want to return to the world above. It would be easier to stay here, in the shadows with her, then to live in hope and dreams that my life may one day be beautiful. Everything I ever valued was gone.

I felt lost, lonely, broken, shattered. At times I wanted to destroy myself completely. At times I wanted to stay in an alcohol and drug induced coma and never wake up again.

But I couldn't be that selfish. Even through it all; through all the deaths, through the loss of friendships, through the loss of myself at times, my heart knew I had to stay alive. There was a world for me out there that I needed to create for myself. I refused to die in sadness. I refused to die for anything less than my absolute potential and fulfillment.

I felt as though by sitting in the darkness with my shadow sister, without judgment, without compassion, without anything, as I had absolutely nothing left within me, I was able to dwell in a place of complete humbleness.

I almost felt as though because I had nothing left, yet the fact that I was still alive meant that I could start again. I could not re-write the past, as the past is always there, never to be erased. But I could re-create my future because all the 'things' I valued were no longer. I could re-write my own story future – however I wanted to. This moment wasn't a sudden epiphany. It wasn't that all of a sudden things started working. It was more of a subtle glimmer of something. It was a little point of golden light that I could see in the distance, and it was so fascinating and enchanting, it gave me something to focus on. It gave me something to dream on, to look forward to.

~*~*~*~

On a dreary day after Adam died, I sat down with a bowl of pasta and watched my favourite childhood show – Rainbow Brite. There was something about the part where Wisp, who was the little ordinary girl set out to restore colour and hope to an evil, dreary world, came across a baby – who ended up being the very significant 'spirit of light'. The baby was stolen by the king of shadows and even though she was taken from Wisp, she was the key that made the colour back. She gave Wisp the courage to stand up to the shadows, to reclaim colour and hope for the whole world. This is Adams legacy to me. I felt as though the end of his life was a catalyst for mine to step up to its potential, to look at my strengths and power, to reclaim my own magnificence and to make a beautiful difference - to myself, my community and my world.

Over time, and with other events in my life, I began to feel that I wasn't destined to howl in the dark, putrid walls of the underworld. I started to believe that I was actually able to live a life of love, happiness and fulfillment and that although I had felt so stripped bare, like everything was taken from me, even human lives, I still had something to offer. I still had something to live for. I was worthy. I allowed myself to grieve as I needed to. If I had days where I howled with sorrow, then I would. If I had days where I wished I had a turtle shell armor to protect me so I wouldn't get hurt, then I would wrap myself up in a blanket and listen to music, drink some hot milo and stay warm. And on the days where I felt ok, I would go outside, close my eyes and put my face in the sunshine. I would feel the moist soil under my feet and I would smile at little things, knowing that I am worthy and am able to manifest myself a beautiful, inspiring life.

I love you Adam. I miss you.

## *Eternal Love, a story of Miscarriage*

Told by Kerry Baulch

For all women the feeling is different and we all cope in various ways, this is my own personal experience of losing a precious little baby angel.

I'm now a happy mother to three children but between my eldest and middle children I have my angel baby. My partner and I in the year 2007 were planning our wedding; I was studying and raising our first born. We decided about 8 months before our wedding that we wouldn't wait until married before we tried for our second baby. We tried, but as each month came along with another period I became more depressed and angry at myself and my body. We got to a point where we felt that we were just having sex to procreate and it no longer felt special or as fun. Realising this, I created myself a space and was able to talk it through, relax in life and enjoy our love again.

We took it easy and reveled in planning our wedding and enjoying our family and allowing the cards fall where they may. It was still hard for me to just let life be but I eventually started to not think about babies all the time. I knew I wasn't thinking straight as whenever I saw a baby or heard of a friend having a baby I would cry and die a little more inside. I didn't think I could feel worse than I did, but as it tends to happen, life throws curve balls all the time and I had a lesson to learn sooner than I thought.

 About Three weeks before our wedding I just felt a little off and decided to do a test to see if I was pregnant. Sure enough I was. I decided to keep it a little secret and surprise my new husband with the news on our wedding night. The smile couldn't be wiped off my face and I walked with my head in the clouds with excitement dreaming and making big plans for my growing family. Little did I know that the fate of my baby was not what I would have ever wanted.

One day, on my way home from placement, I remember the traffic being bumper to bumper and people just seemed to be in bad moods, rushing past, cutting you off. I remember that a car cut off the car in front of me and I had to break suddenly. As I did, I had an instinctive feeling that the car behind me just wasn't going to pull up in time. It seemed like forever but was only mere seconds while I watched in the rear-view mirror and heard the brakes lock up, I braced myself for the impact and sure enough it came. The guy apologised and swapped details while I just went through the motions of getting his info my mind was elsewhere and I just wanted to get home. I felt so sick with worry and spent the whole time driving home holding my stomach protectively while talking to the little babe growing on the inside. I still at that stage didn't tell my partner about the pregnancy as he was already worrying so much about getting the car repaired in time for our wedding.

Later that night I had some strong pains across my lower abdomen and told my partner It was probably just some whiplash and that I needed to soak in the bath. My bath lasted for a while as I spent most of the time crying, upon getting undressed I noticed I was now bleeding and it wasn't like normal, nothing felt right. It was all wrong. Needless to say, a very restless night full of bad dreams and horrible feelings, I was realising my fear was coming true. I was miscarrying and there wasn't a thing I could do to stop it.

The next day while I was alone, everything I feared happening was confirmed for me. The accident the day prior caused me to lose my growing baby. I felt like my heart had been ripped out of my body and thrown on the highway for all to drive over. I had no choice now but to tell my partner what had happened. He didn't know how to react and I didn't make it any easier on him. My emotions took over and all logic went out the window to the point I even wanted to sue the other driver for emotional damages when it was just a freak accident. I have never felt like that, I was in such as low place; it seemed like anything that anyone said or did would make me snap and so unhappy. While it hurts me to admit it, I started to resent my partner and myself because something that happened so easily first time around and certainly wasn't planned had worked but the baby that we tried so hard to get was ripped away from me.

I didn't want to be held or cuddled or touched by my partner which frustrated him because he needed that for his comfort. I knew he wasn't coping very well with it either but I didn't care at that stage. In the end I pushed on and put a smile on my face for my family and

# The Wild Rainbow

friends as the wedding got closer. While they all talked about hair, makeup, flowers and cake, I sat there smiling pretending but cying inside.

I thought I was doing a great job of hiding my feelings; however my mother asked me the night before my wedding what the hell was going on. I told my Mum it was just pre wedding jitters. That night I didn't cry and something seemed different in me. I had the realisation that although nothing I could do would change the outcome, I could still love my baby and have a happy life. I no longer needed to travel the downward spiral. I could live my life now and be the best mum and wife that I could be for my daughter, my husband and any future children.

It was still hard but one day in a ritual of letting my baby go, I wrote many words on paper about how I felt and then ripped out and burnt them, releasing them, saying goodbye to my lost angel.

I didn't share my story with anyone for a very long time not even my mum or best friend. When I did let my mum in on what had really happened she said she felt like I had lost a precious babe but didn't want to push me risking more damage. She wanted me to open up when I felt the time was right. I know that my mum and all my friends would have been there for me if I had have let them but I felt like it was something I had to deal with by myself. My best friend was shocked. So now, in my healing, I share my story with you. And as I do, I feel a kind of sense of weightlessness and feel my lost angel is proud of me to open up and share.

Each year at the same time that I lost my babe, I sit and read to the air and dream about the games we would be playing and lessons we would be learning. I will forever miss my angel baby but realise that there is now another person in the spirit world taking care of me from above. I only hope that for anyone going through the loss of a child that you deal with it as you can but remember that there are many arms there to catch you when you're ready to share your story.

## *The One Who Steals The Innocent*

When I was little and I was scared of monsters, my Mum would tell me "Don't worry bubs, monsters aren't real, they are made out of paper".

But I remember the day I met a real life monster. He was disguised as a human, wearing a human mask.

He took many things from me. Things that could never be returned. Things that could never be replaced, fixed, made whole, bought back or apologised for.

The monster was so dangerous, with no self-control. He had guns under his bed and knives on his wall. His prey were the weak, they were the women and the children, the scared, lost, vulnerable. He will never know love, as he grew with a violent, sick and twisted heart.

He used to always come and steal precious things from my family. He pretended to have a pretty face but I was never fooled by his mask. One look at his eyes and I could see what he was, how he worked, what he wanted from us. He reeked of hatred. He reeked of blood stained hands and torment and he was disgusting. He laughed at our pain. A corner of his lip would lift up in a smirk of satisfaction when he would see us. A knowing in my heart would make it beat faster and I felt the need to run, to hide, to escape his hate. He was physically too strong for me, and my brother and my mother. Our torment, our tears, our broken, vulnerable selves were his fuel and energy that kept him going.

One day, when I don't know if I was feeling defeated or courageous, I looked at his face and stared into his eyes. And in that brief moment of time, when his clouded, cold, demon eyes met my soft, young, emerald eyes, I realised he was scared of me. He was scared of beautiful things. He was scared of small things that held great power. He was scared of gentleness and kindness.

The monster is gone now. He died and he is buried away from our family, where he can't see us or hurt us or take anything from us. He lives in a place where he can't close his eyes, because when he does, he sees what he has done. He is surrounded by fear and he knows the noises he hears in the night are his own ghosts.

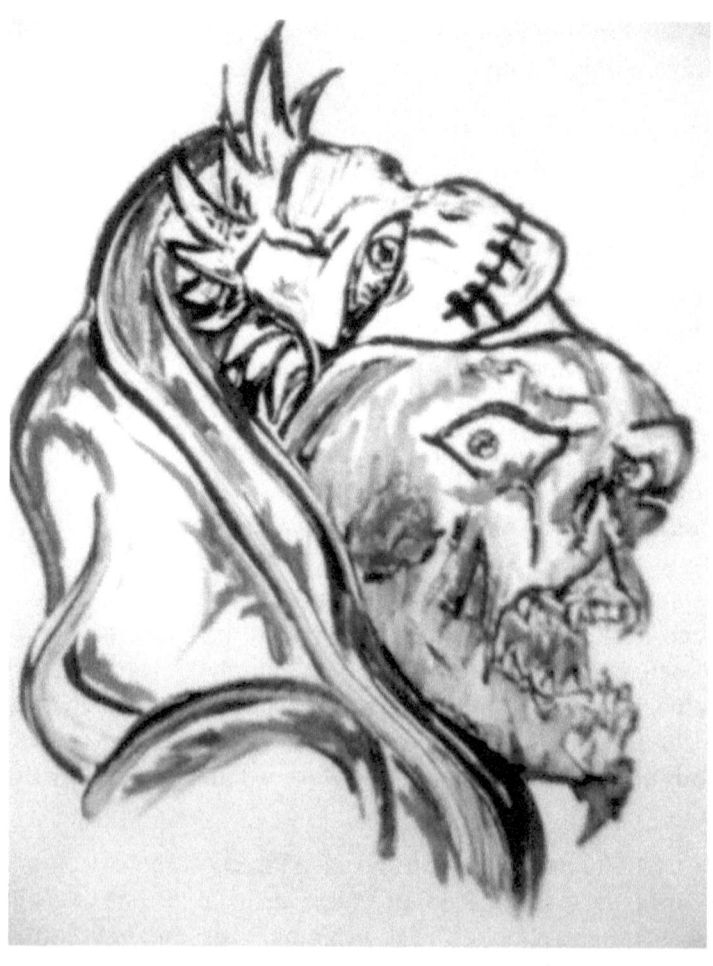

*"Monster"* – Artist: Star Davis

## *Human*

The month has shown me many faces of life.

It has shown me the full spectrum of birth, life, death and rebirth

Lives of 2 people I know have been taken

There has been a new baby roared Earthside

Many of us are in between

Some of us are lost in a lingering place of hopelessness and despair

Some of us are in ecstatic bliss

It has just reminded me to slow down, to stop and smell the roses

To watch the Earth, be in the Earth and love her

What does my heart want?

To be free

Today I am feeling very human

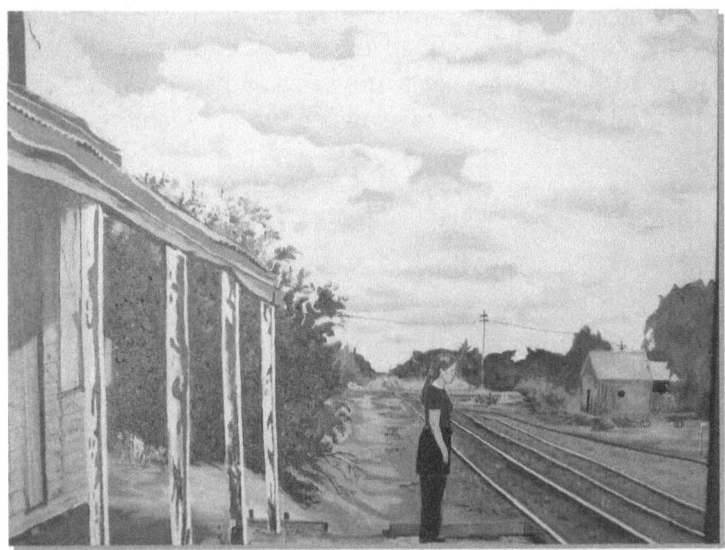

*"Memories"* – Painting: Annie Joy

## *Woman: Honouring the Sacred Wound*

It is believed by many that the 'wound reveals the cure'. If we focus on the problem, we can find the answer and be on our path to wholeness, to our potential.

When I was undertaking a year long journey of Shamanic Midwifery with Jane Hardwicke Collings, we were asked to write a fairytale, based on an exercise by author Jean Houston, called the 'sacred wound'. We were asked to journey to a trauma that happened early in our lives and experience it again by writing it out like a fairytale, but finding magic in it and creating a happy ending.

Once I had picked a particular event and written the story, reading over it, I realised there was a pattern that I play out through my whole life. It wasn't just this one event in my life, but all of them. I found a pattern that I follow where I react exactly the same to any situation I feel scared or threatened in. Once I realised this, I was able to notice when it came up in my life and react to it accordingly, in a different manner to how I would previously. I am more able to face situations that make me feel uneasy or threatened. I felt as though by creating a happy ending in my story, I was finally giving myself permission to rewrite my story, to give myself the happy ending I deserve and to stop the pattern repeating again and again and again. By noticing what my wound is, I am able to release my stories and recreate a new world for myself.

> "The wounding becomes sacred when we are willing to release our old stories and to become the vehicles through which the new story may emerge into time. When we fail to do this, we repeat the same old story over and over again."
>
> - *The Search for the Beloved,* Jean Houston,

## The Wild Girl – A Sacred Wound Story

*Once upon a time a wild woman was born.*

*She grew up in a land of magic with her brother. They spent their days playing in nature, understanding and living within the Earth cycles and communicating with the plant and animal realms. Their hearts were wild and free, they knew no boundaries, as boundaries don't exist when your heartbeat echoes that of The Great Mother.*

*One day as the Wild Children grew; they were taken against their will and placed into a cage. They were put into this cage with a large group of Others. All the Others looked so different to the Wild Boy and Girl. They all had neatly groomed hair, blank eyes and foul mouths. They all stared at the Wild Boy and Wild Girl. And they teased them. It started off with simple teasing – name calling and teasing them as they walked passed. But then it got worse over time. The violence endured by the Wild Boy and Wild Girl was unspeakable, even their dreams were cruel and violent to them.*

*This continued on for many, many cycles of the moon, until one day the Wild Boy and Wild Girl couldn't take it anymore.*

*"Let's wear masks and costumes, so we look just like them" said the Wild Boy*

*"Yes, and brush our hair, dull our eyes and close our hearts" said the Wild Girl*

*So, a pact was made and the journey began. They brushed their hair, made masks that looked like those of the Others. They spent days on costumes and days on scrubbing themselves. No dirt to be seen, no spark in the eye. For their survival, every part of them that was wild, was now tamed.*

*The day came for The Wild Boy and Girl to finally step out into the world of Others. As they did the reaction was massive for them. The Others turned around and welcomed them. The Wild Boy and Girl were weary at first, but one breath at a time, one move at a time, they moved closer and closer into the world of the Others. By the end of the first evening, they were accepted. The Others poured wine, they* danced, laughed, shared stories with them.  The Wild Boy and Girl could barely believe it, it had worked! They were finally accepted and welcomed.

This laughter, acceptance and friendship of their new life continued on for months. There were many merry moments and things felt good. So good in fact, that The Wild Girl suggested to her brother that perhaps they should take off their masks. She felt that because they were accepted now, that that wouldn't change if they revealed themselves.

The Wild Boy was weary, but could see where his sister was coming from so reluctantly agreed.

That night, Wild Boy and Girl took off their masks at the Gathering of the Others. They revealed themselves – their hair untamed and their eyes wild. The Others all looked at each other, and then back to the Wild Ones. Their eyes glazed over and turned a furious red. They were so outraged.

One of the Others got a spear and threw it towards the Wild Ones. It went straight through Wild Boys heart and tore it apart. The Wild Boy died.

Wild Girl was so frightened that she turned into a chameleon and ran away. She spent the next many years, wearing masks, changing shape, adding on layer after layer after layer so that she could not be recognised. To be recognised is to be killed. She travelled to many a strange land and adapted by talking the talk and walking the walk, wearing the masks and costumes that were necessary for her survival.

One day on one of her journeys, she was walking through the scorching hot desert; the heat was so intense that one of the masks melted off her face. She felt terrified of this and tried to hide. But where could she hide when she was surrounded by nothing but a hot ocean of desert sand, a blazing sun and scorpion's? She was out in the open – vulnerable and exposed.

So she did all she could do in a situation such as this. Breathe. And take one step at a time, one foot after the other.

The day continued on and the sun roared even hotter. The ground burnt her feet, it was so hot that layers of her costume kept melting off her. One mask slipped away, and then another, then another. Then her costumes did too. She continued to just breathe, and step, through the desert sun.

By the end of the day Wild Girl was exhausted. She walked as far as she possibly could before falling asleep, surrendering to the possibility that she may never wake up or she may be eaten by vultures. She slept for ages, hours and hours, possibly days.

When she awoke she could barely believe her eyes. She was surrounded by rose petals and sapphires. People were standing around her clapping and cheering. She looked at her naked body lying on the sand and saw that her scars and wounds had healed. Someone in the crowd yelled out loudly "She is awake! She has awoken! The Wild Girl has returned!" The people cheered harder.

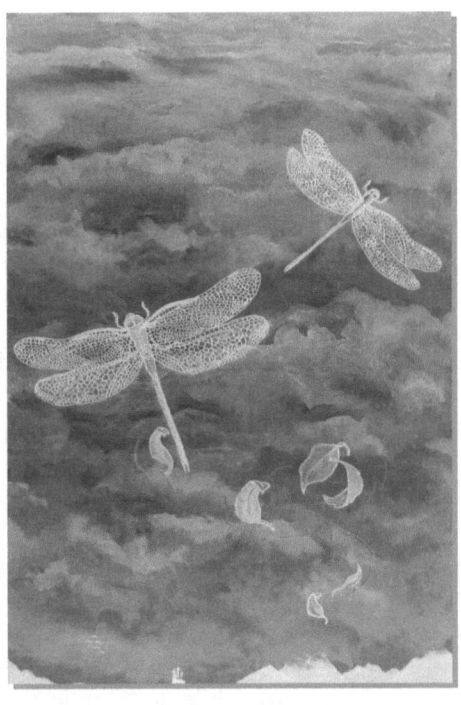

"Dragonflies" – Artist: Annie Joy

Wild Girl stood up, fully exposed, vulnerable and naked, in her own skin, with no masks or costumes. She started to dance and move her snake arms, reclaiming her body. Her wild eyes lit up and she cried with relief. The tears flowed down her cheeks onto the sand ocean – the more tears that fell; the more the desert was nourished. The dancing and the tears continued, it flowed and flowed, connecting her heart to the Earth. Soon, ponds appeared from the tears and many flowers sprung from the ground. Animals arrived and the people cheered even more.

The Wild Girl had returned and taken her place. The Creatrix, the Starwoman, the Storyteller. Her crown was placed upon her head and everything was ok.

Everyone lived Happily Ever After.

## *The Sacred Wound Exercise*

By Jane Hardwicke-Collings,
adapted from *The Search for the Beloved*, Jean Houston

Find a quiet space where you will be undisturbed. This process may take at least an hour, possibly longer. You could start it and then return to it. Read through the whole exercise before you start and decide where you will need to stop if you need to do this in stages. Have your journal on hand to record this process.

- Light a candle and set and intention (decide on your intention once you read though this exercise), smudge yourself and the space, you can use incense if you don't have a smudgestick and again set an intention to cleanse the space and yourself of unwanted energy before you start.

- Call your guardian angel, your power animal, and your guides to be with you.

- Create and altar with your candle and any power objects you want there, call the directions and elements.

- Turn off your phone.

- You can do as much or as little of these things to create your sacred space, the container, as it were, to hold you through your process.

- Using your journal, review the wounding's in your life, make a list.

- Now, choose the one that feels as though it was the earliest in your life, perhaps the first of the ones that followed that had a similar energy. If you can't think of the earliest, then choose the one with the most emotion around it for you, and take time to answer these questions in relation to this experience:

- What happened? How were you wounded?
- What did you feel when you were wounded?
- What were the full consequences of this wounding in your life, for good or ill?
- In light of this, what do you want?
- What does all this mean? What pattern is playing itself out here?
- How does this serve?

➢ Record the answers in your journal.

➢ Building upon these answers, now re-remember your story as a myth.

➢ When creating a myth of your life, you must keep yourself well away from the mundane - something of a trick to do. Allow each figure and situation in the myth to become archetypal.

> *"Thus a soldier becomes a warrior, a young girl is the maiden-to-be-rescued, an animal may become an ally, and a serpent the guardian of the gates. The child is always holy, if unrecognized, the circumstances of birth extraordinary: the family always poor but honest, or of the highest nobility (there is no bourgeoisie in the land of myth); an elderly person is the wise one; the one who yearns is the lover, the one who seeks, the Hero or Heroine."* Jean Houston

➢ Begin your story with "once upon a time..." and take the story past the wounding to the place of transformation. Allow yourself to be whatever your imagination desires - be Brave, Smart, Rich, Loved - this is a myth it's not supposed to be "The Truth"!

➢ And don't forget to let yourself live "happily ever after".

> You can change the details of your story but keep the underlying wound, for example for a past history of sexual abuse, metaphorically present, perhaps:

> *...the princess is kidnapped and taken to a tower from which she cannot escape; she is regularly tormented by her captor until one day she escapes and...*

OR

> *...as a young girl, she had something precioius taken from her...one day when she was searching again, as she always did, she found not the precious jewel she was searching for, but...*

So the idea is to speak of the wounding in the context of the story from a mythological perspective, i.e using archetypal characters (princesses, faeries, demons etc) and larger than life situations that speak as a metaphor for your experience, e.g her father sold her to the local woodsman for firewood so the rest of the family could stay warm. You could use stories that you already know to match yours.

The other point here is to take the story beyond where you're living it now, for example, if you are revisited by painful memories and repeated experiences of your original wound, then write the story beyond that to the place when 'the maiden is rescued by the prince' and remember the prince might be your inner masculine as opposed to an outer male.

> To finish this exercise, give thanks and put out the candle.

To follow this writing exercise it is important to express the energy you have raised, physically. One way to do this is to dance. Put on some soulful music, or whatever feels perfect, and move to it how you feel to. Move with free abandon, as if no one is watching, so that your expression is unguarded and real. Move with the intention of shifting any energy you have inside you that needs to move 'for your highest good' or energy that 'no longer serves you'.

Movement at this time also allows for the physical expression of a previously un-actioned fight or flight response that may have been instigated with the original wound and for one reason or another was never acted out. This expression, at last can in itself be highly healing, with a feeling of finally letting go instead of feeling constantly on guard or on edge, or even startled. It takes a lot of energy to maintain a suspended state of fight or flight and one this is released, so too is the energy required to hold it. This new sense of space enables the individual to be more fully present and to be free to learn and grow. Shifts such as this can also be facilitated by Kinesiology.

After your experience of movements be sure to notice how you feel and reserve that as your new baseline, your new 'default' as it were, for the issue. Being with your sacred wound, honouring its soulcrafting 'gifts', daring to look the pain 'in the eye', and take responsibility for it, and then unraveling patterned behaviour is what raising consciousness looks like.

*"Doing the healing work with your sacred wound can provoke an encounter with the soul itself. Your wound holds a key to your destiny in this life. As you struggle with the grief's and horrors at the heart of the wound, no longer distracting yourself from what you uncover there, you may find yourself, one day, staring straight into the deepest truths of this lifetime"* - Bill Plotkin

# Journeying as Mother

> There is something
> wonderfully bold and liberating
> about saying yes to our entire
> imperfect and messy life.
>
> –Tara Brach

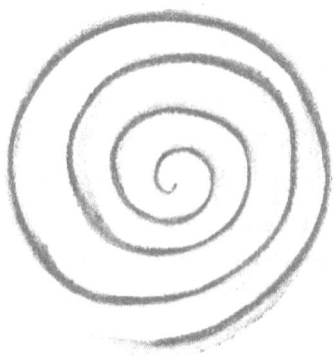

## *My Whirlwind, Explosive, Fast Ride into Motherhood*

I was pregnant at 19 and I was ecstatic. I found out this news 3 months after my brother had died. I was at a point in my life when I felt as though there was no point to life except to die. I was starting to feel as though the universe was against me and that it enjoyed watching everything be taken from me. So, the thought of new life was exciting. Not only new life, but new life that I was creating - I was the Creatrix in this. I was the woman who was able to grow a human life within her body and bring it forth into existence. That was an incredible feeling. My pregnancy with my baby was so exciting. I loved the way my body changed. I loved feeling my baby move. I didn't even mind the sore back, the swollen ankles or the heartburn. It was all wonderful to me. At the time of my pregnancy I was doing my year 12 at a VCE for adults program. My teachers were incredible, encouraging and trusting of me. It was such a supportive environment where I was able to thrive. This baby was the first grandchild on both sides of our families. Everyone was excited. Everything felt good.

It was on Easter Sunday and the day of a big blue moon, I was awoken around 3am with twinges that felt different to the Braxton-Hicks I had been having in the weeks previous. I knew the journey to meet my baby was beginning. Throughout the day I laboured gently with contractions. They were regular but mild and spaced far apart. Steven called his Mum to say we won't be joining them for Easter lunch because we had more important things to attend to on that day. In her excitement, she came over with her sister and dropped us off some Easter eggs. They didn't stay long; just long enough to share in the excitement and wish us luck before they left for their home to celebrate Easter and the impending arrival of our baby.

We decided to go into the hospital after I had laboured gently at home all day as we had no idea of what we were supposed to do. Around 7pm we arrived at the hospital doors. The nurse in Emergency said I don't look like I'm in labour because I look too calm, but she will take me up the the labour ward anyway where a midwife would assess my progress. I didn't let her bitter approach towards me hinder my excitement. Once on the labour ward I was put in a small cubicle and waited for a while for someone to see me. Around 7:30 a midwife came and we listened to the babies' heart rate, she palpated my tummy to feel for contractions and then she asked if she could do a vaginal examination to see what my cervix was doing. I agreed to this and once the vaginal exam was over I was disappointed when she told me that my cervix was still quite posterior and had only dilated 1cm. I was hoping that all that gentle labour at home would have done something a bit more to my cervix. I sighed and then gathered myself for the fact that labour is happening, but no baby will be coming soon. I had a moment where I giggled at the idea that my baby was going to be born on April Fools' Day.

I stood up off the bed so that I could get off my back and once I did, a warm, full gush of fluid poured all down my legs. It was actually like a scene from the movies. There was so much of it, and it was so warm. I remembered that it smelled like moist, damp, nutrient rich earth. I stood there in a puddle of amniotic fluid and turned to the midwife and said 'I think I broke my waters'. She laughed and said 'yes, you most certainly did!'

The midwife left the room to tell the In-Charge what was happening and when she came back she informed me that the best decision to make at the time is to augment the labour with the artificial hormone oxytocin, called syntocinon. Because my labour was 'slow' – my cervix was only 1cm dilated, that the longer I was in labour for with my waters broken, the higher my chance of infection would be to both my self and my baby. I wish that I had known that that was such a ridiculous thing to propose to me. I had no high risk factors, I was healthy and my baby was healthy. And yet here I was agreeing. I guess it is when they mention the word 'baby' in with words like 'risk' and 'death', you just nod your head and agree with what they say, so I consented for my labour to be augmented with an artificial hormone in the hope that it would make my contractions longer, stronger and more regular.

I was moved into a bigger room. It was an actual 'labour room' now and not a 'preparation room'. By about 8:30pm, they had found my vein, inserted the needle, hooked me up to an IV drip of syntocinon, pressed 'commenced' and away we went.

Within 15 minutes of the IV running through my veins, my contractions picked up. They were no longer gentle and rhythmic. They were forceful and harsh. The syntocinon charged through my body intensely. It didn't feel as though it was my body doing its own thing, it felt like I was being controlled by something else. It didn't feel real. The contractions ripped through my body causing forceful, robotic, excruciating pain. I lost all control of my mind and just screamed. It was too much, I couldn't bear it. I asked for pethidine and by the time it was given, the contractions were so close together, many of them were overlapping. I wasn't getting a break. It was just a long pain as my body was chemically opened by the synthetic hormone. An hour and a half after the syntocinon was put up, I got an incredible urge to push. Trying to find a spare breath to speak, I muttered 'push' to the midwife. She looked at me and said 'no, its not time for that yet love. You were 1cm dilated at 8pm and it normally takes 1 cm per hour for your first baby, plus at least an hour of pushing. You know...' Before she could finish her sentence, another contraction ripped through my body and I felt an intense feeling in my vagina and I could feel it tearing from the inside. She looked at me and said 'ok, I can see some of the baby's head. I'm just calling the 2nd midwife in to be present for the birth.'

And then my son was born. The moment I gazed at this perfect human being is one I would never forget. He had a perfect slippery and silky body, his hair was wet and dark, his lips were soft and pink and he was all mine. I had never felt love like this before. He lay on my skin and I was oblivious to the damage that had happened to my body and the panic that was present in the room.

Because of his fast, explosive entrance into the world, I had suffered 3rd degree tears as well as lacerations up the vaginal wall and there was blood everywhere. I was hemorrhaging. A doctor tried suturing some of the tears to stop the bleeding but without anaesthetic, it was excruciatingly painful. I had to leave my freshly newborn son with my man while I was taken to an operating theatre. I was given a spinal anaesthetic and they were able to stop the bleeding and do the suturing without me feeling pain. It was uncomfortable and my legs were up in stirrups for hours, which have led to hip problems for me years later.

I have a memory of them suturing me and talking to each other as though I wasn't even there. It was as though no one recognised and honoured the fact that I had just given birth to my first child. I was a mother now, where a time just before, I wasn't. I had just been initiated into motherhood and this was my experience of it.

In the operating theatre, it seemed as though I was just a nameless person. I was just a body. I wasn't even a body. I was just a broken vagina that needed to be repaired. They were talking about sports and what happened on lasts nights' episode of their favourite TV show. Every now and then one of them would look at me and tell me I am doing well and then they would go back to small chat with their colleagues while they spent 2 hours stitching my poor, swollen, torn, battered vagina. 'Welcome to motherhood' I thought. What sort of initiation was that!?

The months leading to my pregnancy, the pregnancy itself and then the birth were such an incredible time of change. I felt as though it was such a fast, whirlwind, chaotic ride into motherhood and it was one that made me question many things in my life. Why did his labour end up like that for? Why wasn't I supported? Why were those caring for me during that time so uncaring and robotic in nature? Why wasn't I honoured as a woman who had just given birth to her child? Shouldn't every woman who goes through labour and birth be showered in love, honour and respect? Birth is a mammoth event and one that women remember to the end of our days. It is a time where we are so vulnerable and opened in every sense of the words and we surrender to the power and presence of what being a god is – creating life and bringing life into flesh and existence.

My fast, chaotic, traumatic and scary transition into motherhood was another significant transition in my life that changed who I was. I remember being on the postnatal ward and the midwife wanted me to bath my son. I felt as though I couldn't do it as my body felt so weak but when I voiced this to the midwife, she told me that I sound like every other teen mother and that I need to just get over it because this is what my life was going to be like from now on. It turned out that I felt like that because my iron levels were so low from all the blood I lost (which was a result of them interfering with nature in the first place) and I needed to get a blood transfusion. The lack of compassion and love that was shown to me in the hospital changed something deep inside of me. I remember thinking to myself 'being with a woman while she brings her baby into the world is one of the most sacred, magic, amazing things you would ever witness. How can you be so robotic and judgmental in a job such as this?' I remember thinking 'I could do this job way better than any of these midwives here'. And with that thought, I started the next phase of my life. I had made the decision to continue with my year 12 and go to university to become a midwife. I could do the job much better than the women who cared for me. And so I did. The path of that seemed chaotic, fast and uncontrollable was becoming a world of beauty and hope.

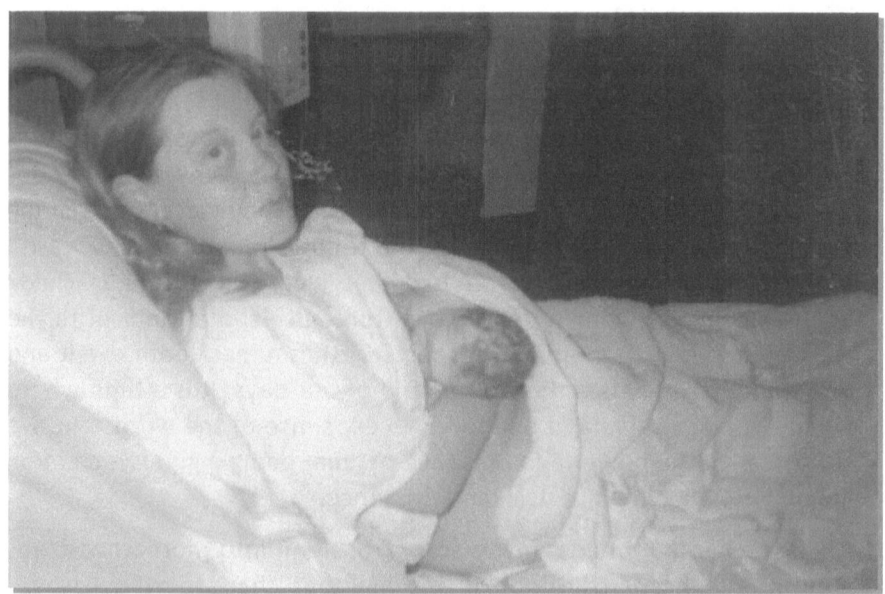

*"Sheree and Baby Caelan"* – Photo: Steven Booth

## *My Gentle Birthing & New Ways of Being.*

With the knowledge I had gained over my training to become a midwife, my search to find others like me and through the birthing my own children, I thought that I had pregnancy, birth and parenting down pat and all under control. But of course, as the case is, the journey never ends and new beginnings and ways of being are continuously unfolding as we evolve more and more into our potential. The journey with my 4th baby bought me to a new level of awareness and consciousness that I had never experienced. It was so primal and instinctual.

Even though I had had 3 previous children, so 3 previous births and two of those were considered 'natural birth' as I laboured and birthed with no drugs, I believe I didn't have a gentle, conscious birth until I birthed my 4th baby. And when I did, it was mind blowing. I feel like it rewired my brain. It changed my whole life.

The timing of becoming pregnant with my 4th baby was in a time of my life when there were a lot of changes were happening. I had just finished my graduate year as a midwife working in a large tertiary hospital where many births I was a part of were harsh and very medicalised. I was feeling so overwhelmed at being a midwife, not yet not feeling like one. I was feeling as though the world around me was falling apart and feeling like an illusion, I left the country for the first time, on my own, to Ethiopia, Africa. I rode my push bike 450kms from Addis Abeba to the remote highlands, where a hospital was, that provided emergency care for women in pregnancy and birth. My time in Ethiopia shifted my perspective; it was another time of a perfect reminder that I have to follow my heart, always, and always do what I feel is right.

Coming home, I quit my job, followed my heart and found *The International College of Spiritual Midwifery.* Just the name of the school made my heart sing. I looked up their courses and I wanted to do them all! I started off going to study the work of the doula. I was intrigued as to what a doula was; they seemed to be like a lay midwife. The philosophy was around 'mothering the mother' and it was about supporting the mother during her pregnancy and birth, however she chose to birth with and with whomever she chose to birth with. This stirred my heart, and I felt my head nodding in agreement with everything one of my sweet, gentle teachers, Sunderai Felich, was saying. This is what I wanted to do! This is what I want midwifery to be! I was so excited about the ideas and philosophy that the College offered.

I ended up doing another course through *the International College of Spiritual Midwifery*, which was *Rebirthing, Breathwork and Cellular Memory Release*. This 14 day intensive course completely opened me energetically. The healing process uses a simple, relaxing, gentle breathing rhythm. It is powerful in dissolving physical tensions and emotional traumas and restores the power of the breath to revitalise and energise the mind, body and spirit. The result is an expanded sense of self-love, creativity and joy.

Rebirthing is based on the understanding that how we think affects how we experience life. Thought is creative. Combining breathing with high quality thoughts can produce positive and lasting changes in our lives. Nurturing our positive thoughts supports us and expands our joy and aliveness. Rebirthing helps to identify and release negative, suppressed thoughts and feelings and allows us to experience self-esteem and love.

From doing this work, I was able to re-create my birth story, I was able to let go of trauma that I had held in my body (for years, and that I didn't even know that I had) and most of all, I felt clarity, peace and contentment. Things felt clear and my life seemed to have more direction and purpose.

So, in the pregnancy with my 4th baby, I felt deeply connected with my body and had a deep trust in the way it worked.

Most mornings, before I started the day, I would lay still in bed and breathe deeply into my womb. I would visualise entering my womb and meeting my baby. In these times, she would tell me what she needed, what I needed and would give me messages.

As a midwife, I had understanding and knowledge of pregnancy and birth, but nothing quite prepared me on how much I already knew about my own baby, my own body and its innate wisdom. I just had to be still and listen to it.

With feeling so connected to my body and my baby, I made a conscious choice to birth at home unassisted, which means a birth with no midwives or doctors present. I felt like there was nothing that a midwife could offer me that I needed or wanted. I had the knowledge, wisdom and trust that all would be well, and if it wasn't, that I would know what to do.

This pregnancy, which had no medical input at all, was the pregnancy that I felt most connected with. I had no experts, machines or institutions' telling me what was happening to me, to my body, to my baby. I had no experts, machines or institutions' telling me what is right, average, recommended, normal. No one was telling me what I was supposed to do or not do. I took the responsibility of my baby and my body all on my own and this made me research, it made me go inward, it made me use my intuition.

For the first time in my life, I fell in love with my body and its capabilities. I trusted it. I learned how it worked. I was so in tune that I could feel my uterus, I could feel what position the baby was in without having to palpate my tummy, I knew what her sleep/awake cycles were in utero and I knew when I needed to rest, to move, what to eat and what not to eat. All this was done by consciously tapping into my own innate wisdom.

When it came time to birth, I knew I wanted water, and that I would most likely birth in the water. I bought myself a birth pool and when I went into labour, I stayed in the pool the entire time, which was around 3.5 hours. We didn't regulate the temperature, I would just say 'more hot' if I wanted it warmer.

I had 2 doula's at the birth of my 4th baby. I wanted doula's because I wanted their emotional support, and I also wanted extra pairs of hands for our children. I had these two women present because they made me feel safe. They loved me and trusted me, and I wanted only people in my birth space that felt that way about me and my choices. And I trusted that they wouldn't intervene.

Whilst in labour with Sage, I listened to how my body wanted to move. I stayed so inward, and didn't open my eyes the entire time I was in labour. The first time I did was when my babys' head was born, and I turned to one of my doulas' and opened my eyes and said 'her heads out'. She grinned and nodded and I closed my eyes again. In transition, I swore a lot. It hurt so much, and swearing helped! I also spun around in the birth pool as it eased the intensity somewhat. I felt to be very hands on with the birth, aware that my first 2 babies 'shot out' and I didn't want to tear. I had a hot facecloth to my perineum and gently guided out her head. It was all instinctive and intuitive, and my baby and I worked in a beautiful conscious partnership.

In the month after she was born, my baby and I didn't leave the house. We stayed in, mostly tucked in bed with people bringing us meals. It felt imperative that we regained our strength. Birth is such an opening, and this makes you so vulnerable after birth, physically, emotionally, psychically. So we stayed in, stayed warm. I took Chinese herbs, ate medicinal foods and we regained our strength before we went back out into the world. I remember hearing a story about a tribe whose women have a stay in period after birth. When the 40 days is up and the woman is stronger and the baby is strong enough to meet the new world, an elder comes and paints the mother and babies skin and they go out of their hut into the village and the mother and baby are welcomed 'home', with song, dance and feasting. This really resonated with me, and even though my body wasn't painted, it felt like when I went out into the world a month after my baby was born, it was very much a recognition, an acknowledgement, a 'welcome home'.

So even though I had had 3 previous birth experiences, 2 of them classified as 'natural birth', it was my pregnancy and birth with my 4th baby that changed my whole life forever. I feel as though it is because I took responsibility for myself, I was able to stop listening to what the 'outside' world was saying to me, and I was able to focus in on my own self and listen to my body. Being sovereign to your own body gives you an incredible sense of empowerment and I wholeheartedly believe that because of the physiological nature that Sage's birth was, that my brain was re-wired. I have NEVER been the same since her birth. I am more intuitive in how I parent my children and how I care for myself, and I am more instinctive in the way I react to what my body is doing.

Gentle and conscious birthing has enabled me to become a more fulfilled, whole and realised human being.

Thankyou Sage, my wise daughter.

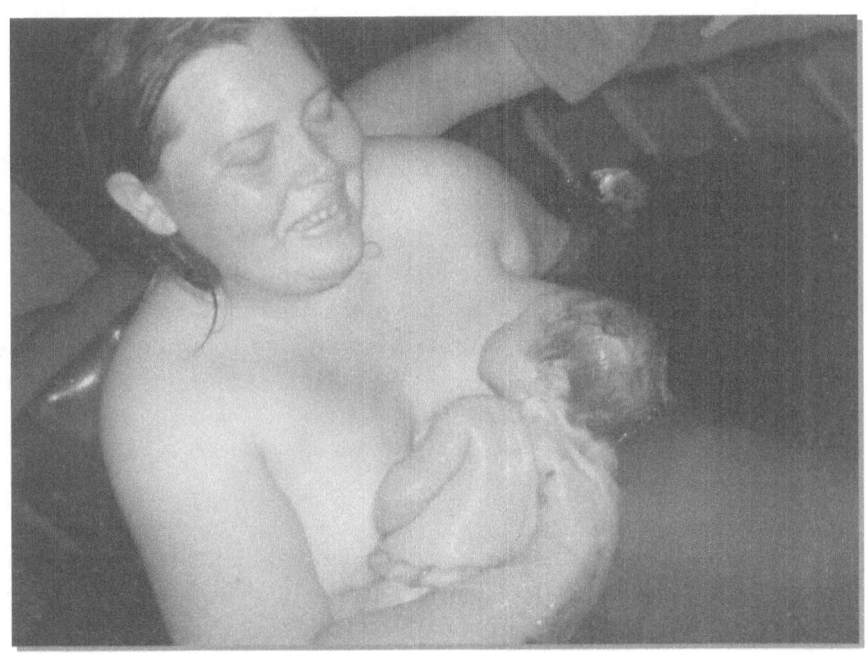

*"Baby Sage"* – Photo: Anna Urbanski

## *Honouring the Mother*

Supporting and honouring the woman in her journey through pregnancy, labour, birth and the early post-partum days is imperative to her overall wellbeing. If she feels strong enough and well supported, then she will be able to better care for herself, her baby and her family. Her body will recover, her mind will be stronger and her heart will be full.

In times gone by, and in times still occurring in many cultures around the world, women gathered and supported each other through their childbearing journey. The wise women, the women who had birthed before, the medicine women, the younger women who needed to learn the women's mysteries, the sisters, the wives, all gathered as a community to support the pregnant mother. A baby was / is considered a valued and important part of the community. Because of this community mindset, women all helped each other out. Each new life was a community event, everyone helped and supported so that their community would grow and thrive with decent human beings.

Honouring the mother can be as simple (yet as powerful) as listening to her needs, or as involved as attending her birth and involving yourself in the care of her children and her household.

I like to create rituals to honour women in transitions they undertake in their lives. A woman who is pregnant is in a huge transition. She is embarking on a journey that stretches her entire being on all levels. Rituals are a way to hold a space that enables the mother to feel supported and empowered as she travels her roads.

The following pages contain a few rituals that I like to do with women who are pregnant, as a way to honour them and to bring community to her heart so that she knows that even though she ultimately travels the road to birth alone, she is still surrounded by sisters.

## Blessing Way Ceremonies

Native American wisdom has always resonated with my heart and when I was pregnant with my 4th baby and first heard of a the Native American blessing way, I knew I wanted one. Traditionally, a blessing way was a ceremony dedicated to someone who was about to undergo a big transition – so, this was often done for women about to traverse the world of labour and birth. She was surrounded by 'elders', i.e. women who had birthed before, therefore had the sacred women's business knowledge, and blessings would be given, stories would be told. The focus was honouring the mother and the blessing way was dedicated to the pregnancy and birth being normal and natural and healthy.

In our current western culture, we place emphasis on the baby, and the mothers need are often unheard and her needs unmet. We have 'baby showers', where the emphasis isn't on the mother at all, it is all on the baby and the mother is gifted with many presents for the baby. There is generally very little, or nothing, that honours her journey as the one that is going to birth and nourish the child for the rest of its life.

Sometimes when women voice their needs and wants, they can be undermined or undervalued by those around her. We tend to just 'put up' with pregnancy complaints and our fears around birth are often silenced with a 'well, you're in good hands' or 'you've got good people looking after you'. Also, caregivers don't usually attend to or meet our emotional needs until it's too late (i.e. PND already happens) and they certainly don't take into account our energetic or spiritual needs. Our physical needs can be met with referrals to different specialists, i.e. physio-, osteo-, chiro-. But our emotional, and spiritual needs seem to not be valid in the process of pregnancy and birth. We aren't often offered a space where we can talk and be heard. Or where we are offered blessings and love for a beautiful birth. Where offerings of beautiful words and food are given. And love, respect and honour are shared. Where the woman feels validated and valued.

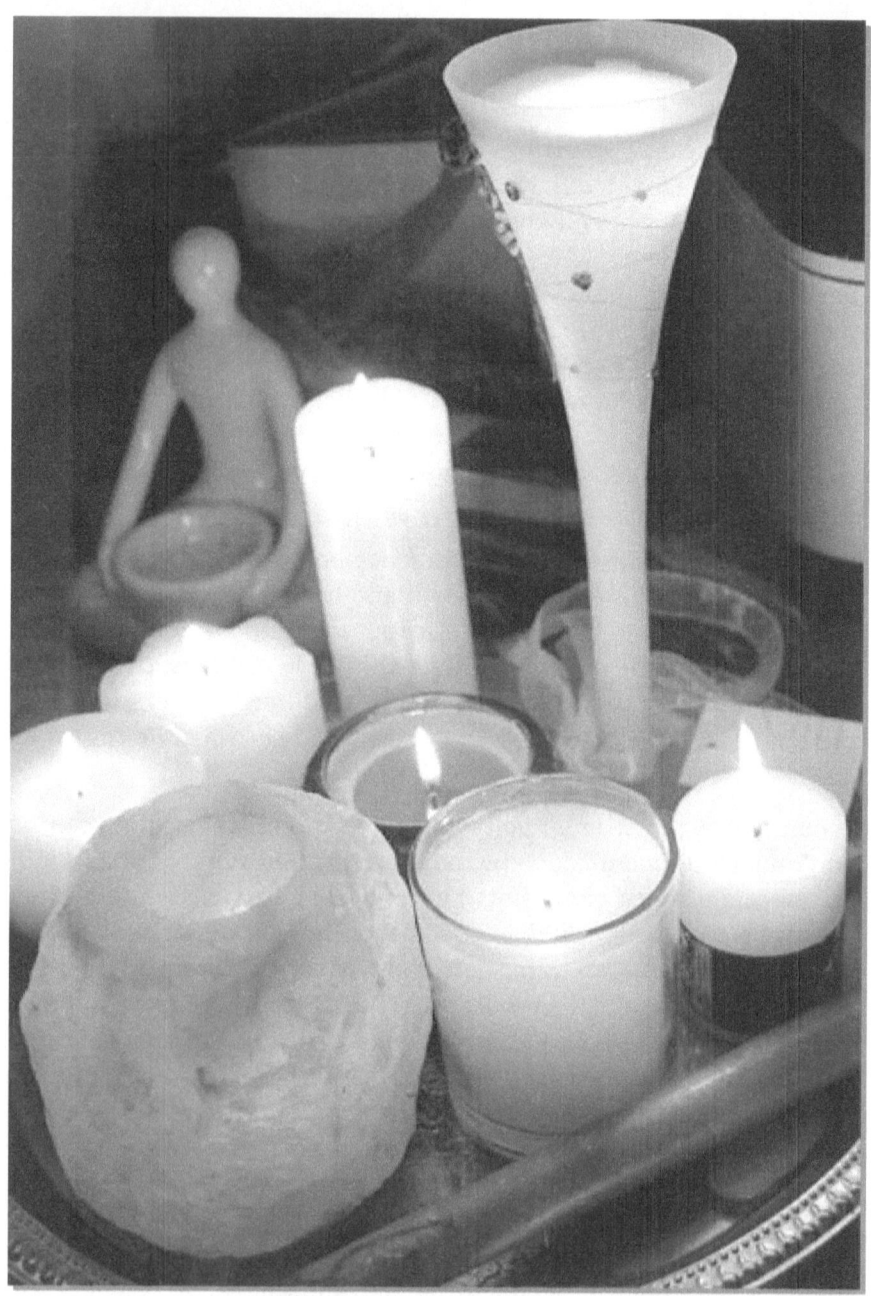

*"Blessingway Candles"* – Photo: Brooke Patel Photography

Pam England, beautifully states in her book 'Birthing From Within' (p15) that *'even though the rituals surrounding birth have changed with the advent of technology, birth itself has not changed. You, as a mother, still need to be prepared, nurtured and "mothered" by other women'.*

I think this is why Blessingways are so beautiful.

Typically for a Blessingway, there is a 'host'. Someone who the mother loves and trusts who 'holds the space' and runs the ceremony. She does the organising and the preparing and the cleaning afterwards. She holds the space for others to talk, for the mother to talk, and she nurtures the mothers needs and wants.

Blessings are often given, positive stories around birth and breastfeeding and the early mothering days are shared, candles are given for the mother to put in a special place and beads are given and created into a necklace which is to remind the mother that she is loved and supported. All the beads that are strewn together on the necklace remind her of all the love and support her, and that she is held safely in the arms of these women who have gone through birth before her.

*At the Blessingway of my 5th baby, I was given blessings and candles. Each woman also made me a small flag that they created themselves, decorated with love and care, which I strung together and made myself something similar to the Tibetan prayer flags, to hang in my birth space. After the round of blessings, I was told to go in the centre of the circle and lie down with my eyes closed. As I settle in feeling comfortable, the women started to make sound, creating a 'sound bath' and the sound of each woman harmonised with the one another. The circle I was in was filled with sounds of nurture and nourishment and I was bathed in it. It consumed my whole being and I felt so blissed out. As the sound bath ended, I felt a hand touch me, and then another, and then another, until all 12 women had a hand on me. I was so held and cradled, I will remember that moment forever. I felt a cool softness on my lips and as I opened my mouth, a sweet friend hand fed me a strawberry. I don't think it was possible to be any more blissed out! We then feasted and laughed and had a beautiful time. I loved it so much. It really prepared my heart and soul for the journey of birth. Knowing I had that much support around me eased my fears and made me feel strong and capable.*

~*~

*"When I was pregnant with my 4th baby, I invited a small circle of people I loved and trusted to join in my blessingway. My doula held the circle with love and it was such an intimate, gentle ceremony. After our blessings, beads and candles were given; we feasted and drew together with chalk pastels on a large piece of calico. We called it 'the river of life' and once finished, placed it on the wall in my birth space. Every time I looked at it I felt connected and supported by those women who contributed to the piece"* Wisp

~*~

"Some of my closest women friends joined me in my home this weekend to celebrate my Blessingway. I felt so incredibly loved and nurtured by each and every one of them. Together we created birth flags for my birth space, gathered beads together to make my necklace, tied wool around our wrists to join us together, and ate lots of yummy food! Having these women join me in my home, in my space, to celebrate my pregnancy and life I am creating was truly beautiful and a day I will remember always." Tamara, Mumma to 3

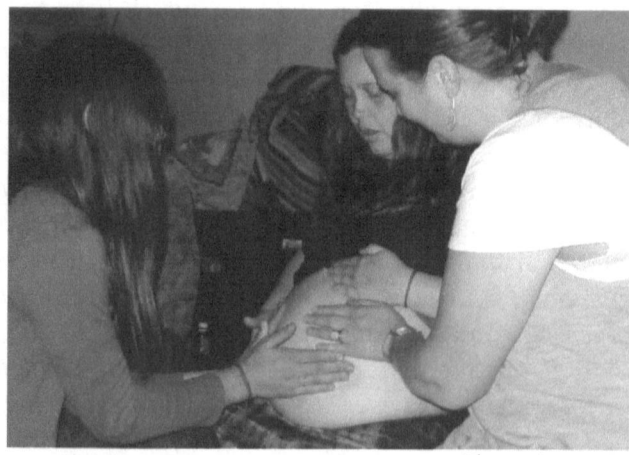

Photo: Steven Booth

## *Ideas for Blessingways:*

*Creating a Tibetan style prayer flag* for the mother to hang in her birth space. All you need to do is get everyone to have a piece of fabric (say A4 size) and get them to decorate it in any way they wish. They can embroider, sew, paint, use crayons, glue pictures on, anything goes! The mother can then sew them together (or get someone to do it for her) in a Tibetan prayer flag style.

*River of Life art piece.* Get a long piece of calico, and draw two blue wavy line up either side of the fabric. Now you have created a river. Next, get the loved ones to draw / paint on it together. A bunch of women, listening to music, with the pregnant mother in their hearts, the patterns and pictures that come out are always beautiful.

*Get your belly decorated with henna!* It is not that difficult and it looks beautiful!

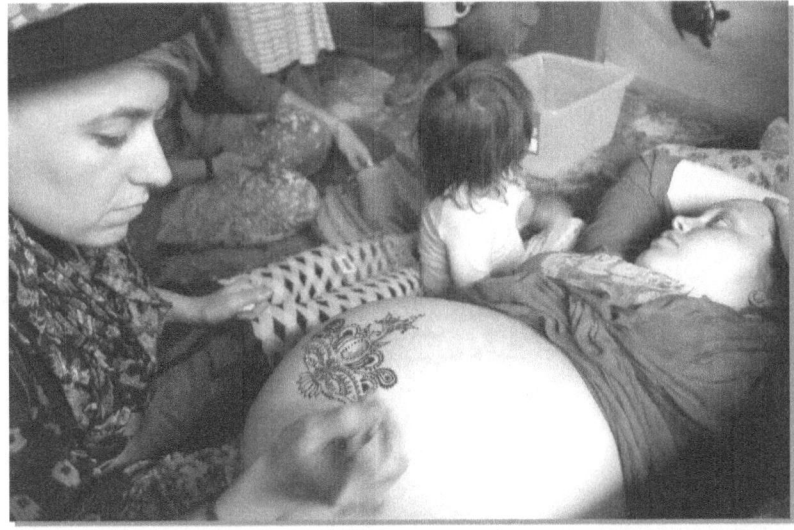

Photo: Beth Stewart-Nichols

## The Wild Rainbow

*A foot* spa with rose petals and delicious essential oils. Clary sage, jasmine and orange are my personal favs.

*A sound bath.* You lie in the centre of the circle and get comfortable, closing your eyes. The people you love are around you and they start to make sounds with their voices. The voices all harmonise and you feel extremely relaxed and blissful. When I had a sound bath at my blessingway, I felt it resonate in every cell in my body. It felt very healing.

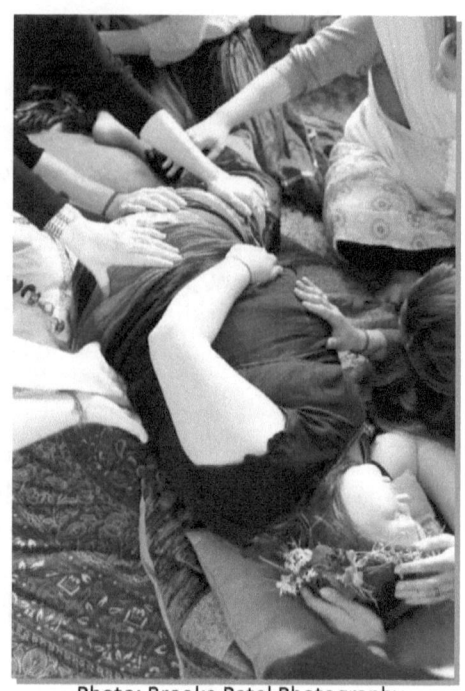

Photo: Brooke Patel Photography

Photo: Aaliyah Stewart

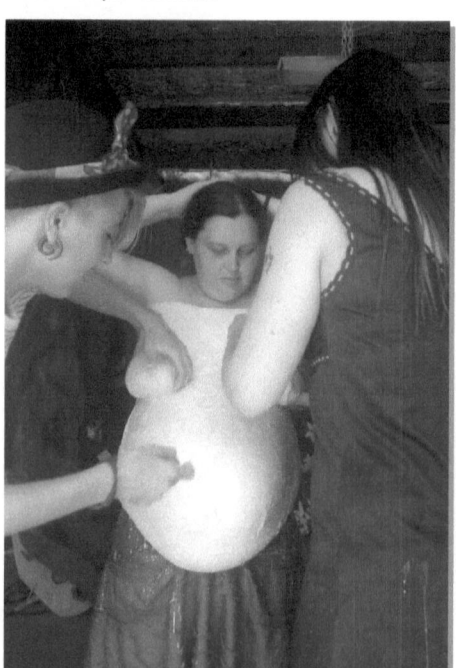

*Get massaged* with scented organic oil and get your hair brushed. It is nurture and nourishment to the max!

*Do a belly cast.* It creates a beautiful, physical memory of an important time in your life

*Some of my favourite poems for Blessingways*

**Before God became a man**

I've known birthing
Before creation
And older than the labour of mankind
My womb is the mother of life
I carried Adam when seeds
In the garden were gestating
I pushed the head of Cronos from
Between my legs and swaddled Him in the Sands of Time
I was midwife to the moon and
And made her crib in my lodge
I wailed with Demeter's chorus
When armies stole children
Killed the land
And I've seen her barren lap
Turn poppy red with birth
In the spring
I've known birthing
Before God became a man

By Margaret Arabella Kenney

### *Chant of the Pregnant Goddess*

*I am the mother of the moon*
*Sister of the Stars*
*Child of the light in your eyes*
*I am powerful*
*The geometry of my shape*
*shifts*
*from gently curved lines*
*to expanding circles*
*earth, moon, sun*
*I am powerful, I am strong*
*the tempo of my vibration quickens,*
*increasing from butterfly wings*
*to floundering fish*
*to beating drum*
*to erupting volcano*
*The rhythm as old and constant*
*as the cycles of the sun*
*and the turn of the tides*
*I am powerful, I am strong*
*I am beautiful*
*I hold the hope of my ancestors*
*The knowledge of my time*
*The fate of my future*
*I am powerful, I am strong*
*I am beautiful*
*I am mother*

By Jana McCarthey

*Willow Tree*

I am a willow tree,
Strong, yet fluid
graceful.
I can bend with the wind,
but my roots are tough,
indestructible.
Opening to birth my child
is flowing with the wind:
from a soft and gentle breeze
to a stormy gale
back to a soft and gentle breeze.
My body is strong, but flexible.
It is my friend, it knows how to open.
I am a friend to my body
eating well, walking, and loving myself.
I shall birth safely, freely, openly . . .
among my loved and trusted ones.
I am the willow, flexible
beautiful resilient
endowed with the power of surrender
to the wind rustling through my leaves,
my branches.
My roots reach deep into Mother Earth
Anchored in Her strength
I bring forth life
In joy!

Anonymous

## *Monsterways and letting go of fears*

I first heard about the term 'monsterway' from reading through some of the work of yogini, midwife and herbalist Jeannine Parvati Bakers. It is traditionally a Native American Ceremony for the men before they go to war. It is about expelling fears. Jeannine thought of how this ceremony could be linked in to pregnant women and the fears they have around their upcoming birth, their labour and parenting their baby.

I, too, think it is so important to be able to have a space for the mother, where she is able to share with one or more significant people in her life, all the fears she has around her journey with her baby.

Imagine being able to feel free to talk about you fears, and ways of stepping through them in a safe, sacred circle held for you with a small group of those you love. Imagine being able to get all the time you need to say these fears out loud. You are heard and validated by those around you. No one tries to 'save' you from your fears. They let you speak them, and they hold the space and listen.

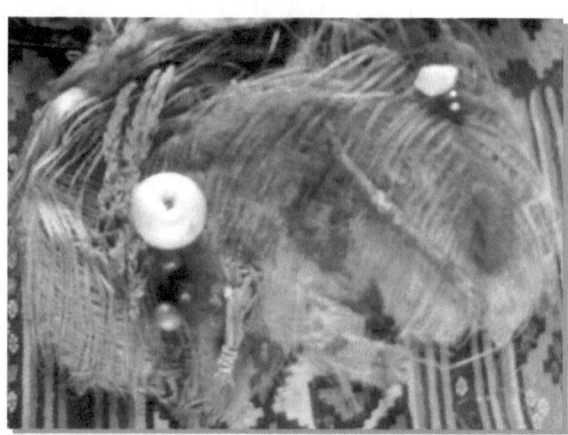

*"Winter"* – Photo: Sheree Stewart

In my heart, I feel that following the talking of the fears, a ritual to 'let go' or 'be rid' of them may benefit, and will add another layer of strength the mother, as well as helping those fears she spoke of be released in some form.

A fire ritual is always a powerful way to burn away our fears, as is a burial – burying our fears in the ground, where they are transmuted and changed into another form. All you would need to do for this is for the woman to write her fears on a bit of paper and then throw them into the fire and watch them burn or dig a little hole in a place she has chosen and bury the fears she has written down on a piece of paper. I believe Monsterways would empower the woman to voice her concerns, feel supported, validated and empowered.

During the pregnancies of my 4th and 5th babies, I did some hypnochildbirth work with MummaDoula, Denise Love. She has the belief that women need to have the space to share their fears, to talk them out loud with people they trust in order to move on. She has 2 wonderful sheets about fears that you fill out during your pregnancy. One is around facing fears and ways to overcome them, and the second one is one you reassessing fears, and is based around looking at your fears in a few months from when you did the first.

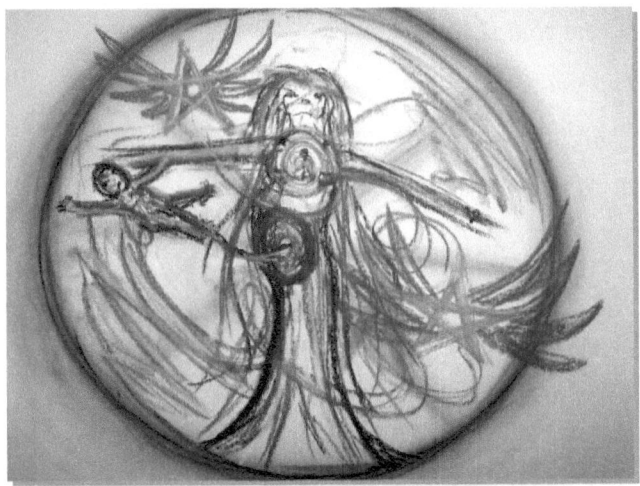

*"The Unnecesarean"* - *Art* Therapy: Star Davis

## *Looking at fears*

- ➢ *My fears about pregnancy are...*
- ➢ *My fears about the birth are...*
- ➢ *My fears about the baby are...*
- ➢ *My fears about being a parent are...*
- ➢ *Positive ways I can work to overcome these fears are...*

## *Reassessing Fears*

- What I really care about is….
- What ifs…
- Secret Fears…
- Things I am scared to think about….
- Every time I think about going into labour, I think…..
- I am so scared that…..
- What if my partner…
- What if the baby…
- I don't think I can….
- I'm not good at …
- I wish I could…
- Help me with…
- When I think of being a mother, I…
- My Mother was…
- Children are…
- My baby is…
- My partner is…
- I need to…

My own fears that spontaneously arose for me when pregnant with my 5th baby gave me insight to not only what I was feeling and experiencing, but it gave me a space to write down things that I was too scared to talk about out loud, in case it was too taboo – it gave me a place where I could reflect and see what I actually wanted and needed in my life

*'Reassessing Fears'.*

*What I really care about is....*being supported, loved and encouraged to be the woman I am and the mother I need to be for my children

*What ifs...*
>What if I can't cope with so many children
>What if I am alone
>What if I lose trust in myself
>What if I die or my baby dies

*Secret Fears...* that no one will support me during labour and birth

*Things I am scared to think about....* I am scared to think of how will I cope if I have a baby born sleeping?

*Every time I think about going into labour, I think......* 'wow' this is going to be big! and also that I need to try to remember to step into the eye of the Goddess and totally be consumed and surrender

*I am so scared that.....*I won't be able to cope with the waves or that my baby will be in an awkward position that will make labour longer and more painful

*What if my partner...*pisses me off?

*What if the baby...*gets stuck?

*I don't think I can....* handle being alone in this labour. I feel it needs to be a celebration and that I need my close friends by my side holding me to their heart.

*I'm not good at ...* transition

*I wish I could....*birth in the bush amongst the trees and butterflies

*Help me with...* coping in the chaos of transition. Hold me and remind me you are there

*When I think of being a mother, I...* feel the connection between me and my mother, to all mothers around the world and to mother Earth

*My Mother was...* strong

*Children are...* our future

*My baby is...* from the stars, soon to arrive on Earth

*My partner is...* strong and protective like a bear

*I need to...* chillax and breathe

# The Wild Rainbow

### *Overcoming Fear – the birth of Aaliyah*

> "Birth, like love, is an energy and a process, happening within a relationship. Both unfold with their own timing, with a uniqueness that can never be anticipated, with a power that can never be controlled, but with an exquisite mystery to be appreciated." –Elizabeth Noble

My wild, creative, unique daughter who does things in her own way was born at 42weeks +6 days gestation, compound presentation, natural hospital birth

At 36 weeks pregnant, I had just finished a 3 week stint of night shifts as a student midwife. If being so heavily pregnant wasn't draining enough, I was also witness to many brutal, violent and traumatic births at the hands of some of the doctors there, one in particular. With these experiences fresh in my mind, I was feeling terrified of giving birth. Even though I knew birth was normal and natural, my mind couldn't sit still with these images of violent births playing out in my head.

I went to 43 weeks gestation, I believe because of all the fear. I had lied to the birth centre about my dates so according to them I was 9 days 'overdue'.

So, at 42 weeks and 6 days, my labour started at one am. The feeling of the first wave was distinctly different to the few braxton hicks I had had the week or so previously. I felt both nervous and excited and woke Steven to tell him what was happening.

We were booked into a birth centre and we were aware of the need to call Steven's Mum, who was coming to take care of our eldest 2 children, whilst I laboured and birthed our baby. Steven gave her a call, just to give her a heads up (she later told us she never went back to sleep!) and that we would have a baby today.

At around 4, the contractions were getting stronger. The stronger they were getting, the more nervous I was feeling. At one point when I was in the shower, I checked my own cervix and was 4cm's dilated. Knowing that my last 2 births were quick, I felt it was time to go to the birth centre.

At 5ish, Steven's Mum arrived and she looked at me with sympathy and said good luck. The trip to the birth centre was ok - the contractions had slowed down, I suppose because I was so nervous travelling in the car to the birth centre. I remember getting one contraction in the car and all I could hear was Crowded House's 'Distant Sun' playing. It was somehow soothing and made me focus on the music rather than the pain. I really didn't want to feel the pain, I really wanted to be removed from it.

We got to the Birth Centre and were settled into a room. All I remember was that it was so big and open and bright, even in the early hours of daylight. The midwives stuffed around to put a cannula in my hand, because I was GBS positive, the hospital I was at has a very strict policy regarding the treatment of GBS during labour. One midwife couldn't put the cannula in my hand so she went to find someone else from another ward to do it. They fiddled for ages, talking about mundane things that I had no interest in. Once it was finally in, I went and locked myself in the bathroom. It was the only place that was dark and quiet enough where I felt safe. The midwife was lovely enough. She went and got me some mats to kneel on and asked me if I thought I was going to birth in the shower. I just yelled out 'no!' as I couldn't be bothered talking to anyone.

The contractions got more intense and the more intense they got, the more frightened I was. At one point I was swinging off a bar / rail that was along the shower, I felt it helped me bring her head down during the contractions. All I remember was feeling scared. Sometimes when I would feel another surge some, I would clench up my bum, trying to make it stop. I didn't want it to hurt any more. I really wanted to be removed from experiencing pain.

Every now and then the midwife would pop her head in and say 'you're doing great' and then leave again. Really, at that point, all I wanted was for someone to hold me, and rock me and stroke my hair and tell me how awesome I was. Instead, I felt really isolated. The

## The Wild Rainbow

birth centre was full. Every other woman who was in there was a 1st time mumma and I felt as though the midwives left me alone - 'the competent multi'. Steven was great. He was really present and incredibly supportive. I just felt so frightened.

Around 10ish, the midwife came in and said that she would like to do a vaginal exam to see how far dilated I was seeing I had been in the birth centre 'for ages' (it was about 4 hours) and I said yes as I was hoping to have made some progress and thought that knowing would give me some incentive to get on with the job of birthing. At that point I was 7cms and bubbies head was still quite high. The midwife told me that I need to move around and get babies head down. All I wanted to do was lay down and sleep. So, once she left the room that is exactly what I did. I dozed off. Steven must have too. No one must have checked on us for around an hour, when I heard the midwife say 'come on, wake up, don't lose these contractions now'. I looked at the clock and realised that I had been asleep for an hour! It was just after 11 and I felt a little more refreshed and remembered where I was and what I was doing.

I hopped up and went back in the shower. I had a moment to myself where I said 'just do this. Then it will be over. Then you can sleep more. And meet your baby'. As soon as I said that the contractions came on again, so strong. I swore, I swung off the rail in the bathroom, I stamped around, I rocked on the birth ball with Steven supporting me, I kneel across the bed, I leaned on the wall, I swore and swore and fucking swore some more.

Just after midday my water broke when I was on the birth ball - a big gush of warm light pink fluid, all over the ball, the floor and probably on Steven as well.

One of the midwives at the desk must have heard one of my roars, as she came in a hurry and asked how we were going. I remember Steven saying 'her waters broke' and she said 'where is your midwife?' and we said 'we have no idea!' She went out in a hurry and came back soon with the first midwife we had.

At that point my mind was lost in the frenzy chaos of transition. It hurt so much, I thought I was going to die. I hopped on all fours on the bed. I swore some more. I lay on my back. I swore some more. I lay on my side I swore some more. And then that familiar contraction that takes your whole being over happened - that deep long rooooooooooooaaaar of a birthing woman who is pushing started to happen. 'Oh fuck, is it going to be over soon?' I asked. The midwife looked at me and smiled and said 'yes, not long, well done'. I pushed so slowly with this baby. On my birth records it says I pushed for 21 minutes (which is a long time for me!!!) I think I asked with each contraction that passed 'is it nearly over?' and they were so encouraging. They used hot facecloths to my peri which felt like heaven. I hated that feeling of the stretching - that ring of fire that burns your body.

With one big contraction my baby's head was born! She was compound presentation, which means that her hand was above her face - she looked like superwoman coming out, ready to save the world! The contraction stopped and her head was born, just sitting there on my peri, when all of a sudden she opened her eyes and started to cry!! It was really quite surreal! It felt so strange! We all had a little giggle about it. A minute or 2 later with the next contraction, her body slipped out of mine and she was placed on my chest! Although, her cord was really short, so really, she was placed to my belly button! About 15 minutes later the cord stopped pulsing and was cut and I put her up to my chest for a snuggle. She was so beautiful and chubby and she fed straight away. Life as a family of 5 was just beginning and I felt as though by birthing her I overcame many fears I had surrounding birth.

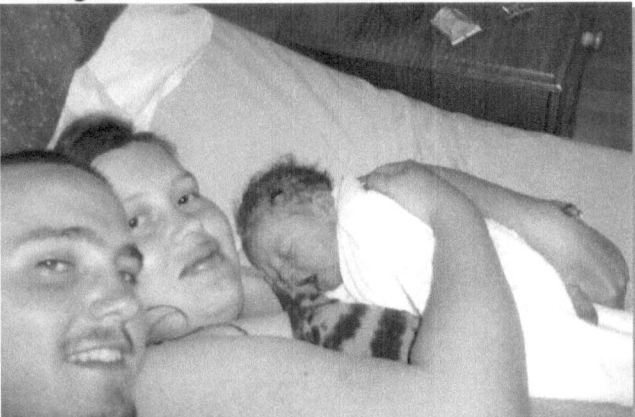

*"Baby Aaliyah, Self Shot"* – Photo: Steven Booth

## *Mamatoto Connections*

Connecting to our babes in womb is a natural, instinctive response that all of us as women have access to. Unfortunately, the industrialisation of childbirth means that childbirth has become a medical event, and with all the technology available, we are able to constantly look outside of ourselves and to machines to find answers. Women's instincts are often ignored or undermined and as a culture we are more looking to CTG machines and ultrasounds for answers and solutions, rather than following our 'gut' feeling or being in tune with our organic reality and the innate wisdom it naturally has.

If we allow ourselves to stop and slow down, to connect and tune in with our bodies, we will be able to see quite quickly and clearly what our bodies and babies need. It actually isn't as difficult as it may seem. Even If you find that you are too busy, if you don't know where to start, if you don't have enough time, if you don't believe in yourself, have a little read through this next section. It can give you some ideas and stories from other women who have stopped to connect and reclaim their own body medicine. Even if you are working long hours, have a 'to do list' that is a million miles long, if you have deadlines to meet, you can still drop in to your body each day and feel into what it needs.

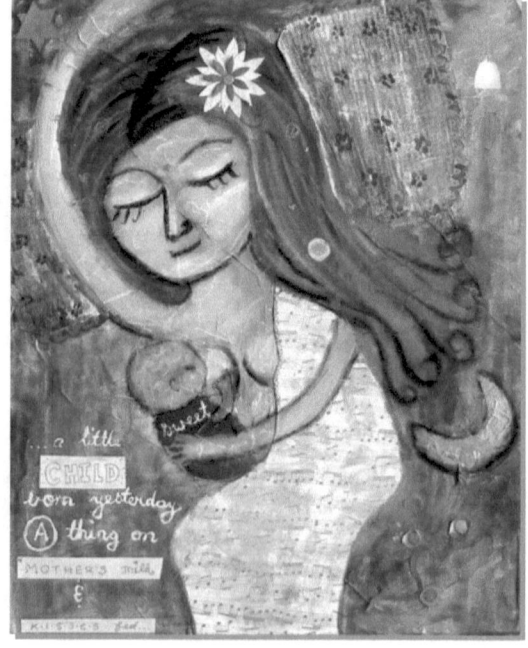

*"Secret Life of Mother"* –

Artist: Daisy Mabel

## *Dance*

Dance during pregnancy is a beautiful way to connect to your body and your baby. Even simple movements can create awareness, self love and connection. It can remove fear; make you feel more confident and radiant and transmute energetic blockages. If you allow yourself to feel the pulse of your body and allow yourself to move with it, you will find yourself feeling more free and intuitive to what your body desires and needs.

I always wanted to dance in my life, but often just felt too shy. When I was pregnant with my 6th baby, I ended up going to Dance For Pregnancy classes, hosted by a dear friend of mine in Melbourne, Nicola Eddington. She was so gentle and encouraging, making me feel open to move as I needed and connect in with my baby and womb heart space.

During pregnancy, give yourself the gift of dance. Dance with your baby, either alone, with your partner, with friends, or other pregnant women. Spiral your hips, move slowly, move deeply and see what it is that you find.

### My experience of ecstatic dance while pregnant

As I entered the quiet state of stillness, I connected to the baby in womb.

I could feel him in there, but he was quiet.

The music played in the background, and I instinctively moved. Slowly at first, and low to the ground.

Lots of deep spiralling of my hips. Lots of rocking back and forth.

The longer the music went for, the deeper I went inside myself, the deeper I connected to my baby.

We danced and moved for an hour and a half.

My eyes were closed for the whole time. I saw colours and patterns. I saw flashes of his birth.

It was the same birth vision that I keep seeing again and again and again.

I am standing up with my husband supporting me as I lean into him and my woman with tears in her eyes, down below, catching the baby into her hands.

When she passes him up to me, my husband notices the sex and yells out 'it's a boy!' and we all laugh in bliss.

The music slows and my big, swirling movements become quieter.

The baby tells me that the squatting and spiralling movements will help him be born.

I lie in love as the experience of connecting to my baby through dance washes over me.

## *Journeying with the drum*

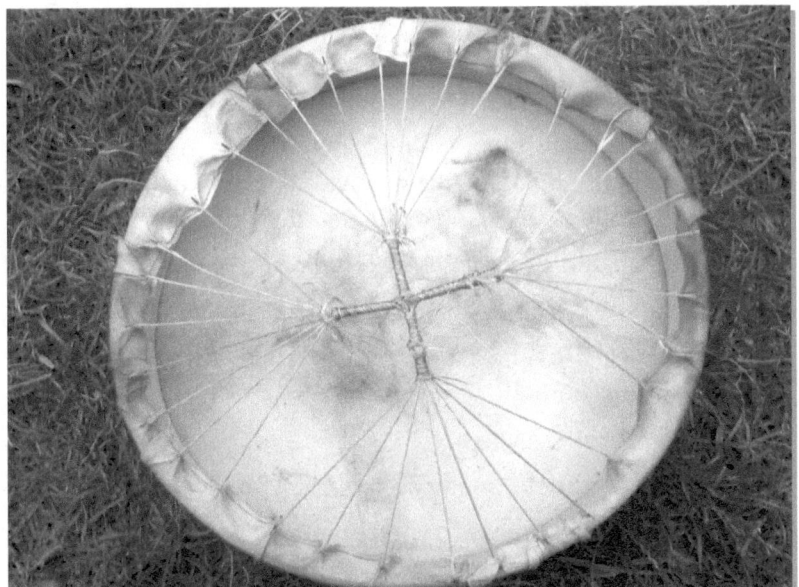

"My Deer-hide Drum" – Photo: ShereeStewart

### *Drumming During Pregnancy*

By Jane Hardwicke Collings

Pregnancy and birth are shamanic experiences, deep inner experiences that are transformational. In the shamanic drum journey a mother can access her inner knowing and strength and seek and find guidance and support via the shamanic realms, through connection with the Divine Feminine, her Guides, and Power Animals. She can connect with her baby during pregnancy via shamanic journeying and use this connection to communicate with her unborn one at all times.

This is a potent process and the connection formed often brings great healing. Valuable tools and information for the labour and birth can be accessed by the mother as well as such things as the baby's name and advice on who should be present at the birth.

Shamanic journeying during pregnancy offers great preparation for labour and birth as both are best approached from a similar altered state of consciousness.

### *A Shamanic Drum Journey into your womb to meet your baby*

> To begin, cleanse yourself of any negative energy. This can be done by smudging or through wilful intention by speaking the words "I cleanse myself of all negative energies".
>
> Lie down and cover yourself for warmth.
>
> If you are in the company of others, be careful to not touch anyone else – you may go on the same journey if you do!
>
> Relax your body
>
> Melt into where you are
>
> Check your body for any held tension and let it go.
>
> Take your awareness to your breath
>
> Deepen your in breath
>
> Slow your breathing down
>
> Relax
>
> The drumming will be at a rapid rate
>
> Focus on the beating of the drum
>
> If you start thinking, or getting distracted, just bring your focus back to the drum beat
>
> Single pointed focus on the drum beat.
>
> For the journey into your womb to meet your baby you will need to take your awareness to your vulva, enter, travel up your vagina, checking it out on the way, make friends with your cervix, know where it is, what it looks like, and arrange that you will be in communication during your labour as you open to bring your baby earth side.

Then go through your cervix and enter your womb.

Once inside your womb, call out to your baby -

"Mummy's here" Call the baby to be with you tell your baby what you want to tell them

Ask them questions – how can I best help you be born?

Where do you want to be born?

What do I need to know for our journey together?

Enjoy their company.

You may get information visually, with pictures or hearing sounds or voices or by feeling, and probably a combination of these

You may travel to other realms

if you encounter anything on your journey that concerns you, or you are not sure of, ask it "are you for my highest good?" if it is, it will stay and you can ask it a question, if it's not for your highest good it will disappear.

When the journey is over and it's time to come background

The drumming will change from fast to slow

At the point say Thank you and say goodbye, perhaps arrange another meeting, and retrace your steps, coming back the way you went in.

Pay attention, and enjoy the journey.

State three times to yourself:

"I am travelling to my womb to meet my baby"

Now take your awareness to your vulva and enter.

*drumming starts -*

When it is time to return from the journey, you will hear a call back through the change in the drumming rhythm.

In preparing to leave, say thank you and say goodbye, arrange to meet again

As you return from your journey it is important to retrace your steps back to your body in this world, so back down through your cervix, your vagina, out your vulva and back into the world.

Once back into your present moment awareness, wriggle your fingers and toes and take some deep breaths. Write down what you can remember in your journal.

Remember you can return to your journal writing again at any stage. Often you can recall more details later after you have written down the initial entry.

If you feel a bit shaky or faint, drink some water, splash some on your face and eat something. If you are still not feeling fully present and in your body then lie down on your belly on the earth and if necessary have someone shake a rattle all around you.

~*~

*If you would like to read Jane's full article around Drumming During Pregnancy and for Labour, it is available on her website http://moonsong.com.au/drumming.html*

*You are also access The Shamanic Drum Journey into Your Womb to Meet your Inner Goddess and is downloadable for free and the Four Shamanic Drum Journeys and A Shamanic Drum Journey for Pregnancy to Meet Your Baby, and Drumming for Labour which is available for purchase.*

*http://moonsong.com.au/shamanic_drum_journeys.html*

## My drum journeys to meet my baby

I went into the drum journeys many times when pregnant with my 6th baby, with the intentions of getting some information or messages from my baby on what to do, what we need to do/know. The pregnancy of my 6th baby was unplanned and I went through some pretty big emotions coming to terms with what was happening. I was shocked and struggled for a while on what to do and how to cope . Each drum journey bought me closer to my own truth and empowerment.

### Drumming in early pregnancy.

Listening to the drum, I made my way to my cervix, which when reaching it, I paused to honour it, calling it 'the gatekeeper of life'. I lit a beeswax candle and created an altar at the os.

I saw my baby in his embryo form, then he changed into his baby self, then his toddler self, then his child self. He looked like my brother with wild white hair and blue eyes, with a tall slender build, but strong shoulders.

"what do I need to know?" I asked him

"that I will be born on the eclipse, that you need to feel supported, that you are supported, you just need to open your heart to those around you" he replied.

As he said that, images of people came into my head, whom I knew where meant to be in my support circle. Some of them were obvious, two of them surprised me as they were people I wouldn't have necessarily thought of. They were both people who I recently reconnected with, but neither of them were really close to me at the time of the drum journey. But as time passed, those people did end up coming more closer into my life and became a part of that support circle of people who nourish me.

I asked if there was anything else I needed to know, but my baby started fading out and I found myself saying thank you and goodbye and travelled back out of my cervix, vagina and vulva and back into the room.

I felt clear headed and happy and felt as though I was given vital clues to what and who I needed in my life in that time.

**Drumming in late pregnancy**

Travelling up into my womb, I sense the womens mysteries, the wildness, the power of what being a creatrix is. In my womb, I smell the same smell I have had all along whenever I go and visit my baby. It is the smell of wet soil, of damp Earth, of fertile ground that is rich with nutrients and life force.

My waters are clear and through them I can see the umbilical cord. It sways like seaweed in the sea, being rocked and motioned by my very own ocean, my amniotic waters.

I look at my baby, who is growing so well. I don't get a sense if it is a boy or a girl. I see beautiful thin dark hair and when the eyes open, they are green like the green you find in the deepest, most secret parts of the forest. As I look in my baby's eyes, I see the reflections of ferns and they are unfurling.

I am reminded 'in my own time and in my own way and everything is perfect'. My baby looks so healthy and robust. Chubby arms, a strong mind, an inner strength. I notice a small birthmark. It is on my babies chest, on the left, just higher then where the heart is.

I ask my baby "show me what I need for preparation for the birth"

I see an abundance of food. There is particular food this baby needs. No citrus, but lemons are ok. No cows' milk. There are bananas, dates, avocado, coconuts, sweet potato, sweet corn, honey, cashews, brazil nuts, black beans, red kidney beans, peas, eggs.

I get told that I need to do daily meditation where I connect and draw energy from both the sky and the earth, drawing it into my solar plexus, stirring it around, keeping me full. This is will give me energy for birth I am told.

"Birth is steady" baby said, "But not too quick. It's not ferocious, but it moves steadily. The last contractions before I am born, you will need to be standing. Between doorways, in the place where there is lots of movement in our house."

My husband is standing behind me, holding me in all the right ways. I have a friend who is in the background, sitting in the lounge-room on the couch simply being beautiful. Holding the space and trusting the process. Mish is holding me from the front. I never look at her, but I feel her gazing at me lovingly and I feel her hands on my belly. I feel safe and loved.

The baby is born while I am standing and he cries straight away. A fierce little dragon cry and he turns pinky red immediately.

We notice he is a boy and we all cry. The placenta comes away easily, the blood loss is minimal and we are all feeling blown away, opened and our hearts are full as we all gaze lovingly at this new being who has joined us.

The drums begin the beating and I know it is time to return back to the world to prepare the space for my baby. I say thank you and goodbye to my baby, feeling excited to meet this new person, face to face in around 8 weeks. I leave my womb smiling.

## *Mandalas*

Mandalas are a physical representation of our subconscious. When we draw a circle on paper, and allow our creative selves to 'fill in' the circle with paint, pencils, chalk, pastels etc., we are often left with a piece of the puzzle, an answer to our question or a message.

According to psychiatrist Carl Jung, *a mandala is the psychological expression of the totality of the self.* You can use mandala's during pregnancy as a way to connect in with your baby. You can gain information, insights, messages and instructions from your baby.

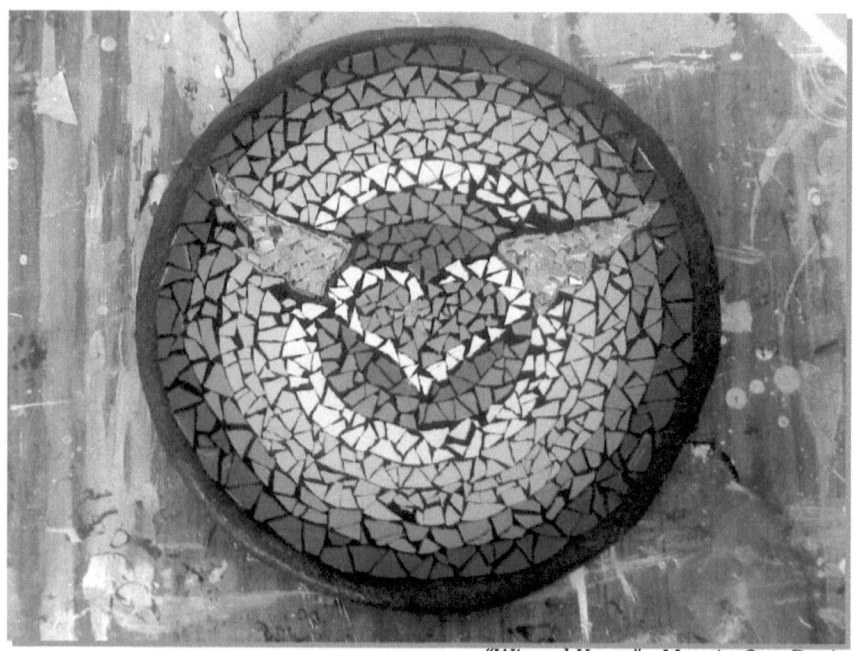

*"Winged Heart"* – Mosaic: Star Davis

## *How to create a mandala*

- Find a quiet space, where you won't be disturbed.
- Have your paper and art supplies ready
- Get comfortable, close your eyes, and start focusing in on your breathing
- Connect in with what you are feeling
- Take your awareness to your heart, then to your womb, then to your baby. Connect them together with love
- Big, deep conscious breaths. This only needs to be done for a couple minutes. Once you have soften and connected, then ask in your mind and to your baby a question that you want an answer to. It can be simple, yet important questions, such as 'what do I need to know?', 'how do you want your birth to be?, 'what can I do to optimise this experience?'
- Open your eyes and don't think. Start intuitively drawing, don't think about the colours, just pick them out. Start creating what needs to be created in the circle.
- Once you have finished look at what you created for a while. What do you see? What colours did you use? How does your heart feel when you see it? What is the message? Give your mandala a title – what is it called?
- You can turn your mandala around, look at it from all angles. What else can you see? You can record this information in your journal or on the back side of your mandala.

*"When I was pregnant with my 2nd baby I drew many mandalas. It was so simple yet a powerful way for me to gain insight into what was happening and what I needed my do. My subconscious gave me many messages when I allowed it to! Powerful, beautiful, insightful"*

*- Zara, mother of 2*

## *Meditation During Pregnancy*

Jane Hardwicke Collings

Pregnancy is a time when a woman is more naturally in touch with her body and her inner self. Introducing a meditation practice can enhance the experience by creating a "way in" to her mind's inner sanctum, she can then see deeper than her mind's chatter and fears and connect with her calm inner core. Once she has established that connection, she can return to that place as desired or as necessary.

During labour, when women are acting intuitively and free of fear they choose to withdraw and focus internally, finding their calm inner mind space. The hormones flowing in her blood stream at that point support, enhance and co-create this experience. If a labouring woman in this harmonious natural state is disturbed by others or disturbed by fear, her hormones change, she loses her focus, her labour may be prolonged and or more painful and her baby may be jeopardised.

Using meditation as a tool, she can again access the appropriate mindspace that supports and is necessary for natural labour, and improve her experience and the outcome of her labour and birth, making it safer for her baby and herself. The implication of this for childbirth is that a woman can choose to create a state of consciousness that is associated with a quicker and less painful labour and birth.

When a woman in labour is undisturbed she focuses internally and has reduced beta waves. If she is disturbed by people asking lots of questions or her own thoughts or fears then her beta waves will increase, and the hormones in her body will change. She will be on alert, and will experience an increase in adrenaline. Adrenaline inhibits oxytocin, and therefore slows down labour.

To best facilitate the natural process of birth the labouring woman needs to feel safe, and have her physical and emotional needs met. Once in this situation, she can relax her mind as per meditation, be in an aroused or relaxed body state and access deep levels of consciousness.

Then she can connect with her innate body wisdom and give birth in a blissful painless state of complete awareness - the evolved mind state. This is the biologically intended space from which to give birth. All that is required to access this state, if she is not already there, or comes in and out of it too often (increased beta waves) is a method of creating alpha waves such as:-

- focus on the breath
- making constant deep sounds (toning)
- constantly staying physically and mentally relaxed (letting go of body tension and thoughts or fears)
- reduced mental and sensory stimulation - a darkened environment, being in water and undisturbed

The work of French Obstetrician, Michel Odent supports this. He suggests women labour in an environment that is quiet and dark, with access to water. The basis of this is to reduce the neo-cortical activity of the brain, by reducing mental stimulation, so as to enable the Reptilian brain (the part of the brain responsible for non-thinking automatic natural normal body functions) to "get on" with the function of labour and birth. Neo-cortical stimulation (producing beta waves)-like answering questions and thinking of any sort, disturbs the natural process that births the baby.

Women need to be protected and cared for in labour so that they can quietly retreat to their inner world. Labour and birth are about letting go, and to give birth a woman needs to let go in the same way that she does to orgasm. A quiet, focussed mind, such as meditation reminds us of, is the best mindspace to labour and give birth from.

A woman who is being fussed over or who is in a state of fear (her own or others projected onto her) will not labour as efficiently as she might without that and her baby will be at risk of distress as a result of the adrenaline hormones that are released. Women often stop labouring until they can move back into a calm quiet space without distraction.

In labour, when a woman flows with the energy of the contractions, withdrawing into herself, she will focus - single pointedly on the physical sensations, the pain, her breath or a visual image - creating the alpha bridge to the other brain waves and therefore access theta and delta waves.

In this brain wave state she can experience the deep knowing of delta and feel as many women report - a connection with all women who have or are giving birth. This gives a great inner strength and often much less or no pain. This will only occur when the woman is undisturbed. Women who meditate in pregnancy have reported easy birth experiences, often painless and often ecstatic.

It seems that when birth is approached from a place of trust it can unfold in its natural way and be a positive initiation into motherhood. If this is possible for some women it is possible for all. A meditation practice can help one understand the way their mind works.

By bringing awareness to the process of thought, one is able to choose to control the "chatter" and in so doing, isolate from the thoughts, the fears. Fears can rule over an individual's life, creating whatever it is that is feared. Acknowledging fears is the first step to being freed from them. Fears are simply thoughts, they carry with them emotion and are retained and maintained by choice. As is well known, birth from a fearful state results in an inability to 'let go', long labours, intervention and increased morbidity (damage) and mortality. The way birth is managed in our modern culture is a reflection of the beliefs and fears held about women's bodies and the natural process of birth.

The pregnant woman encounters everyone's opinions and viewpoints on the matter and is often subject to procedures that have unwanted side effects (often these are not known to her) without her informed consent, using fear to get her to agree to them.

In the birth setting, if she has not chosen who will be present (such as for a home or birth-center birth) she will have people in attendance who will not necessarily be aware of the effect they will have on the natural unfolding of her unique birth experience. However, by simply focusing on her breath, and other easy meditation techniques to be discussed, she can alter her state of consciousness enabling her to connect with her intuition and body wisdom.

This will best facilitate the natural process as well as reveal to the woman obstacles such as fears or the adverse presence of someone, that may be inhibiting her from letting go and giving birth.

## Meditation Experiences

During my meditation, which was a journey to my womb, I went to a lake, and hopped in a boat. It was long and golden and it rocked gently as I moved across the lake. It entered a dark cave and I called out to my baby, hoping to get information or messages to bring back to my everyday living.

I could not see anything, but could smell the dark cave. It smelled like damp, sweet earth and I could almost taste it in my mouth. It was so moist and full of nutrients and life force.

When I looked up, I saw my sweet Mish's face. She was holding my hand, and continued to do so for the whole time I was in the cave. She just held my hand and didn't let go.

When I saw my baby, it was the boy. Each time I do a drum journey, I always see a dark haired blue eyed girl, or a blonde haired green eyed boy. There were no words spoken this time, just a connection.

I got the sense of creating my whole home into a sacred space. Creating little altars around the home. And doing movement. Some sort of creative dance or movement as this day is constantly moving in my womb and I feel a constant need to shift energies, thoughts, feelings, colours.

I asked about the birth and I got images of
- Water and stones
- Flowing water
- Big river stones

I came out of the meditation with the taste of earth in my mouth and a desire to create beautiful things.

~*~*~*~

> *I meditated a lot with my 2nd baby. I felt calmer through the whole pregnancy and I owe that to the meditation practice. I also did quite a lot of visualising. Visualising made me feel connected and I felt as though I got a lot of answers to what my baby needed. I remember having visions of birthing while on all fours. I was in that position with my first baby and it was intensely painful and I thought 'no way am I doing that'.*

*However, at her homebirth, I was side lying on the lounge room floor when her head was out. Her shoulders felt heavy and I didn't know if I could get them out. My midwife asked if I could turn over on to all fours. About 30 after doing that, I had a huge contraction that expelled her shoulders and body and she came our screaming. I now trust my body and the wisdom it gave me for my daughter's birth and I am now conscious and aware as a human being because of it. – Antalia*

~*~*~*~

*I decided to try meditation during pregnancy because I had anxiety issues in the past. I did 5 minutes every day in the morning before I got out of bed. It made my whole day more positive. I felt calmer in my body and mind or more connected to my baby. - Chloe*

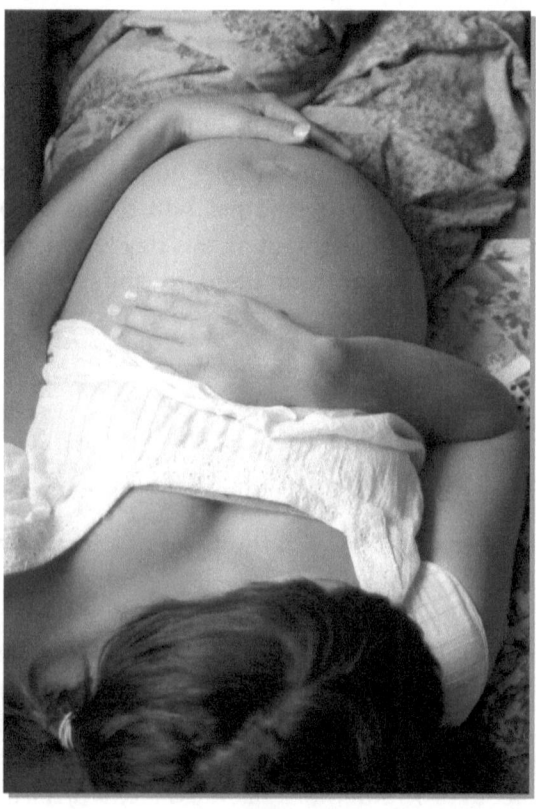

"Hailey" – Photo: Shea Bresnehan Photography

## *Pregnancy and Birth*

Choosing where to have your baby is a very personal choice. Currently in Australia, over 97% of women birth in hospitals. Birth Centres' and One to One Midwifery led hospital based programs are becoming an increasingly popular option for women. Homebirth is not a main stream choice, but it is a valid, safe choice for women if this is what makes them feel safe and comfortable.

When I was pregnant with my first baby I had no idea of any options available to me. I was of the idea that you book into the closest hospital and that was that.

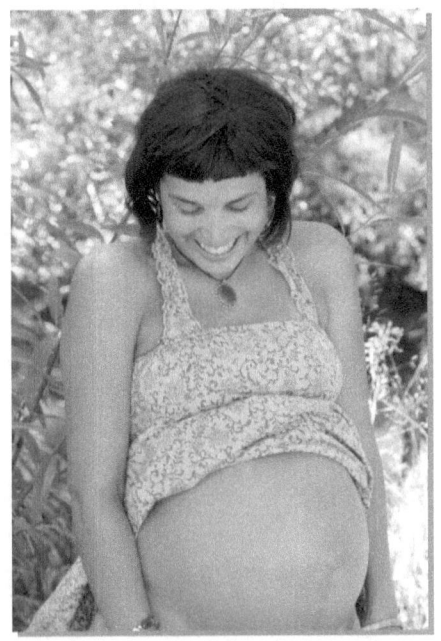

"Beautiful Hailey" – Photo: Shea Bresnehan Photography

When you are thinking of where to birth, it is important to ask questions that arise in regards to the practices and rates of intervention that your care provider gives. This way you can make an informed choice about where you want to birth your baby

Here is a list of things you might want to ask and consider:
- What is your caesarean rate?
- Do you have a bath? A waterbirth policy? Will I be supported if I choose to birth in water?
- Do you support the role of a doula?
- What is the policy around who can be in your birth space? Are children allowed?
- What is your induction / augmentation of labour rate?
- If it is in hospital, is it an Australian Breastfeeding Association registered Breastfeeding Friendly Hospital?
- What is the rate of instrumental births?
- What is the rate of episiotomies?

### Birthing Rhiannon

*The birth of my 2<sup>nd</sup> child, a natural birth in hospital*

I was 39 weeks watching Neighbours on the TV when I felt a rumble across my belly. My body tingled inside as I realised this was the beginning of my daughters journey to be born! Steven was busy with Caelan when I went and announced to him what was happening. I went to the toilet and felt pressure, as though her head had dropped. I didn't have a show, my waters hadn't broken, I was just having gentle ripples across my belly.

My plan for my baby was to birth in a hospital that was close to Steven's Mum so that she was able to look after Caelan. We had no other support so we had no option but to do this. We decided to drive to her house now, so that I could get Caelan settled and then call the hospital to go in. The drive was around 40 minutes; the ripples were coming and coming, but not too painful. Of course once we got to Steven's Mums house, the contractions stopped. So we made the decision to just go to bed and see what happens.

We must have slept for hours; it may have been around 4am that I woke with the contractions. I was weary of labouring in my mother in laws house and understandably not feeling comfortable to do so, so told Steven I wanted to go into hospital. When we were in the car, I told Steven to just keep driving for a bit. It was nice to be 'nowhere'. I wasn't in hospital; I wasn't at my mother in laws. I was able to just relax in the car and listen to music. We drove around for a bit until Steven said he can't keep his eyes open much longer so we went to the hospital. My contractions were not that painful at that time, but I felt like I had no option but to go in.

Once we went in, I was taken to the labour room where the midwife wanted to do a VE to see how far dilated I was, which I agreed to. I felt so down when she said my cervix is posterior and 1 cm. I said I couldn't go home, we had to organise Caelan and the thought of coming back and forth was distressing. She agreed that I could stay on until morning staff and they could assess what was happening, but I may have to go home if labour doesn't take off.

Within the hour, the contractions picked up and labour established easily. I went into the shower for some relief, and whilst in there closed my eyes and tried some meditation techniques I had learned. Breathing in and out, envisioning warm blue and purple light showering over me, protecting me, guiding me. It helped me slip in to my own space, in to labour land. When I was in the shower I felt so much more in control, yet also able to surrender.

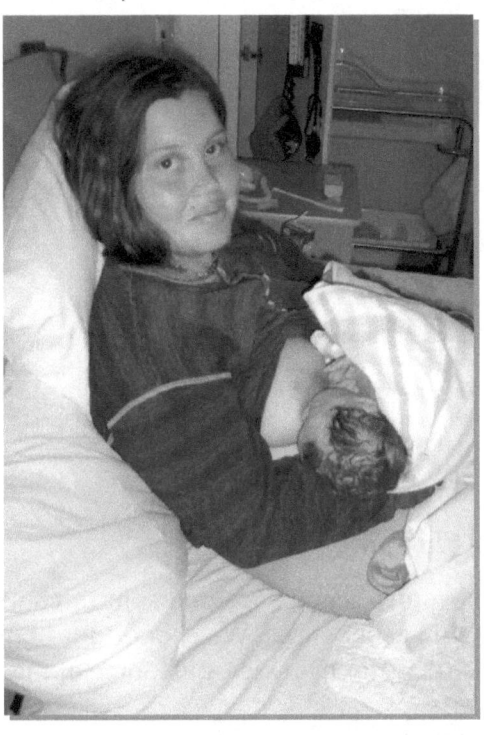

"Baby Rhiannon" – Photo: Steven Booth

Transition was so difficult. The chaos that builds up in my body is so intense, I feel like I am going crazy. I remember screaming, and grabbing onto Steven, squeezing his hand and digging my nails into his hand. I couldn't open my eyes because the room was so bright. The midwives got me on the bed and I remember writhing around, feeling so out of control and a stern bossy midwife came and told me to get on the bed more. She felt so threatening, I was just struggling so much. And then the urge to push came. It was such a different feeling and my mind switched from chaos to determination. I knew I was near the end. With one of the contractions, I remember thinking to myself, 'actually this is ok, this feels ok'. The pushing gave me focus, it was easy. Within 15 minutes of pushing, her sweet little head, and then body was born into the hands of the midwife and then passed to me. I was so excited, but so incredibly tired that I held her and fell asleep in about 10 minutes with Rhiannon in my arms. It was so amazing to see this little person who I always dreamed of. She looked just like she was in my dreams, with dark hair, soft pink lips and long eyelashes.

I felt so proud of myself for doing it naturally, doing it drug free. I now had one son and one daughter to journey with. It felt wonderful.

## *Choosing Homebirth*

By Janet Fraser

Birth, like sex, can be an intensely exhilarating, intimate and empowering experience. The women who report feeling this way in Australia are most commonly women who have chosen to give birth at home.

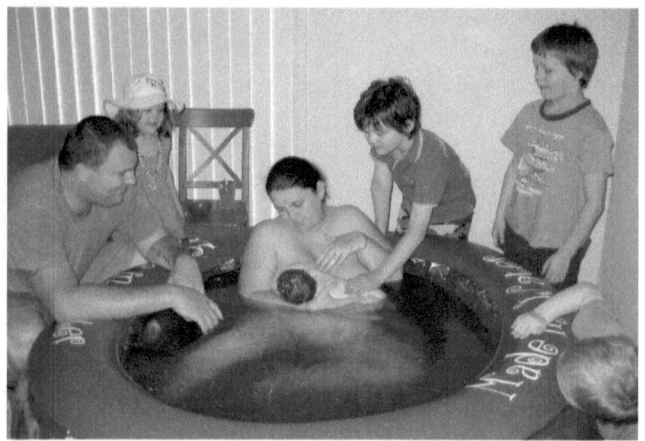

*"Clares Family Birth"* – Photo: Julie Bell

## Choosing homebirth

Women who choose homebirth come from a variety of backgrounds and experiences. We choose our homes as the place to welcome our babies for many reasons. Some of them are:-

<u>Safety</u> - high routine intervention rates in hospitals and birth centres have made birth potentially dangerous and traumatic for women and babies. Spontaneous, normal, physiological birth is the safest way for babies to be born and very difficult to achieve in a medicalised setting.

<u>Natural Birth</u> – natural birth is important to us and we see how difficult it is to achieve normal physiological birth in a medicalised setting. Midwives carry medical equipment the same as most birth centres but it is rarely required in an unhindered birth.

<u>Birth after caesarean</u> – planning a vaginal birth after previous surgery is fraught with stress and difficulty in hospitals. Because homebirth midwives provide evidence based care, birth after caesarean is viewed no differently from any other birth. Our birthing potential is in no way

diminished by previous caesareans and many women birth beautifully at home even after several surgeries.

<u>Midwifery model of care</u> – we choose a model of care which asserts pregnancy and birth are normal physiological states not medical emergencies. Your midwife should promote and maintain an evidence-based practice. Regardless of the model of care you choose, remember to always remain a consumer and advocate for yourself and your baby.

<u>Experience</u> – we choose to have the most personal, intimate moments of our lives take place in our homes where our children are conceived and surrounded by people we know, trust and love. This might also be very important to us if our children were conceived via methods like IVF which can be impersonal. We want to be the first person to hold our babies and have them on our bare skin from birth without any interruption.

<u>Avoiding trauma</u> – we choose to remove ourselves from the medical system which may have traumatised us and our babies at previous births or choose to avoid trauma with our first baby.

<u>Community</u> - we choose a midwife who is part of our local community network and who will sometimes continue to be an important and cherished part of our families after the birth of our children.

<u>Breastfeeding</u> - women who birth at home have greater support and better experiences with breastfeeding. We also establish breastfeeding from birth as our babies are not taken away from us and the hours after birth are crucial in this process.

<u>Siblings</u> - we may want to have our children at the births of their siblings thus including them in the ordinary miracle of birth. This is a loving gift which will stay with them the rest of their lives.

<u>Knowledge</u> - we choose to be active and proactive in how we labour and birth and learn as much as we can. We take the power of knowledge with us into birth instead of giving others responsibility for our care, choices and outcomes.

<u>Health care crisis</u> – we see that our hospital system is in crisis partly because of an unhealthy emphasis on birth as a medical event and that the funds spent on unnecessary interventions and obstetricians would be better placed giving women access to midwifery care. The

outcomes of other countries, like New Zealand, where midwifery care is the norm are significantly better than those in Australia.

<u>Gentle parenting</u> – we want our babies to enter the world gently, without harsh lights, unnecessary intrusive procedures and strangers. Our relationship with our children gets off to the best possible start when the natural processes of labour and birth are unhindered. Babies are designed to birth, they are not designed to cope with unnecessary drugs and surgery.

<u>Control</u> - we want to have complete control over the environment in which we birth without having to negotiate with strangers who have timetables and ideas about birth that don't match our own.

<u>Continuity of care</u> – we see one primary midwife through our entire pregnancy, for monthly appointments of up to, or more than, an hour. Some midwives visit our homes each month; some will alternate between their office (often in their homes) and ours. Some women hire a second midwife who arrives towards the end of labour. Our primary midwife will visit a number of times in the weeks after the birth of a baby as well to monitor our wellbeing and that of our babies. She will also be on call through this time. Many women also like to have a doula or birth attendant as well. Some women choose to only have family members present at their birth.

<u>Memory</u> - we want our memories of birth to be of hard work with passion and accomplishment. We remember how we first met our babies for the rest of our lives so we owe it to us, and them, for that to be on our terms and as beautiful as we can make it.

## *How to choose homebirth in Australia*

You need to find a midwife in private practice with whom you feel comfortable. Just as you engage any other professional to provide you with a service, you have the right to interview, ask questions and meet a midwife face-to-face and make sure she is the right midwife for you. In the unlikely event that you choose to transfer to a hospital, she will provide you with information to help make the decision and will also accompany you. There are publicly funded homebirth programs in some states but these are only open to a small group of women. You need to book in early and fill strict criteria to access them.

## *Support*

Contacting your local homebirth support network will help you meet other women and families for whom homebirth is an important and normal part of life. They can also talk with you about choosing your special birth companions. Joyous Birth meets all over Australia.

## *Learning about pregnancy and birth*

Your midwife should be able to share a great deal with you such as videos, books, journals and experience so you can begin to gather all the vital information around you for achieving a homebirth. There are a number of groups in Australia which provide excellent classes and discussion groups on homebirth and natural birth and you can easily access these as well. Both your support group and your midwife can give you contact details. The Joyous Birth forums are chockfull of information to ensure you achieve the safest and best birth for you and your baby!

*This article was written by Janet Fraser for Joyous Birth*
*© Janet Fraser 2004*
*Joyous Birth Forums: http://joyousbirth.info/*

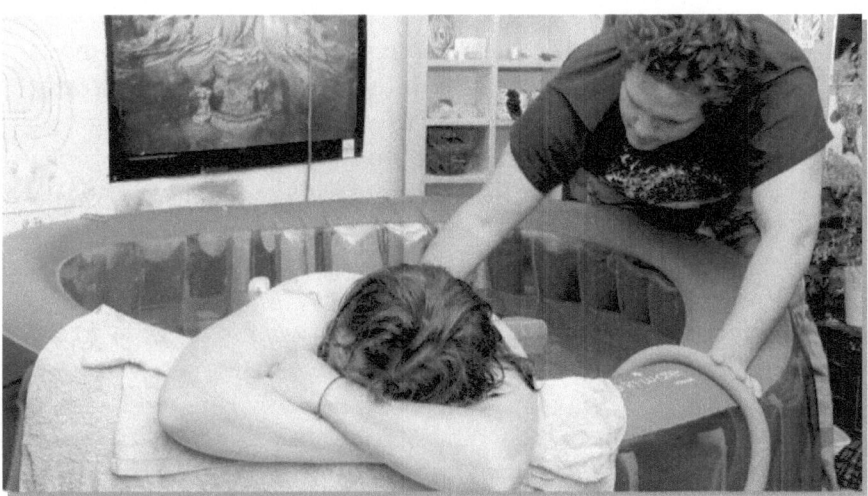

Photo: Brooke Patel Photography

## *Women Choosing Homebirth*

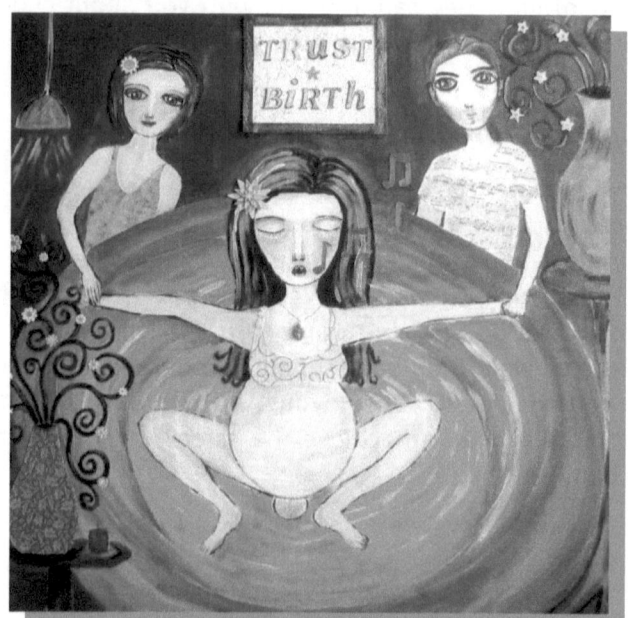

"Birth Song" – Artist: Daisy Mabel

*I chose homebirth because for me it was the safest, most comfortable option. I was able to labour at home, undisturbed, with whomever I pleased and with no restrictions or limitations placed on me. I was sovereign to myself, in tune with my baby, and able to have the safest, most satisfying experience possible.*
*- Whisp*

~*~

*I trusted my body and my knowledge and wanted my baby to be born into hands of love rather than a stranger. - Rebecca Lush*

~*~

*I loved that I could have the opportunity to really form a relationship with my midwife that she cared and understood our family and values, mostly though, so I was in charge of my birth.*

*I did not feel I could call the shot so to speak of I was to birth anywhere else* – Kirra Bird

~*~

*Our first homebirth was with baby #4. We had experienced private, public and birth centre before him, in that order. Each birth I learnt more about what my body was capable of doing, and just how awesome it really was in birth. Each birth also lead me deeper within myself, and needing less and less of others. I chose homebirth because it was what I needed to be able to labour quietly and birth our baby.* - Clare Peterson-Morrissey

~*~

*I chose homebirth so I had the best chance at a physiological birth with the cocktail of wonderful birth hormones that are released. Nature created this process perfectly and I was not one to want to mess with it, I surrendered to the birthing process. At home I felt safe, secure and comfortable. There was nothing that could inhibit the release of those hormones and I became perfectly in tune with my body, knowing exactly what I needed to do, what position to birth in, giving my baby and I the best chance at a safe birth. It was by far the most incredible thing I have had the honour to experience; I can't wait until the day I get to experience it again.* - Bridgette Mansfield

~*~

*Home Birth was the right decision for me and my family. I know it is not for everyone, and I do not think that all women should home birth, but I believe that all women should have the right to birth their babies the way they choose to, not the way someone else thinks you should.* - Johanna Metcalfe

~*~

*I chose homebirth because even after 2 c-sections I had to believe I was not broken. I needed to heal and I needed to do what my heart told me I could. It was like breathing to me, natural* - Crystal Sauceda-Dodson

~*~

*When it came to my second pregnancy, homebirth was the only option. My daughter chose me at a time in my life when I could make empowering choices on how to birth, raise and love my children and I had the support around me to follow through these. It only seemed true to homebirth, to give her the slow, natural, raw, private birth she was entitled to.* - Courtney Gale

~*~

*Because it's the way women have been birthing their babies longer than they haven't!* - Melinda

~*~

*I chose homebirth because it is a safe option.* - Red

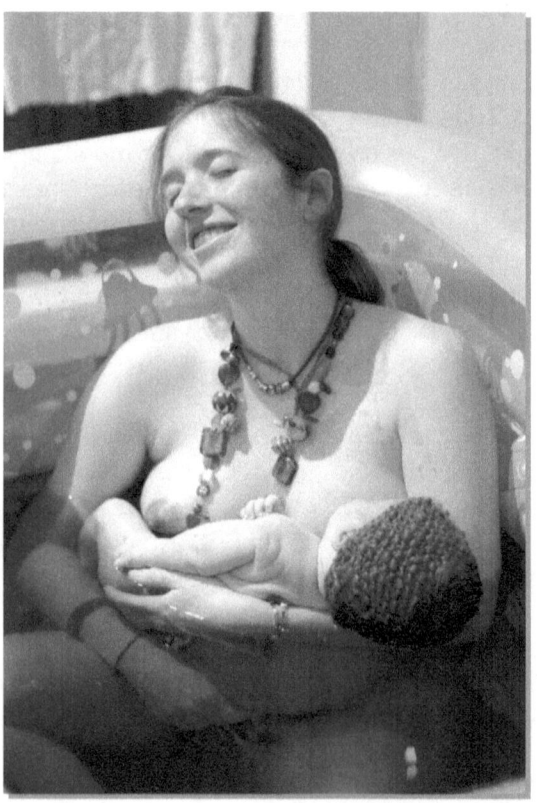

"Billie and River" – Photo: Billie's Partner

## *Finding My Power*

### *Bree's Home Birth After 2 Caesareans Story*
told by Bree Downes

My first son was born in April of 2006. I had self-induced with castor oil at 41 weeks because I had planned to birth in a birth center and I was worried if I went too overdue I'd be transferred out. I really didn't want to birth in delivery suite as I didn't believe I would achieve a natural birth in that setting with the cascade of interventions that come with that system. My waters broke the next morning and my birth then unfolded with very little natural progress over 48 hours, moving into drip augmentation, epidural, and at 3cm dilation and 65 hours after my waters had broken, my only option was a cesarean birth. The classic 'failure to progress'. After my son was born they did tell me that he was in a posterior position and that my cervix was swollen.

My second son was born in Feb of 2009. We planned a homebirth this time, having done my research and realising that my best chance for a successful vbac was at home with an independent midwife, rather than in hospital. I did everything I knew to do and talked to many birth professionals and took all their advice. I was very hopeful that I would get to birth naturally at home. I learned about optimal fetal positioning and made sure my baby was in an anterior position this time, however at 38 weeks he had other ideas and turned posterior which I could then not get him out of. This time I wanted to avoid all interventions and let my baby choose his birth. At 17 days overdue on Black Saturday, I awoke in labour. My labour started and stopped over the next 3 days. I'd have a night of intense contractions 2-3 min apart, and upon sunrise they would all stop. I felt like I was constantly 'resting' yet not getting any rest! On the 3rd night it was incredibly draining and intense. A short lull in contractions at 6am followed by a whopping contraction and a pushing urge, gave myself and the midwife a pleasant surprise, thinking it had been transition and that I was now ready to push. I hopped into the birth pool and the pushing urge continued with each contraction. After a while my midwife suggested I hop out of the pool so that she could check me. I was 6cm.

On one hand that was great news as it was a lot further than the 2-3cm I got with my first labour, but it was a long way off the 10cm that I thought I was. So why the pushing urge? My cervix had swollen and it could have been pressing on a nerve? I had to try not to push with every contraction, otherwise my cervix would not un-swell and I wouldn't dilate. I spent the rest of the day trying not to push, which was incredibly difficult and it took everything I had. I couldn't eat as I felt so nauseous and I wasn't drinking nearly enough given how hot it had been. At around 10pm my midwife checked me again and I was still 6cm. My midwife and doula said that it was time to either break my waters to get this labour moving, or to transfer to hospital for a assistance. The baby was still high so there was a concern of cord prolapse if my waters were broken. I also didn't want to interfere with my son's birth as I had promised him he could choose his own birth. I was so exhausted and had very little energy left to burn, so I made the gut wrenching decision to transfer to hospital. He was born at 2:24am by emergency cesarean, 92 hours after my first contraction. A strong and healthy 4.1kg.

My 3rd pregnancy was a complete surprise. My second son was only 8 months old and I was using an IUD. My husband and I had literally just had the 'no more kids' conversation. Once the shock of being pregnant passed, I was then faced with what choices I was going to make for this baby's birth. A big part of me felt like I'd been through the emotional and physical wringer with my son's births, and I wasn't sure if I could do it again. I was still breastfeeding and I felt incredibly drained. For a brief moment I did consider having an elective cesarean. But something didn't sit right with me about it; I felt it was the easy way out. I felt that if I didn't at least give natural birth a go, I'd never know if I could have done it or not, and that would have haunted me for life. I knew it was my birth right as a woman to experience giving birth. I'd looked forward to that day since I was a little girl, and I knew I would forever feel empty and unfulfilled if I didn't at least try.

So I decided to attempt another homebirth VBAC. I did everything I knew and felt right along my path to succeed. From counselling, bodywork, acupuncture, exercise, and I chose a team of women that I felt would nurture and hold my inner child as I felt that who was running the show for my first 2 labours, and her needs didn't get met. So this time I made sure my 'little Bree's' needs were met with support. My labour started at 6am, 2 days past my due date. My baby was anterior which I felt so relieved about after my 2 posterior boys and it gave me some hope that things were starting different. I spent the whole day in pre labour pottering at home with my husband, his parents came and picked up our boys in the late morning and I baked a cheesecake. We got the house ready, listened to some of our favorite music, I ate plenty of energy building foods and had a nap. My contractions were about 10 min apart for most of the day and I was rather enjoying them and loving feeling my body working. I went to bed at 7:30 that night thinking I would try to sleep while I still could, but I only got about 2hrs sleep before waking up to an intense contraction and I needed to get up. I sat on the fit ball and spiraled whilst watching a movie, then made my way face down into a bean bag where I was sleeping in between contractions that were now coming every 4-5 min.

At midnight there was a knock at our door which gave me a fright. It was our midwife, we had spoken to her earlier on but she decided to come even though we didn't feel we needed her yet. As soon as she arrived things seemed to rise in intensity, I obviously did need her there and felt free to let go knowing we were now supported. She checked me and I was 2cm, which I'd guessed before she checked. A sign that I'm in tune with my body. I felt very calm and peaceful, almost like in a dream state, looking back at the video now I look completely out of it.

At around 2am I went to the toilet and had a contraction with a pushing urge. I immediately knew something was wrong; it felt exactly the same as the pushing urges I had in Reef's birth. I knew I couldn't be 10cm yet. In my head I thought it was all over, it's happening again. I thought "This means my cervix has swollen again and I won't be able to dilate, they should just take me to the hospital for a caesar now". My midwife came in and I explained to her what was happening, I felt very disheartened. She said to me that we have come to that fork in the road again where we can do nothing and wait, and potentially end up with the same result as last time, or we can take a different path and break my waters and see where that leads us. I decided I wanted to break my waters and perhaps that will allow enough pressure on my cervix for it to thin out and for these pushing urges to stop. She went to get her hook out of her bag and I was to get off the toilet after the next contraction that was almost due. With the next contraction my waters broke on their own. I couldn't believe it! I felt this was a sign from the baby to trust and surrender, to completely let go of control. Another internal exam and I was about 4cm, but my cervix is very thick and swollen. My husband fills the birth pool and midwife calls my doula to come, it's now about 4:30am. The next hour is very intense with pushy contractions coming hard and fast. I'm desperately trying not to push but at times I can't help it and then I get distressed as I know when I'm pushing It's swelling my cervix. I honestly believe it's not going to happen and I feel everyone else has more hope and trust than I do right now. I can't understand why no one is packing me into the car and heading down Eastlink! I even say to Keith "I think I need help".

My midwife gave me homeopathics to help relieve the swelling on my cervix and she checks me again thinking I'm around 6cm but still very swollen. My doula arrives at 5:15am and kneels down with me and we do some pant style breathing through the contractions for about 45 min, I seem to regain some focus and energy from her arrival and support. My midwife inserts ice into my vagina to try and reduce the swelling on my cervix and whilst doing so, feels my cervix is completely thinned and gone except for an anterior lip. She kisses my husband on the forehead and says "she's going to do it" but I am so out of it I don't register, and in my head I'm in the back of the station wagon and on the way to the Womens' hospital. I feel immense pressure in my hips and start raising them in the water, the pressure in my bottom is so full on I say, "can someone do something about my bum?" Then I feel myself tear and I declare, "I'm tearing, I'm tearing!"

My midwife gets her torch and shines it in the water and says "we've got head on view!" I'm baffled by this and don't believe it to be true as I'm sure my cervix is still swollen? They tell me to reach down and feel my baby's head, which I do, but that's not a head, it's my insides exploding out of me isn't it? My doula realises I'm not computing anything they are telling me and says, "With the next contraction, you can go with that pushing urge". The penny drops. "Are you serious?" I say, and with that comes a contraction and I didn't even have to push, I just didn't hold back and my baby shot out of me like a rocket across the birth pool. Time stood still. "There's your baby, pick up your baby Bree," they said. I scooped up the delicious body and brought this little soul to my breast. "Oh my god" is all I can mutter. I am in complete shock at what I have done, at what my baby has done. After a moment to soak this all in, I decide to check the sex of the baby. At first I see the umbilical cord and in the low light briefly think it's a penis but then move it aside to discover my divine little girl. At 5:45am in July 2010, after approximately 6 hours of 'active' labour, I got my vaginal birth, and I got my girl.

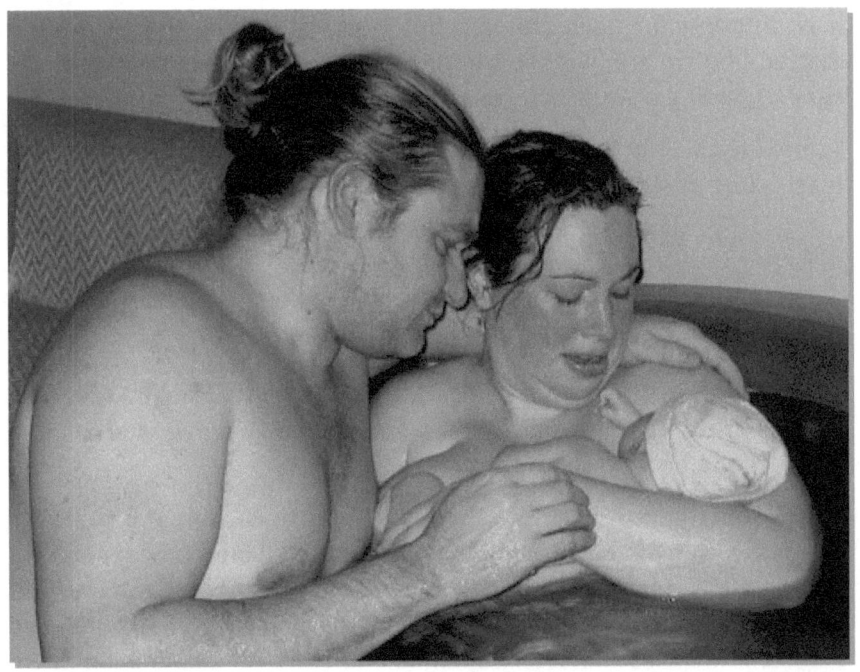

"Beautiful Bree" – Photo: Rhea Dempsey

## *Finding Your Birth Team – feeling safe and loved.*

> *"If you are birthing in a hospital, you automatically become of that system. A woman's intolerance of labour pain may not be to the pain, but to other peoples responses to it"*
> - PAM ENGLAND (Birthing From Within, p202)

Choosing the right people to attend your birth is a huge thing. I am often asked, "How do you know who should be at your birth?" I guess it is different for each woman, but I honestly think that it doesn't matter who we are, we need to find those who we feel confident will keep us feeling private, safe and undisturbed.

Some things that I asked myself, and I recommend all women ask these same or similar questions to themselves, are:

- Who do I connect with?
- Who do I feel safe with?
- Who can I be vulnerable in front of?
- Who is it that I am so comfortable with, that my body is able to do its thing, and open my cervix and vagina wide enough for a baby to come through?

I think sometimes it is easy to forget what birth is. Sure, it is the birth of a baby. But the birth of the baby is an incredible body experience that gets a woman in her primal state, her fierce, animal self and this involves contractions that feel like nothing you've ever experienced before. It involves the cervix opening and the baby descending down the vagina, and the vagina stretching to capacities that you may never thought possible. It is an extremely powerful time and also an extremely vulnerable time. Having people you know and love at the birth can help you feel less self-conscious and more safe, relaxed and confident. Having people who you are not comfortable or familiar with, or having too many people in the room can increase your anxiety, make you more stressed which leads to more adrenaline being produced which can prolong your labour and make the experience of pain for greater.

- How do you feel about giving birth in front of strangers?
- In front of a man?
- How do you feel about students coming in to the room, needing to practice on your labouring body?
- How do you feel about the idea of having several midwives whom you've never met attend your birth? Depending on how long you are in hospital for, you may see several midwives as they change shifts.

As women, as humans, we don't normally allow people close to us to see our vagina or our anus, let alone strangers. If someone walks in on us on the toilet, we are normally embarrassed, as is the person that walked in on you.

- How do you feel about a stranger looking at your vagina and anus, when it is opening, expelling fluids and blood, and then a baby and placenta?
- How about if they put their fingers in there?
- Or wipe your bottom?
- Or hold a facewasher against your stretching perineum?
- Or shine a torch on it?
- Or put a mirror on the ground underneath you so they can see it all from a different angle?

I am asking such intimate questions on purpose, because birth is such an intimate process. We know that other mammals go and birth in privacy, in the dark, away from others. When they are disturbed, their labour stalls or stops until they feel safe again. We are mammals too, so we are no different. Dr. Sarah Buckley so beautifully says that all women during labour need to have our mammalian needs met, and that is to feel private, safe and undisturbed. So, a darkened space, the mother not being disturbed by ANYONE and her feeling safe, which can be assisted by her having people there that she feels comfortable with. Bright lights, unfamiliar care providers and the mother not feeling as though her wishes and needs are being met are not optimal for a normal, straightforward physiological birth.

## The Wild Rainbow

Dim the lights, keep the room warm, making sure there is access to water, being free to move, and the gentle non-intrusive presence of people you love can help facilitate a gentle, physiological birth.

When thinking of the birth of my last 3 children, but particularly my 6th child, I asked myself all of the above questions. And then I realised that for me to birth, I HAVE to feel safe. For me, I chose people who I felt safe and comfortable with who I didn't mind if they saw me swear, if they saw my vagina, my stretch marks, if I poo'ed in front of them, or if my waters broke all over their feet. If I felt ok with all of the above happening in the presence of someone, then they could be invited into my birth space.

Speaking of all of this, bought back a memory of just after the birth of my 5th child. I was sitting on the lounge room couch with my sweet newborn, and I my husband and birth team were walking past me, each with a bucket of water from the birth pool, that was full of amniotic fluid, blood and all bits of birth, as they took them outside to pour onto the garden, and I sat there thinking *'I knew these people were the right ones for me'*. They did it with smiles on their faces and joy in their hearts. It wasn't a job for them, they didn't have to do it. They just did it, and the birth water didn't bother them at all.

Have a birth team that makes you feel safe, loved, supported and nourished, and it will help immensely in your birth.

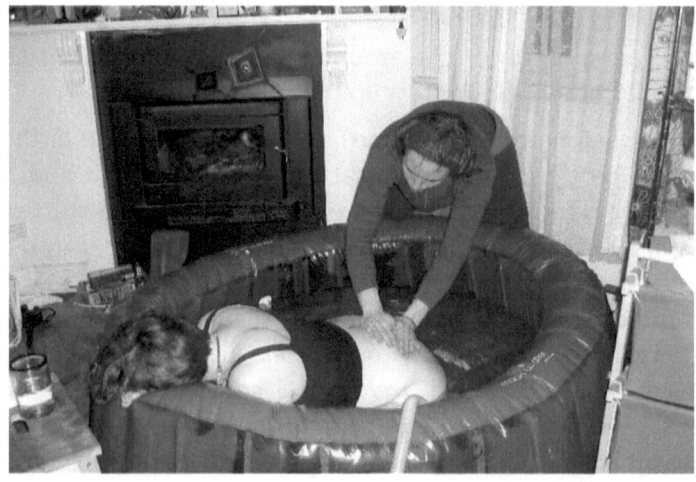

"Courtney and Grace" – Photo: Sheree Stewart

Journeying as Mother

## *The Homebirth Of Lilith*

*told by Lauren Gibbins*

Just so you know who everyone is, Beth and Cath were my housemates/family when Lilith was born and Malachai, Jasper and Tuesday are their kids. One of Liliths middle names is after Beth, she was my biggest source of support, we saw each other through a lot, both with pregnancy, birth and otherwise.

Saturday around 4:30 in the afternoon (the 8th of October and 38 weeks and 5 days pregnant) I was in the shower chatting away to Malachai and I got an incredibly painful rush that lasted for a few minutes and made me have to turn the shower off because the water touching me got really annoying. I thought nothing of it but Malachai told me I was going to have a baby that night so I shouldn't have been surprised when I did. Kids are very intuitive and we always had a special bond.

After I got out of the shower and got dressed I went across the street to pick up some food, the whole 15 minutes I was out of the house I was getting quite strong and uncomfortable rushes every few minutes and half of me was thinking, could this be it? and the other half was thinking, it's probably just wishful thinking.

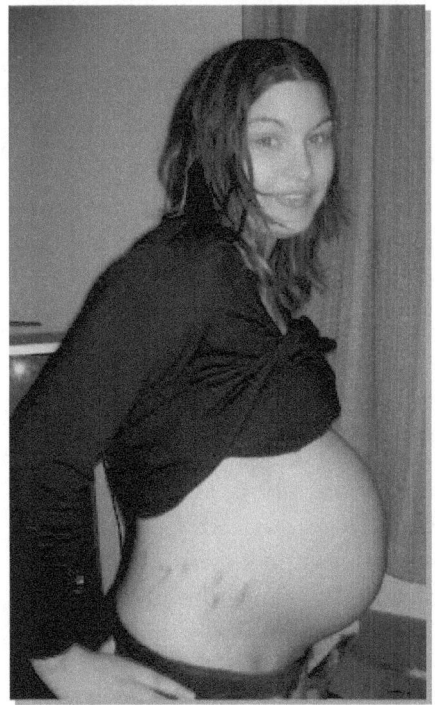

I got home with my food and sat down on the couch and just as I was settling down for dinner with Jasper, my waters broke. I wasn't sure if it was just major incontinence setting in so I went to the toilet and lo and behold, it had a slightly bloody tinge and that distinct earthy smell, it was definitely amniotic fluid.

Photo: Beth Stewart-Nichols

# The Wild Rainbow

For a while I just went about my day, kids jumping on me, playing in the garden, posting on my blog, the usual. The rushes started off coming every few minutes and I think lasting for a couple of minutes so within the hour it was hard to focus on anything but having a baby.

I was freezing but couldn't stand the thought of wearing anything so I just had the heater next to me and up really high the entire time. Every rush I had to lean over onto something or someone, first a chair and then as things progressed either Beth or Cath. One of my biggest memories of labour was having my head buried in Beth's breasts breathing and swaying.

I jumped into the shower and made the fascinating discovery of my mucous plug coming out even though I had been 4 cm's dilated and able to feel the membranes and her head for a couple of weeks, it was so good, the water felt amazing and every time I had a rush I arched my body over and leaned on the side of the bathtub, it was like heaven. Unfortunately the hot water system gave up on me for the first time ever so I had to get out.

I was pacing for quite a while, making humming noises and twisting my hands around which felt like it was releasing energy from me.

Once Cath had the birthing pool half full I hopped in and had to lie down so the water entirely immersed my body, this felt great between rushes but while I was in the midst of one I had to sit up.

After a while I made Beth jump in with me and she sat in front of me while I squatted and then when my knees got sore we stood up and I leaned on her swaying and toning my way through rushes.

By this point the rushes were constant and there was no break in between. I felt so in control for most of my labour, the entire time there were only 1 or 2 times when I thought, I am over this, need to sit and relax now, maybe take up smoking again.

I could feel her moving down during some rushes and at a point I decided kneeling in the water seemed like a good idea, so I was kneeling resting my bum on my feet, my legs and knees on the ground and spread really far apart (hard position to explain) and leaning on Beth, my face so far down it was almost in the water and my arms resting on her legs.

All of a sudden there was a stop and I felt like I had consumed copious amounts of opiates thanks to the sweet, wacky birthing hormones. This lasted awhile and then suddenly I felt my body contract and this roaring noise forcing itself out of me and as soon as I let the noise out I felt her moving down, beginning to make her way out.

I didn't push at all just let this noise out and then the rush stopped and I had another long round of opiated peace then the same thing happened and I felt her move down a little more, it felt like the roaring was responsible for moving her down, I wasn't pushing at all. Best of all it didn't hurt in the slightest.

This went on for a long time (an hour, hour and a half) and then finally I got really boiling hot (Cath had to start pouring cold water into the birth pool and I had a freezing washcloth on my forehead but was so hot). I roared and I could feel her coming out and I tried pushing but it seemed to push her back in and it hurt for the first time so I gave up that idea and just continued to breathe her out.

After asking if I wanted birth pictures and me being so focused I didn't, I got Cath to jump into the birth pool and get behind me so I could lean on her (which was so incredibly comfortable) and I squatted and just breathed her out, I could feel pressure but it didn't hurt at all, I was just working with my body roaring her out.

I could feel myself opening up and Beth was saying to me that she could see her head and the next thing I knew there was this intense pressure and my entire body felt like I was going to explode from the intensity (but still no pain, I didn't have an orgasm but I totally understand the term orgasmic birth, it was the sweetest release) and at 12:06am on the 9th of October she was out.

Beth caught her and handed her to me, she had her eyes closed until she was in my arms, then she opened them straight away.

I could feel the cord warm and pulsing and she was just looking around quietly taking in her surroundings and blinking, then she started making little kitten noises and I started crying and was just in shock.

After losing a baby and this incredible journey of learning to trust my body, that I could birth without any 'help' or intervention, reclaiming every single ounce of self-respect, woman pride and strength that had ever been torn from me, I was reborn.

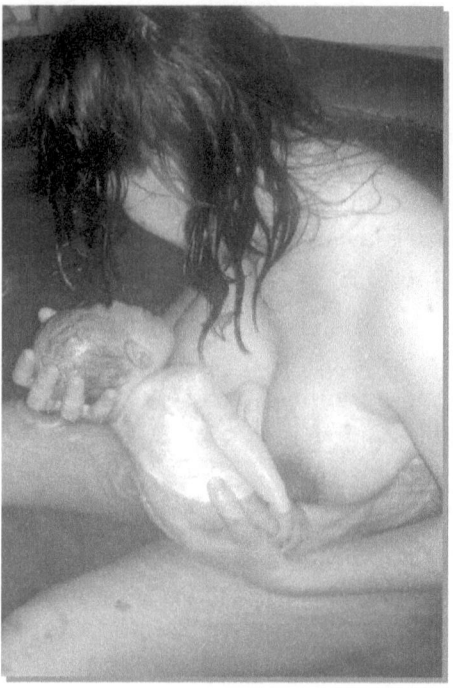

Photo: Beth Stewart-Nichols

I started getting contractions again and then the placenta separated but didn't come out. At some point I got out of the water and about an hour or so after the birth (or so I've been told, I had no concept of time, it felt like 5 minutes) it came out.

I really wanted Malachai to be there but he wouldn't get out of bed and then afterwards got really upset about it (all the kids slept through her birth).

After this we went and snuggled up in bed and she had her first breastfeed (first of thousands, she still is rather attached). I felt so whole and changed.

## *For The Love Of Doulas.*

My experience of having doula's

What I really, really love and what really worked for me was having a doula. The love and support that Doula's bring to your care is incredible.

I had doulas for the pregnancy of my 4th and 5th children. Our chats and never ending cups of tea go for hours! Each Doula has such unique and varied knowledge. So many of them work with their intuitive knowledge.

When I saw them for my pregnancy visits, they bought food, they made cups of tea, they played with my children, and they did my dishes. I got foot massages! One of them hosted my Blessingway when my belly was round and full. They listened to me as I shared my birth visions, my fears, my dreams, and my nightmares. They don't look at their watches because time is not important to them. I am important to them. If I wanted to cry for 2 hours, then they will hold the space for me to do that. They use the reboso to relax me, to help me reconnect to my body, to help the baby whose head is in an awkward position to move a bit!

During labour they sat still and held the space. They tend to the needs of my children so was fully able to get on with the business of birthing! They lit the candles from my Blessingway and reminded me that all the women in my circle are thinking of me and are sending me love and strength.

They knew what I wanted because we have spent hours and hours together.

They wiped my brow with a cold face washer and they passed me hot washers that I could put on my stretching perineum as I was birthing. The passed me drinks before I even had to ask.

They tell me I look beautiful and they tell me I am safe. I can melt into them because I can trust them so much.

After the birth in the early post-partum days they organised family and friends to bring around meals for our family. They did what they can to make me feel loved and supported and well rested so that I could recover from the birth as quickly as possible and that I could bond with my new baby. The massages continue and so do the long chats and endless cups of tea. If I wasn't up for talking, they would watch my children while I caught up on some sleep.

We laughed together and cried together and carry a bond that lasts forever. To me, it felt so real and primal and right. It is like truth in action, like this is how it is just meant to be. I am supported in love and trust.

*Dedicated to my birth teams over my last 3 pregnancies and births - Anna, Grace, Courtney, Brooke, Lauren, Star, Mish and Lucy*

If you like statistics, here are proven benefits of having an experienced birth attendant:

- 50% reduction in the caesarean rate
- 25% shorter labour
- 60% reduction in epidural requests
- 40% reduction in oxytocin use
- 30% reduction in analgesia use
- 40% reduction in forceps delivery

*Mothering the Mother: How a Doula Can Help You Have a Shorter Easier and Healthier Birth*, Klaus, Kennell, and Klaus (1993).

## *The Freebirth Of Imogen*

*told by Tamara Travaglia*

Imogen's story began around the middle of October 2011 when we saw two dark pink lines. At first I was nervous and worried about this pregnancy because just a few weeks earlier I sadly lost my angel at just 6 weeks gestation and I was not done grieving. The first 12 weeks of my pregnancy was a nerve wrecking, but really exciting time for me. I voluntarily requested frequent blood tests to make sure my levels were rising as they should have been, and of course they were. The next two months went by without any issues. At 21 weeks I became a single mama, which left me frightened, lots of crazy thoughts would go through my head "How could I possibly manage 3 children on my own?" and "Oh my god! I'm going to have a toddler AND a newborn" were the main ones. I doubted myself a lot.

I had 4 weeks to find myself and my two children a house to live in, because we had to be out of our current place. So I spent many weeks packing and house hunting, with 2 children and a growing belly in tow, every step of the way. We finally found our home and moved in on 2nd April and immediately my stress levels went right down. Everything was falling into place, finally. I knew my new home was going to be my baby's birth place. I spent the rest of my pregnancy enjoying lots of little (and big!) kicks and rolls from within. I made sure to enjoy every moment, because time was going faster than I wanted it to. 25th June at around 10:30pm I messaged my friend Sheree to let her know I've had a few "bitey" surges and that I think my body is preparing to meet this babe, but I don't think it will be too soon, because I was too tired to birth that night. They fizzled out when I went to bed. 26th June I woke up and continued having random not very frequent strong Braxton hicks with a bit of pressure added in.

By the evening they were certainly there, but not frequent or painful so I just continued to think they were just strong Braxton hicks, bringing me one step closer to meeting my babe though, which was very exciting for me. My other friend Courtney came over in the evening and hung my birth flags up in my lounge room for me and we chatted for a while. I told her the surges were coming around 10-15

# The Wild Rainbow

minutes apart, but I was not timing, just guessing and going with the flow. After she left, I put myself to bed and had the best sleep I've had in such a long time, only waking once from a mild contraction (which I was still convinced were just Braxton hicks). 27th June I woke up and started our morning as normal. I made Amelia's school lunch and got her ready for school. Contractions were certainly very present this morning, but not painful and not really frequent I didn't think (wasn't timing them). We headed off to school where I quietly warned her that either Courtney or Sheree may or may not be picking her up from school today, because I was having a few contractions and that I think the baby might come later today, but probably tonight. In hindsight, I should have kept her home today. After dropping Amelia at school I headed out to enrol her into her new school which she will be attending as of next term. After handing the paperwork in for that, Blake and I decided to check out an op-shop on our way home, I was still contracting about every 7-10 minutes (guessing) at this stage, again, not painful, just "bitey". Blake spotted a basket of handmade knitted baby beanies, and he picked out a lovely little dark purple/violet/blue coloured beanie for our baby. We headed home after that and I decided it was time I took my very last pregnancy photo.

At 10:50am I messaged Sheree and told her that the contractions were burning quite a bit now and seeming closer together than they were earlier. I told her I was worried they weren't the real thing, mostly because whilst the contractions seemed strong, they weren't how I remember them with my previous births. I was still able to talk to Blake and tend to him as I needed to. At 12pm I begin to realise that in fact they were the real deal and this baby was going to be born soon, not tonight like I had thought. I wasn't at all worried that I was alone with my 2 year old and getting close to birthing. It all just felt right and normal. I messaged Sheree again and said "coming closer now and strong", she replied back to me instantly and said "Going to get coffee and petrol then head over. Keep doing what you're doing, well done". Her words were reassuring to me. At 12:40pm I messaged Courtney who was to pick Amelia up from school for me. I told her "I think you should get her pretty soon if you can, contractions getting closer and stronger". I wasn't sure whether the school would allow for Courtney to pick her up as she isn't one of the people so I called the school to inform them on what was happening, and it was all fine. The receptionist tried to converse with me about me being in labour and if I thought the baby was going to be born soon. I just wanted to get off the phone.

At about 1:05pm I messaged Sheree again and said "Baby isn't far I don't think", she replied back to me right away and said "That's ok. It's all perfect. I'm almost there". This is when I felt my baby come right down ready for birth. I decided I had better make my way to the front door to unlock it so Sheree could get in when she arrives, because I know a lot can change in just minutes, I may not have been able to unlock it when she did arrive (which was just 5 minutes after her last text), and it was a very good thing that I did unlock the door when I did because just minutes later I was on the floor, asking Blake to bring me my phone and my water bottle while I grabbed a towel out of my birth box to place under me. 1:10pm Sheree came into my home and quickly pottered around, preparing my space with lots of towels and chatting with Blake. She asked me if I wanted her to set up the pool, but I told her I didn't think there would be enough time.

I could feel my baby was very close now, as I begin to feel "pushy". I don't intentionally push as I want to breathe my baby out and go with my body, it knew exactly what to do. Sheree hands me a hot wash cloth to place on my perineum but I either can't reach it in the position I was in, or it just felt too uncomfortable, so she helped hold the cloth for me. My lower back and hips were burning every time I had a contraction. Minutes later my baby's head emerged, still in the caul. I tried to see by using a hand mirror but couldn't get it in a good position to see clearly. Baby's body followed quickly and was born into Sheree's loving hands. Baby was looking very bright eyed and lovely and pink right away. Her amniotic sack was intact right up until her stomach was out. My beautiful baby is going to have good luck for the rest of her life! After her sack broke away we discovered she had fresh meconium in her waters, which was not an issue. If she were born in a hospital setting I am positive she would have been cut from her placenta right after birth and rushed away from me to be checked by a doctor, just like Amelia was at birth due to the same thing. But instead she was kept close to my chest and touched only by people who loved her.

# The Wild Rainbow

Her placenta came around 40-45 minutes later. Amelia and Courtney arrive home shortly after; thankfully Amelia wasn't too upset about missing the birth. I wanted to wait for Amelia to get here before we discover the baby's gender. I thought it would be something special for Amelia, to discover the gender of her new sibling. She tells me "it's a girl" with a huge grin on her face. She always wanted a baby sister, so she was a bit chuffed. Imogen's birth was nothing short of amazing. I was in total control of my body the entire time and I felt awesome. I didn't expect to birth quite so quickly though. I was so sure I would labour all day and birth at night again. Her birth taught me that I should never ever doubt myself, and to always trust my body, which is exactly what I did.

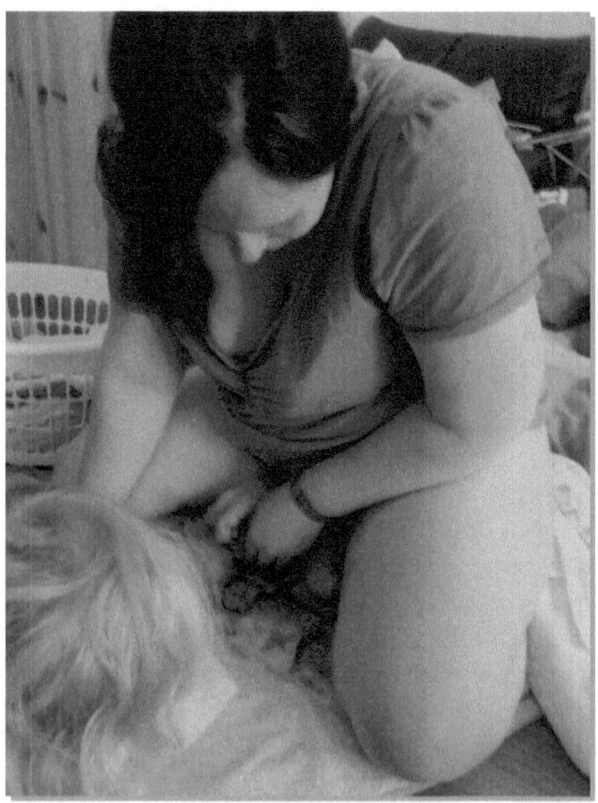

*Tamara, Blake and Baby Imogen* – Photo: Sheree Stewart

## *Siblings at Birth*

When I was planning my first homebirth, pregnant with my 4th child, I assumed my children would be there. I had 2 doulas and the idea was the one of them would always be with my children. Instead, I went into labour and birthed my daughter when my 3 children had a sleepover at their grandmother's house! Also, I was pregnant with my 5th baby, I had chosen the same tactic of having a doula there for my children. My 2 year old stayed with my doula (who was also a close friend), they snuggled each other and she breastfed her while they lay on my bed and kept each other company.

Around the same time of my 5th baby's birth, my then 8 year old son said to me "It's so good there are girls in the world to have babies. It must be so amazing to grow a human inside your body, is it Mum?", whilst my then 4 year old daughter told me "girls have boobies so that they can breastfeed. You can even give booby milk if you have two babies".

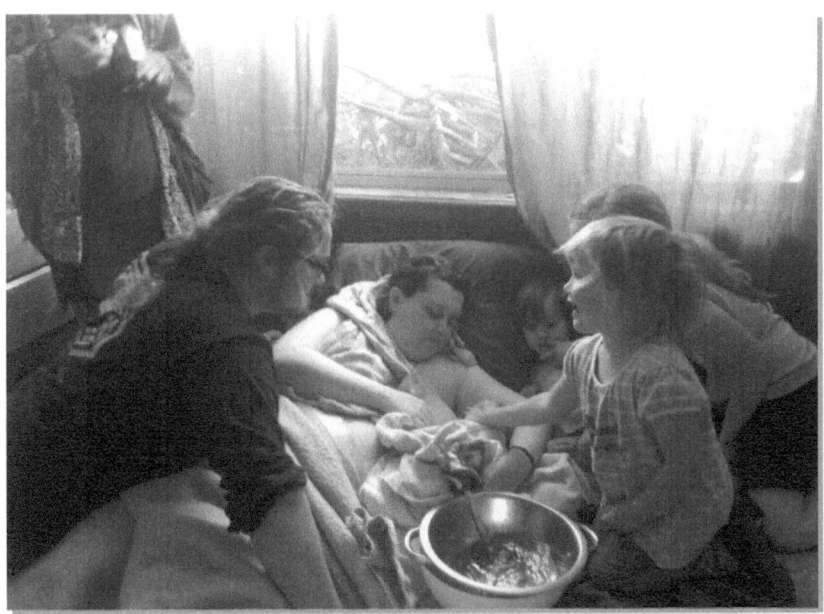

Photo: Lucy Johnston

I have had many conversations with my children around birth. It is a normal part of life. And in my home, with my job as a midwife and doula, talk of birth comes up a lot. My children all have a lot of knowledge when it comes to pregnancy and birth and I sometimes forget just how much they actually know until I hear them speaking to their friends or me about it. One day when Rhiannon was 6 she said to me, "Why doesn't anyone else that's a kid know what a placenta is?" I often hear them talk about the safety and normalcy of birth and of how mothers catch their babies into their own hands. My sons favourite part of homebirth is that you get to stay at home and eat breakfast that is nice, not like the hospital food.

My favourite story I heard my then 4 year old daughter, Aaliyah, tell her grandmother about birth was this:

"When babies are born in the water they know how to swim and breathe underwater. When they are adults they can choose if they want to be humans or mermaids"

## *Stories of siblings at birth.*

> *My little one was present and feeding me a lolly snake just after Roo was born. He insisted. Then he insisted on making me toast. Which he ate himself. He woke up just as I was starting to feel pushy. He came out and sat on the sofa observing me. After a particularly strong contraction and some guttural moaning from me he looked at me and said with a big smile "oh you scared me mummy"* – Billie

~*~

> *My son wore his ear muffs when I started getting vocal. He wanted his torch to point into the water just as our midwife was doing. And he was fascinated with the placenta & learning about "the little house where our baby lived inside mum's tummy". The most precious moment was when he came to the pool side & said "I can hold your hand if you need mummy"* – Nic

## Rory

Julie's children generously shared their perspectives of when their sweet brother Rory was born at home.

> To all the people of the earth
> My wonderful mum has given birth
> It was hard that's what she said
> Soon she will go to sleep in bed
>
> But first we'll celebrate his birthday
> We'll shout out loud hip hip hooray
> You should see the henna on her tummy
> I made a mistake and it looked funny
>
> This afternoon has been so fun
> And to Mummy and Daddy - Well Done!
> This afternoon has been so cool
> My Mum had her baby in Claire's birth pool
>
> Now our family has 6 people
> Rory I think is very beautiful
> The cutest baby in the whole wide world
> And the bestest parents in the world as well.

~*~

"When I got out of bed, Daddy was getting ready for Mummy's birth. Then I started to help. I was so excited. Soon Gaye came to help and then Claire came. When Mummy got into the birth pool I was even more excited. Flicka was very funny, when Mummy had her loudest contraction, she woke up and her eyes went round and she looked very surprised. I was happy the whole time. I nearly cried, but I was too embarrassed to cry in front of everyone. When Rory came out, I nearly cried again. He was so cute he only cried a little bit. When I had my first hold I was superdooper happy. Rory is the cutest funniest best baby I've ever seen. There was alot of blood in the water. That was the happiest Saturday I've ever had in my life."

## The Wild Rainbow

~*~

"When Rory was born, I thought it was taking a long time because I was looking at the wrong place. After a little while then I saw the baby's real head. After the shoulders came out, the body came out as quick as Flicka pounces. After Rory was born, Rory was so cute. Now I felt really excited because now I have got a little brother. After Rory was born, the water was really really red. When Mummy was holding Rory, I patted his head. It felt warm and soft, like wet fur."

~*~

"The day Rory was born: I woke up on Saturday morning and heard the vacuum cleaner. That meant we were going to do lots of cleaning. But why would they have it out this early? I listened a little bit more. Suddenly I realised the noise wasn't the vacuum cleaner. I jumped out of bed and ran into the toy corner. Daddy was blowing up the birth pool. I asked him why he was blowing it up now and he said because Mummy was going to have a baby soon - but i thought he meant in a few days. But when he started to put water in the birth pool I knew that Mummy was going to have the baby today. I was so happy and excited that I couldn't think properly. Claire and Gaye came and Mummy got into the birth pool. The funniest part of the day was when Mummy was having her biggest contraction and Flicka got such a big fright and ran away. I was laughing so much. Soon I could see the top of his head. Then his head stayed there for a while then it just went back in altogether. After a little while his whole head was out. Mummy's waters never broke so the caul was still around his head. It looked like a little bubble around his head. He was born in water in a birth pool. After his head was out the rest of his body came out really quick. When he came out I was shaking from how happy I was. I was so excited when I found out he was a boy. He was so cute and small. Mummy and Daddly named him Rory! I was so happy when I had my first hold. It was one of the best days of my life."

## *Placenta*

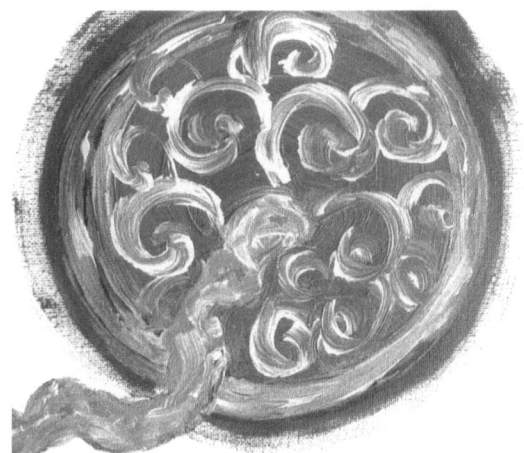

*"Placenta"* – Artwork: Lucy Johnston

**What is 'placenta'**

The placenta is an amazing organ that is often overlooked and under-appreciated! The word placenta means 'flat cake' and is the organ that has many functions which keeps the baby alive in utero. Oxygen and nutrients are carried to the baby via the placenta and umbilical cord and baby's waste products are passed through the placenta into the mother's bloodstream for her to get rid of. It is a protective filter which keeps out lots of bacteria and it passes on antibodies to protect the baby's health for the time in utero as well as the first few months earthside.

In hospitals, once the placenta is birthed, it is put in a biohazard bag and placed in the medical waste furnace to be burned. This distresses me! I feel as though the placenta needs to be honoured in some way – kept attached to the baby until it naturally detaches, buried in the earth or made into medicine and tinctures. I am obviously not alone in this thought, as there is a whole new movement around what we, as women, are doing with our placentas.

Being conscious and aware is the first step.

## *Lotus Birth*

*"We need to relearn what a birth can be like when it is not disturbed by the cultural milieu. We need a reference point from which we should try not to deviate too much. Lotus Birth is such a reference point."* - Michel Odent

Lotus birth is the practice of leaving the umbilical cord intact, which keeps baby and placenta connected until natural separation, which naturally occurs 3- 8 days post birth. Although it seems to be a relatively new practice, it is one that is becoming more common as families become aware of and better understand this option. The reasons as to why families choose lotus birth varies, ranging from feelings of completeness if the baby holds onto the placenta until she is ready to 'let go', for physiological benefits of baby getting the full blood supply from the placenta, to energetic and spiritual reasons. Many families have reported a change in their babies state once their placenta has fallen away. More alert, more willing to be held by people other than the mother, more eye to eye contact with others, more 'ready for the world'.

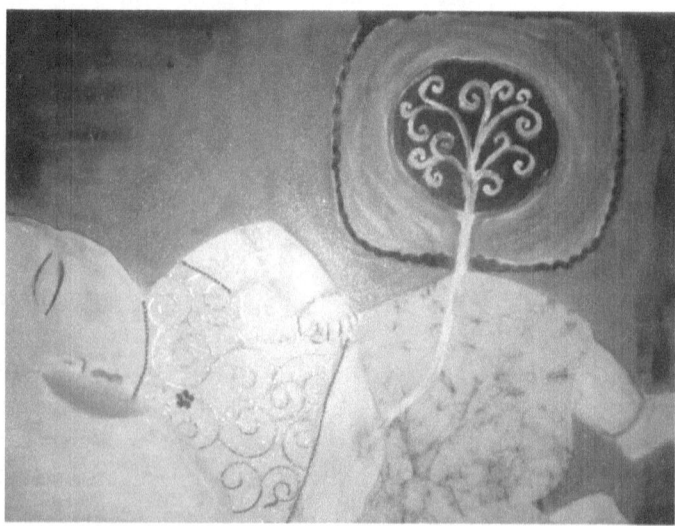

*"Lotus Birth"* – Artist: Daisy Mabel

## Care of the Placenta

*By Shivam Rachana*

- When the baby is born, leave the umbilical cord intact. If the cord is around the baby's neck, simply lift it over.

- Wait for the natural delivery of the placenta. Do not use oxytocin - this forces too much too soon into the infant and compromises the placenta delivery.

- When the placenta delivers, place it into a receiving bowl beside the mother.

- Wait for full transfusion of the umbilical blood into the baby before handling the placenta.

- Gently wash the placenta with warm water and pat dry.

- Place the placenta into a sieve or colander for 24hrs to allow drainage.

- Wrap the placenta in absorbent material, a nappy or cloth and put in into a placenta bag. The covering is changed daily or more often if seepage occurs. Alternatively, the placenta may be laid on a bed of sea salt (which is changed daily) and liberally covered with salt.

- The baby is held and fed as the mother wishes.

- The baby is clothed loosely.

- The baby can be bathed as usual - keep the placenta with it.

- Keep movement to a minimum.

http://www.lotusbirth.net/

# The Wild Rainbow

**Sage's Lotus Birth**

*The lotus birth story of my 4th baby.*

Sage had a lotus birth. We left her umbilical cord and placenta intact. We did this for many reasons, the main ones being my aboriginal background. Many Aboriginal tribes cut the umbilical cord long, at the end of the cord, at the start of the placenta. There were many beliefs surrounding this. I felt lotus birth was an extension of this, and was a way to honour my ancestry.

It seemed a natural progression of the natural, undisturbed, physiological birth that Sage had had. I didn't want to interrupt this by cutting the cord, when everything else about her pregnancy and birth had been so unhindered. It seemed unnatural to start interrupting a natural process now.

It was important for Sage to get all the physiological benefits of keeping the placenta intact, which is giving her own blood supply which her placenta returns to her after birth. Early cord clamping deprives babies of up to a third of their blood supply and I didn't want Sage to be deprived from anything that was rightfully hers to begin with.

Lotus birth gave me and my baby a chance to bond without interruptions. The placenta held a certain quiet space. I am sure many mothers would agree that lotus birth almost forces the mother and baby and family to be still and quiet. It allowed us to stay in contact, quiet contact, and made bonding easy and blissful. We were chemically and hormonally connected and fell in love in these early lotus days, and that will last forever.

In the first day of Sage's life, I felt lotus birth to be awkward, but I still appreciated it. It held a quiet space and it seems to keep the world still and quiet. I savoured the closeness and the bonding that lotus birth bought into our lives.

On the day of her birth we sat the placenta in a colander which allowed the blood to drain. Later in the afternoon, we rinsed it in under warm water to expel the clots. I remember marvelling at this amazing organ that sustained my daughter for 9 months.

I wanted to salt the placenta, to help it dry, as I was worried about the smell (it didn't end up smelling at all). My son picked rosemary and lavender from the garden and together we lay the placenta on a terry towel cloth and sprinkled it with salt, then put the herbs on it. We wrapped it up and it stayed in a bundle, neatly packaged with my daughter.

The next 3 days we followed this same ritual. On the 2nd day her cord had dried out quite a lot. Sage preferred the placenta close to her, especially if it was wrapped up in a bundle with her. I felt the energetic between Sage and her placenta was obvious.

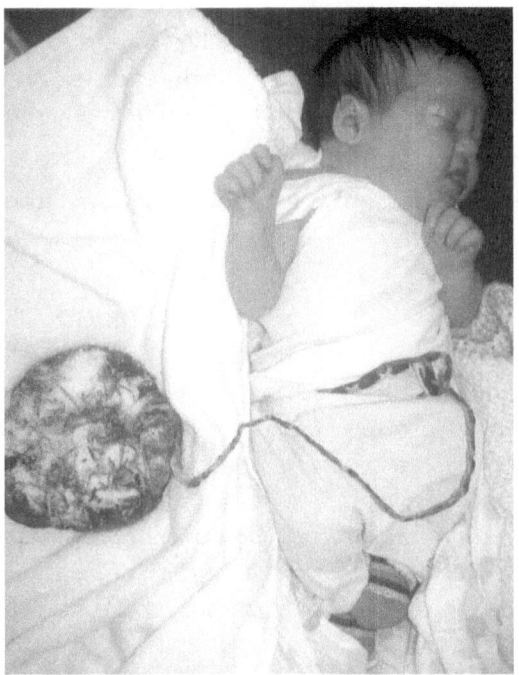

"Sage and Ruby" – Photo: Sheree Stewart

On the 3rd day, the cord was hard and brittle and dark. It had changed so much from the day before. It still looked as though it was pulsing with life, even though there was no physical exchange happening, the energetic exchange was still strong. Sage still needed her placenta that day,

On the 4th day, the placenta had shrunk quite a lot and the cord was very hard. It was the first day that Sage wasn't still. She seemed restless. She was also very alert – usually she would gaze at my husband or I, but on this day she was gazing deeply into the faces of others and of various things around the house.

Around 7pm that night, Sage started crying. It was the first time she cried since birth. I held her as she cried. She cried for more than an hour. At times, she held on to her cord and cried. After an hour, she fell asleep in my arms and I went and lay her in bed. When I went to go and change her nappy a few hours later, I saw that her umbilical cord had detached from her navel.

She was lotus born!

I was so excited and felt a sense of achievement for Sage. She had a full physiological birth and lotus birth and everything that had happened so far in her life was in her own terms, in her own time, in her own tune.

We buried her placenta in the garden a few days later, in a beautiful private family ceremony.

*Lotus Birth is a call to pay attention to the natural physiological process. It's practice, through witnessing, restores faith in the natural order. Lotus Birth extends the birth time into the sacred days that follow and enables baby, mother and father and all family members to pause, reflect and engage in nature's conduct. Lotus birth is a call to return to the rhythms of nature, to witness the natural order and to the experience of not doing, just being.*

- Shivam Rachana

## *Ceremonies for the Placenta*

In Aboriginal Law, after the baby is born, the umbilical cord is cut at the start of the placenta, so the baby has its full length umbilical cord attached. The idea is that that way, the baby will never get thirsty, which is an important belief to have when you are living in desert and arid areas in Australia! The placenta is buried under (or within) a tree – my understanding is for each tribe, or area, there is a specific type of tree where placentas go. Each type of tree holds is own medicine and magic and its believed the tree spirit will guard, connect the baby to the earth mother and keep the baby healthy. This is age old magic and ceremony, and one that is kept alive in some tribes today.

There are other ways to honour the placenta. Ceremonies are emerging from women living from the heart, who feel the connection to their babies and their placenta and who feel the strangeness of their placenta being thrown out and incinerated in medical waste. Women from the heart can feel the call to do something more, to create a connection between themselves and the whole. Below are some ceremonies around honouring the placenta.

## Placenta Prints

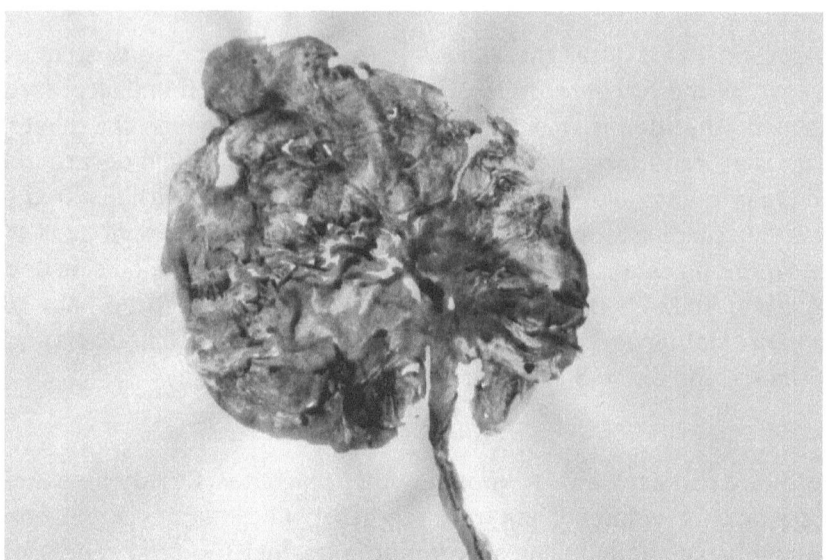

Photos: Steven Booth

After my 6th baby was born, my husband, children and support team gathered together to create artwork with our baby's placenta. It was fun, beautiful and enjoyed by all. By doing this, we have not only captured a magic moment in our lives, but the process itself was a bonding experience for the family.

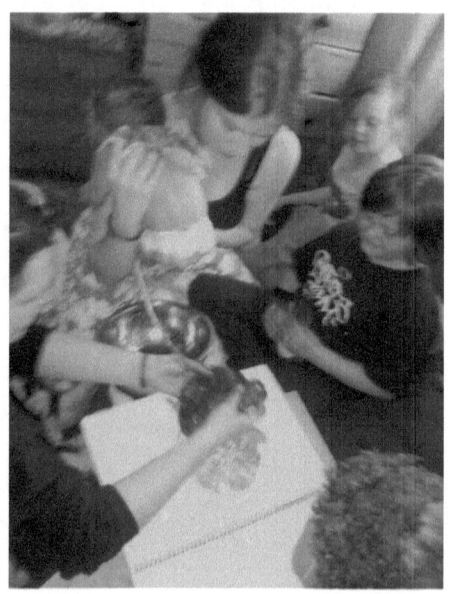

*A guide for making placenta prints*

By Sarah Langford

After my daughter was lotus born we cut her dried umbilical cord from her placenta, wrapped the placenta and remaining part of the cord still attached in plastic wrap and placed it in the back of our freezer to keep. We had planned to defrost the placenta and plant it with a pot plant on her first birthday. During the year we found out about placenta prints and decided we would like to make our own on the anniversary of her lotus birth (the day her cord detached from her belly button).

We made two different styles of placenta prints; the traditional blood print and a paint print on canvas. The following instructions are specifically for those who had a lotus birth and froze their placentas after they naturally detached from their babies. They can also be of use to parents who did not have a lotus birth, disregard steps about defrosting.

~*~*~*~

**Instructions for Making a Blood Placenta Print From a Lotus Born Placenta**

**You will need**
Good quality water-colour paper
Placenta that has not completely dried out and still has some blood on it

**Step 1.** We removed the placenta from our freezer and left to defrost.

**Step 2.** Once defrosted we unwrapped our placenta and found that despite being dry when we first froze it, the defrosting process had made our placenta bloody again and perfect for making prints.

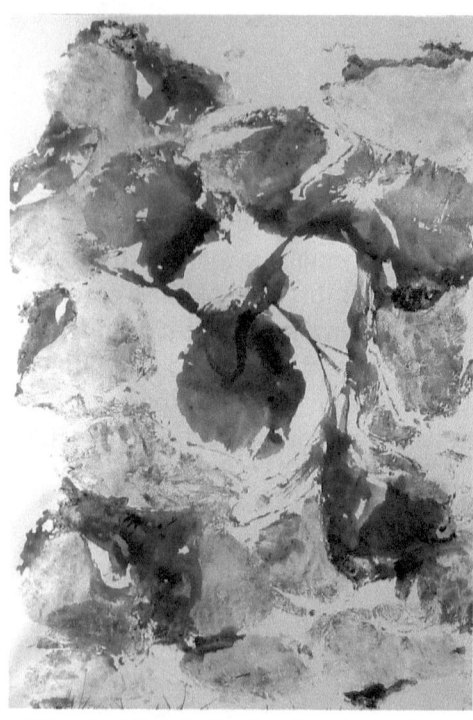

*"Placenta, blood on canvas"*
– Photo: Sarah Langford

**Step 3.** We gently placed the placenta onto our water colour paper and let it sit their briefly, there was no need to press the placenta into the paper. We continued to do this on the page until we felt our image was complete. Alternatively you can lie the placenta flat first and gently press your paper down onto the placenta.

**Step 4.** Once the print is complete you can wrap the placenta up in fresh plastic wrap and return to the freezer until such time as you would like to bury it under your garden or with a pot plant, or you can plant it straight away.

**Step 5.** Wash your hands thoroughly.

**Step 6.** Your blood print will change colour as the blood dries. The bright red will turn to a faded brown. To preserve the print it is a nice idea to have it framed.

~*~*~*~

**Instructions for Making a Paint on Canvas Placenta Print From a Lotus Born Placenta**

This style of printing is ideal for lotus born placentas that are too dry to create blood prints with and for anyone who loves colourful abstract art with a lot of love behind it.

**You will need**
Canvas
Placenta
Paint in whatever colours you would like (we chose to use acrylic paint because it is easy to spread and less expensive than other kinds of paint).

**Step 1**. We removed the placenta from our freezer and left to defrost.

**Step 2.** Once defrosted we unwrapped our placenta. Because you are using paint instead of blood as your main medium it does not matter whether or not the placenta is still bloody.

**Step 3.** Pour your paint onto a flat surface, gently dip one side of your placenta into the paint.

**Step 4.** Gently place the paint covered side of your placenta onto the canvas.

**Step 5.** If you would like to use more than one colour, thoroughly rinse the paint side of your placenta, gently massage the placenta, helping to remove any paint from it. Then repeat steps 3 and 4 with a new colour.

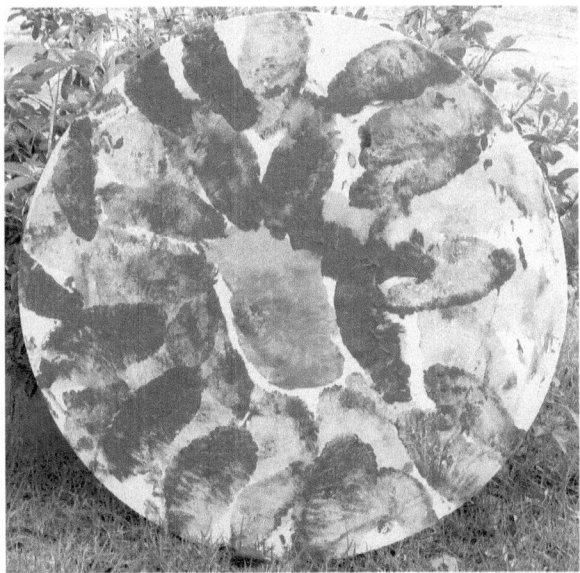

*"Placenta, paint on canvas"* – Photo: Sarah Langford

**Step 6.** Once you have finished using your placenta to make paint prints thoroughly rinse the placenta under running water, always handle the placenta gently. It is important to wash paint off the placenta as soon as you have finished with a particular colour, to ensure that no paint dries to the placenta (in case you wish to bury it later).

**Step 7.** Once the print is complete you can wrap the placenta up in fresh plastic wrap and return to the freezer until such time as you would like to bury it under your garden or with a pot plant, or you can plant it straight away.

**Step 8.** Wash your hands thoroughly.

**Things to Consider**

Work swiftly (but don't rush, always handle the placenta with care) to avoid the blood or paint on the placenta drying before you are finished.

Handling the organ that was once inside you, who kept your child alive for many months, (which in the beginning was made of the same cells as the child you now care for each day) can be quite an emotional experience, especially if you are working with an older placenta just defrosted for an anniversary. Be ready for certain feelings to come up for you while making a placenta print. Make sure that those present for the printing process are sympathetic loved ones who appreciate the significance of the placenta and will honour any feelings you might experience while making a placenta print.

Don't get caught up in making the print look like something in particular. The print will be what it will be. Every placenta is different and so every print is unique. Much like birth, you have little control over what the end product will look like. Rather than focusing on what your art will look like when you're done, stay present to the moment and enjoy gently handling your placenta, reflecting on your child's lotus birth and how far you've come since those early days.

Once defrosted your placenta will smell much the same as it did the day that you froze it. Scent has a powerful way of overwhelming us with memories; be prepared to be taken back to those early days of your child's life.

### Journeying as Mother

***Placenta Burial.***

I know of many families who have buried their placentas in the Earth. It seems to be a beautiful growing trend of women living from the heart, having a sense of duty and honour to connect our babies back in with the earth. Living in such a technological advanced civilisation has many benefits, but it also draws us away from ourselves and our centres. Technology gives us something to rely on, to give us information and tell us what is going on with our bodies. It saves our lives and does many great things. However, if we only rely on this, then we lose our heart. We lose our connection to the great mother, to the cyclical nature of existence and of the greater understanding of how a world works organically. If we are able to sometimes pull back from the technological state of our planet and work intuitively and instinctively, then we will see this connection, feel it and live from it.

*After Layla's birth, we buried her placenta with her brother Jarrah's, which was still in our freezer 5 years later. We buried them together under a newly planted wattle tree, connecting them forever to each other and to the earth.* Jess Krop, mother of 2

~*~

*When I was born my parents and sisters planted my placenta under a honey suckle cutting which had been in a bunch of flowers given to celebrate my birth. My oldest sisters placenta resides in the earth at the house our great grandfather built and the gumtree which was nourished by my middle sisters placenta still grows large and strong at the home my parents built; the home where I was born. On Myles' first birthday, he helped us to plant his placenta beneath a lemon tree. The freezer had turned it golden and it was one of the most beautiful things I had ever seen. It seemed only right that after helping to grow and nourish him, it would help grow and nourish the tree.* Billie Wallace-Yarrow

~*~

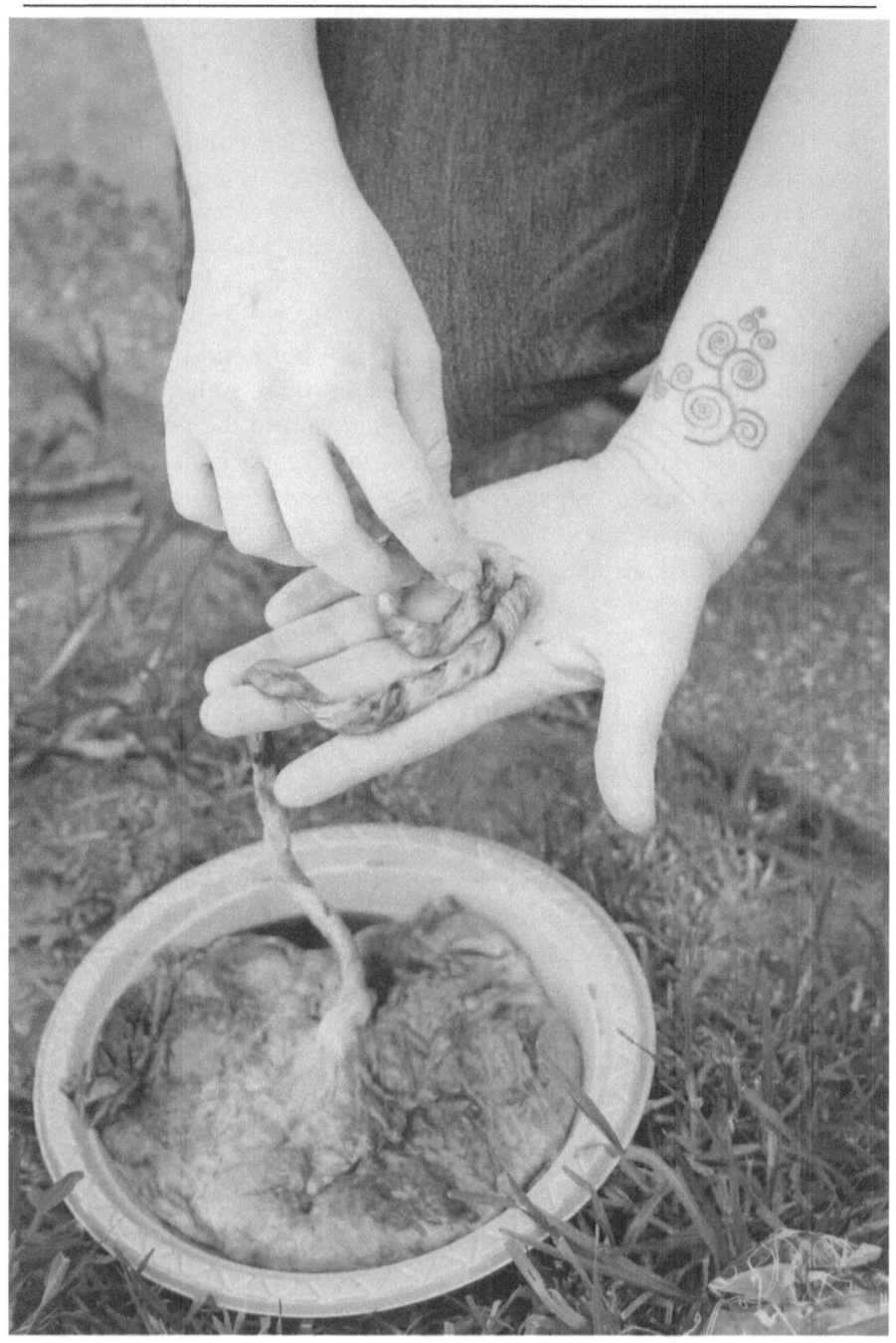

*"Placenta Burial"* - Photo :Billie Button Photography

*We buried Indira's placenta as a family, around her 2nd birthday. We put it underneath a huge ghost gum on Fernleigh trail- a bushwalking trail near our home. We've since moved further west but look forward to visiting for a bushwalk again soon, to show Indira, now 4, her special placenta burial site.* Kerrie Thomas

~*~

*We buried my son's placenta in a pot, as we're renting. I planted a couple of Australian native grasses in that pot and it is the most fertile pot in my collection :)*

*Even after birth, my placenta is nourishing!* Beck Heyfron

~*~

*We buried Miss Milly May's placenta under a beautiful young jacarandah tree in our backyard on National Tree Planting day, eight months after her birth, returning it to Mother Earth. It makes me so sad to think that I didn't have the insight to keep my first two babies placenta's and that they were discarded in hospital waste* Tania Delahoy

~*~

*We buried my son Xylon's placenta in a forest where my husband and I had special memories. A year later we went back to 'visit' and it had been dug up. Presumably by a fox. My son never 'knew' this and as he grew he became increasingly interested and connected to foxes and they are his favorite animal.* Bree Downes

~*~

*We buried Audrey Mae's placenta on her first birthday in a big pot underneath a stunning pink rose bush. When I was pregnant with Audrey, I would tune into her I would see the deep pink rose heart, so the rose is her rose, the name of the rose is called pink delight which also feels right. Audrey helped bury her placenta by placing and playing with the soil. She played near the pot all day long, I like to believe that she was saying goodbye to her time in the womb. When we find the right place we will reconnect the soil and rose to the earth and she will always be able to visit it.* Mara McCleery

~*~

*My daughter was born at home in a rental house, so her frozen placenta moved with us a few times before we bought a home. On her second birthday, it was planted under a mandarin tree with her help and lots of curious onlookers.* Emma Archer

~*~

*After Edith's lotus birth, we buried her placenta underneath a crabapple tree. I think it will be nice to watch the tree grow with her - a fitting reminder of the 'nature' of her peaceful birth at home.)* Tessa Kowaliw

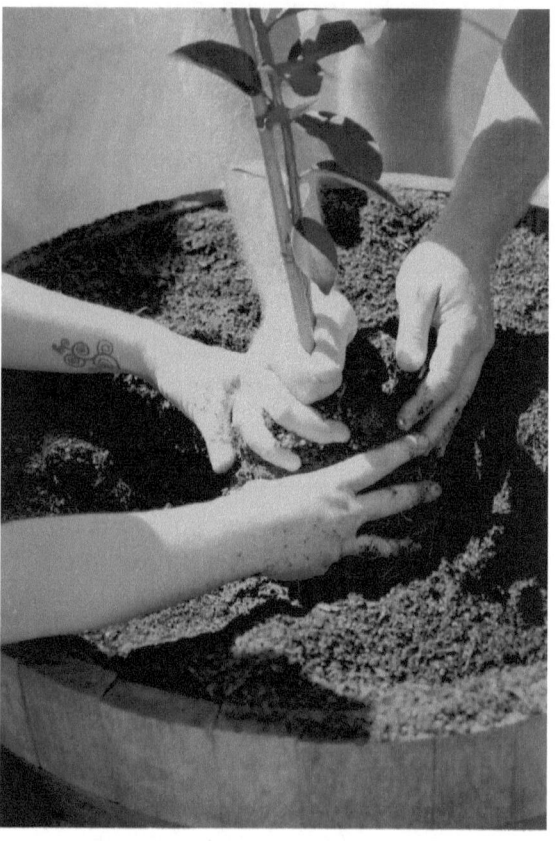

"Planting" – Photo: Billie Button Photograph

~*~

*Tuesday was born at home just before dawn with a true knot in her umbilical cord cord. When her 2 older brothers woke I showed & explained about her rich healthy placenta. Sadly my 10 yr old cat (who had been a wonderful, patient friend to my children even though she came first) died within 2 weeks of Tuesdays birth so we buried Tuesdays placenta over the top of our dearly departed cat in the backyard of our house. Even now when we drive past the old home Tuesday says it was where she was born and where her placenta is... Probably nourishing some strangers vegies.* Beth Stewart-Nichols

**The Placenta Garden**

*(one of my stories, first published in Shivam Rachana's Lotus Birth 2nd edition)*

The following is a story that was written after the birth of my 4th daughter. We decided to have a family ceremony where we buried our daughter's placenta along with the rest of the families substitute placenta's in a ceremony that healed previous trauma and connected us as a family to the Earth.

When my husband Steven and I had decided on a Lotus Birth for our daughter Sage, we talked to the kids about it. I explained what was going to happen – that when Sage was born she was still going to be connected to her placenta by her umbilical cord and that she would let go of it when she was ready to. I showed them pictures of lotus babies, and also explained the function of the placenta and cord. The simple questions from six and four year old lead to a huge 'explosion' in our family, which eventually turned into a huge healing.

Caelan asked what we did with his cord and placenta, and then Rhiannon asked the same. When I told them that their cords were cut straight away when they were born, they looked at me in horror. And when I told them that the hospital staff had taken their placentas away and put them in a fire, Rhiannon was deeply upset.

She looked at me with such a look of horror.

"The placenta is the babies skin, don't you even know that?" she exclaimed.

Before I could respond, she continued: 'that means you let them take my skin away in the hospital and burn it in the fire!'

When she said that I recalled all the problems she had had with her skin since birth. She always has heat rash in the summer months and her skin is 'always itchy'. She wouldn't go to sleep unless you scratched her back. The connection of these things seemed so obvious in the 2 sentences spoken by my four year old daughter.

## The Wild Rainbow

Then Caelan looked at me. "Well, why did you let them do that to me?" He was demanding an answer.

I felt like a child. 'I don't know,' I managed to stumble. 'I didn't know that's not what you do'.

I started to feel nervous and felt as though I had a gaping wound, which of course I did have. My children talking about their placentas', triggered off my own placenta trauma. The wound was my umbilicus, and I could feel the heat on it, and the pus. My own umbilical cord, like millions of others, had been cut at birth and my mother told me that it took weeks to heal. 'It had a lot of pus all the time' she said 'it just wouldn't heal'.

Caelan and Rhiannon were still looking up at me. I felt awful. But then I had an idea.

I remembered that the word placenta means 'flat cake' or in some languages 'mother cake'.

'Let's make a cake,' I suggested. I talked to them about making a cake and allowing that to represent their placentas. We talked about burying it in the ground and asking mother earth to keep us connected to her, to keep us strong, truthful and nourished. Their faces looked so happy! So we decided that once the baby was born, and she had let go of her placenta, that we would have a mass placenta burial ritual and connect us all back into our sacred mother and also reconnect us back to ourselves.

We would all acknowledge our placentas.

It was around a week after Sage let go of her placenta and was lotus born that our family held a ceremony in our garden for our placentas. It was simple, but extraordinarily powerful.

We all each had a cake, and a snake lolly (which represented our umbilical cord). Caelan suggested we all write a note to our placentas so they knew how we were feeling. Everyone in our family ended up naming their placentas as we took them outside. Steven dug a hole and we took turns putting our placentas in the earth.

It was interesting to watch the kids and how they let their placentas go. Rhiannon very gently put hers in the hole and then neatly put the letter next to it. Caelan took a big mouthful from his 'placenta', eating about half of it. He obviously still needed the nourishment and connection that he missed out on after his birth. Then he threw it in the hole and walked off really fast.

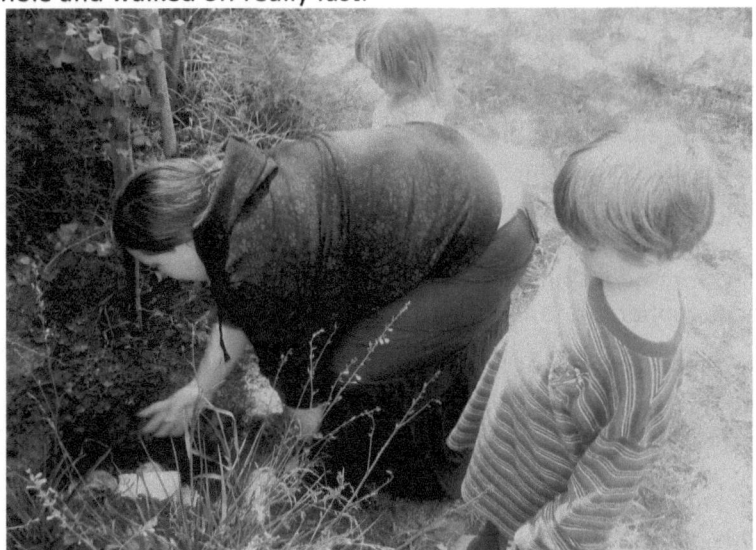

*"Honouring Ruby"* – Photo: Steven Booth

I buried Sage's placenta and felt overwhelmed with gratitude as I looked at it in its placental form one last time. This was a part of my daughter that I knew I would never see again but knew that it played such a crucial role in my daughter's life. In fact, my daughter depended on this. She and Sage had at one point been the same bunch of cells. This placenta had grown, protected and nourished her. I felt and enormous amount of gratitude and love for it, and I had a tear in my eye as I gently placed it with our other 'placentas'.

Once we had all let our 'placentas' go, the kids took turns shoveling sand over the top of the placentas. I felt moved at how such a simple ceremony made such a huge impact on our family.

Our placentas now lie in the earth's soil so that we can continue to be nourished by our ultimate mother – Mother Earth. They lie in the garden next to a ginkgo tree. Hopefully by our placentas being in the earth near the ginkgo tree, we can love and grow from its wisdom, as well as be nourished, since we have finally laid our placenta trauma to rest.

## *Medicinal Placenta*

***Homeopathic Remedy***

By Jane Hardwicke Collings

The placenta can be used in homeopathic medicine as a remedy. Original research into the placental remedy, Placenta humanum, has indicated its benefit in the treatment of conditions where the child's immune system has failed to respond effectively to a challenge or illness. If the remedy is prepared from the child's own placenta, it provides an added individualized boost to overcome the child's own particular inherited tendencies.

Placenta humanum was homeopathically proven in Wales by Biggs and Gwillum in 2000 in order to identify its therapeutic actions and indications for clinical use

When I am with a family and we are starting the process of making the remedy, I always say what was said to me, and that is - when you start this process you unlock the healing powers of placenta. This may be felt in a huge variety of individual ways.

<u>The Recipe for Making a Homoeopathic Placental Remedy</u>

*Select a piece of the placenta*

Quite your mind and feel into which is the right piece to choose, just tear it off rather than using a knife or scissors. Choose a piece about the size of a match head.

*Add 1 part placenta to 9 parts brandy*
say a piece of placenta the size of a walnut to 90 mls of Brandy.
Or say 1 teaspoon placenta plus 9 teaspoons brandy
(You can use Brandy, whisky, vodka, ethanol etc)
Sit for 3 days, or longer (in a brown glass bottle or a covered bottle/jar in a cool, dark place)
Use 1 part of this mixture and add to 99 parts brandy

*Say 2 mls mixture plus 198mls brandy*

*Discard original mixture with the placenta in it.*

*Succuss 100 times*

Put mixture in a well-sealed glass bottle and bash firmly against a phonebook (or the palm of your hand) 100 times, be focused on your task.

*This now creates the 1C MOTHER TINCTURE. 200mls*

Store this in a brown glass bottle in a cool dark place. You can store the remedy as Mother Tincture 1C) and as 5C
To prepare 5C, make 2C from 1C by:
Use 1 part of 1C and add to 99 parts brandy
    *Succuss 100 times = 2C*
Use 1 part of 2C and add to 99 parts brandy
    *Succuss 100 times = 3C*
Use 1 part of 3C and add to 99 parts brandy
    *Succuss 100 times = 4C*
Use 1 part of 4C and add to 99 parts brandy
    *Succuss 100 times = 5C*
Administer 6C
Use 1 part of 5C and add to 99 parts brandy
    *Succuss 100 times = 6C*

10 drops = one dose

## Application:

This will be a constitutional remedy for the baby throughout her/his life. It could be used for many/any constitutional or unusual ailments (except) when specific remedy is appropriate eg arnica for bruising). The placenta contains stem cells so this remedy will be a very good immune remedy.

The placenta contains all one's strengths and weakness so treating the individual with this remedy will provide balance when there is imbalance.

**For more details, see the full article at** http://moonsong.com.au/placental.html

### Placenta Encapsulation

A way of using the placenta as method of healing is through encapsulation, which is making the placenta into a powdered form and then placing it inside of capsules so that it can be taken orally. The process involves cleaning the placenta and removing the membranes and umbilical cord, steaming it, dehydrating it, grinding it into powdered form and then putting it in capsules.

Although this is not a common practice in western culture, there are many benefits as to how encapsulated placenta is extremely beneficial to the mother.

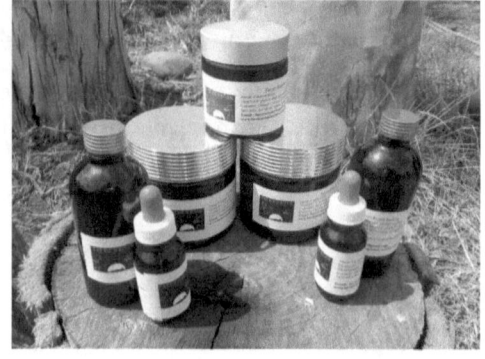

*"Placenta Healing"* – Photo: Kasey Whitehead

The placenta is full of goodness. It has a very high iron content, which will benefit the mother who may have low iron levels post birth. It is good pain relief and full of beneficial hormones which may help recovery of body and mind. Benefits of placenta encapsulation are lessening the risk of postnatal depression, it is a natural pain relief, it replenishes B vitamins, assists with milk supply, replenishes blood loss post birth and assists in stabilising hormone changes.

There are hormones present in the placenta, which, when encapsulated and consumed by the mother are passed to her. Some interesting ones is the presence of Oxytocin, which is known as 'the love hormone' and will help create feelings of love, bonding, attachment, happiness and relieve pain. POEF (Placental Opioid-Enhancing Factor) which helps with natural pain relief, Prolactin, which assists in milk production and Interferons, which stimulates the immune system to fight off infections post birth.

Placenta Encapsulation can be done in almost any circumstances, and this includes with twin placentas, lotus birthed placentas, frozen placentas (up to 6 months in the freezer), meconium stained placentas and placentas with abnormalities (such as placenta previa).

The Encapsulation can be done by the mother but it is a growing trend for Birthworkers to now have training in it, learning about the placenta in depths and how to do the process. I personally find it an honour to be able to create this healing natural medicine for women postbirth.

> "I ingested the placenta of my (6 weeks) terminated Little One. I made a smoothie with exotic fruits and watermelon juice. I did it because I knew it was the single most nourishing and loving thing I could do for my body on every level. It firstly told my body to shut down, stop bleeding, and heal. The endorphin hit was unmatched. Secondly I was honouring the rite of passage of the Little One who came to teach me much and I brought her home. Thirdly I empowered my body, my Self with the ancient Body wisdom of my lineage and my Feminine Being. A sister of my heart, who doula-ed my entire process also took a deep swig! Wickedly palatable brew! She gifted me the truest reflection of what it is to Be With Woman. (I love you eternally Jodi Fagan). My services as a Doula also specialise now in conscious termination support." ~ Nel Da Silva

> "I had Postnatal Depression with my 2$^{nd}$ child and I also had difficulty breastfeeding. I was stressed. When I fell pregnant with my 3rd baby, my doula introduced me to placenta encapsulation. Once I knew about the benefits surrounding milk supply, bonding and depression, I knew I had to do it. I noticed a big change after taking the capsules. It was very noticeable to my milk supply and my emotional health within 3-4 days" – Rebecca

> "Even though I suffered badly from anaemia after giving birth, I hate to think where I would have been without the encapsulation. I have a history of depression and even though I was physically unwell in the first weeks of being a mother, I'm sure that encapsulation our placenta prevented me from suffering from PND. I can't say I was in perfect health but I am glad that I did it. It also felt really good to know that I was still connected to my pregnancy and in a strange way was honouring the value of the placenta itself. i will definitely do it again." - Charity

## Post Birth

### The Early Daze.

The first few weeks of birth pass in a blur of sleep, snuggles, breastmilk and regaining strength. Support in this time both physically and emotionally is vital and will not only nourish you for that particular time, but for the months to come. I am a firm believer of the 'babymoon', a time (for around 4 weeks once baby is born, think in terms of a whole moon cycle) in which the mother and baby are snuggled together, like being cocooned, while they adapt to this new life, establish feeding, regain strength and recover from the birth.

Many countries across Asia have been doing this forever. The mothers are kept warm and nourished, she does no housework. The mothers mother or mother in law comes and stays to do the child rearing and chores. She is given warm food and warm drinks. Herbal compresses are made for the perineum and breasts. Her activity is kept to a minimum. All she needs to do is focus on recovering and allowing her baby to adapt to life outside the womb.

Keeping visitors to a minimum is sanity saving, unless they are actually there to help. Friends and family can be rostered on to come and help with meals, cleaning and playing with the other children. Phones can be switched off. If the mother is nourished, honoured and nurtured post birth, I firmly believe our rates of Post natal depression would be much lower and we would start to see a community of strong, able, nurtured mothers.

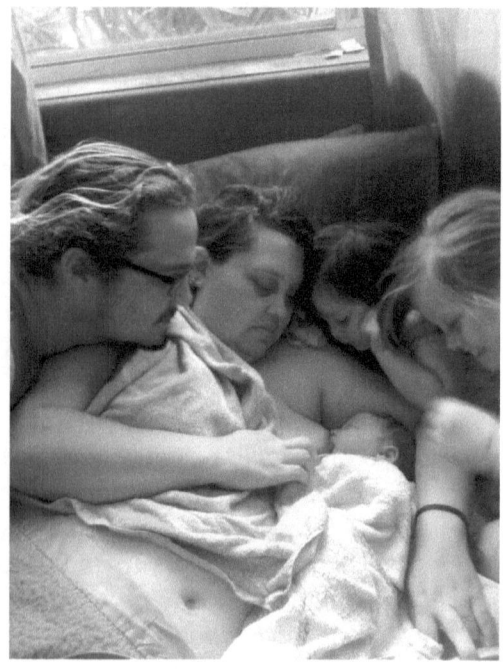

Photo: Lucy Johnston

## *Settling In - the first 2 weeks with my 4th baby*

The first 12 days with my 4th baby was all about settling in. We all needed to learn how to adjust to fit this new baby in to our lives, and to work out how to work harmoniously as a family of 6. Sage was really settled; I expected that she would be as she was snuggled in my hug-a-bub most of the time. I felt ecstatic about my birth experience. It felt incredible to birth with intuition and instinct and to be able to allow my baby to birth 'her way', in her own time, by her own rules and not by the rules of anyone or anything else.

Since her lotus birth, she seemed really alert, awake and present. She interacts with her siblings a lot more.

After Sages birth I was well supported and looked after and thus enabling me to have a rapid recovery. One of my doula's, Grace, organised a meal tree, so in the first 3 weeks, we had people dropping in with delicious food and to see if we needed anything done around the house or if we needed help with the older children.

Friends were so helpful and thoughtful and I know that this is from preparation that I did in pregnancy. I spoke about what worked and didn't work in my previous births and made it clear (which was very difficult, but empowering once it was done!) on what I needed. I had some very struggling times post birth with my first 3 babies, with extreme lack of support and I wanted to make sure that this time we were all nurtured and nourished.

Courtney bought over some craft activities to keep the kids entertained, lent us some of her books and cooked us a big delicious coconut curry! I was given homeopathic remedies and herbal mixtures from both my doulas and I could feel the benefits from both working well and harmoniously in my body. I was given a beautiful postpartum acupressure massage 4 days after birth which made me so relaxed and able to sink deep into bliss. My Mum came down after 5 days and helped with dishes, cleaned the floors and played with the babies when I needed afternoon naps with my baby. Steven kept on top of the washing and he fixed things around the house. Things were flowing harmoniously. It was a beautiful time.

# The Wild Rainbow

The older kids didn't feel left out at all. They got lots of attention given to them. They relished in the arrival of Sage and loved singing her songs and holding her. Nannon would choose clothes for her, Lala forever admires her thumbs (she is a thumb sucker and fascinated by thumbs!) and Caelan always would ask when it was his turn to hold the baby.

Twelve days later, I was still deeply in the birth space. I didn't leave my bedroom except for bathroom breaks for the first week and on the 12th day, I ventured out, we all went for a drive, but it seemed too much. It felt too bright, too open and I felt so vulnerable and intimidated by all the people around, I just wanted to go back home. I was grateful for recognising what was happening, and listened to that instinct of what I needed. It is fine, I didn't need to be anywhere and I had to remind myself it was a different experience to my other children. My first 2 children, I went back to school when they were only 3 weeks old (my first I was in year 12 and my 2nd I just started uni). With all this in mind, I savoured every moment I had with Sage. I knew this time wouldn't last long in the scheme of things, but the importance of this is lifelong. The memories I have of those first 2 weeks are blissful and magic, nurturing and nourishing. I wish every woman the opportunity to have a postpartum experience as this.

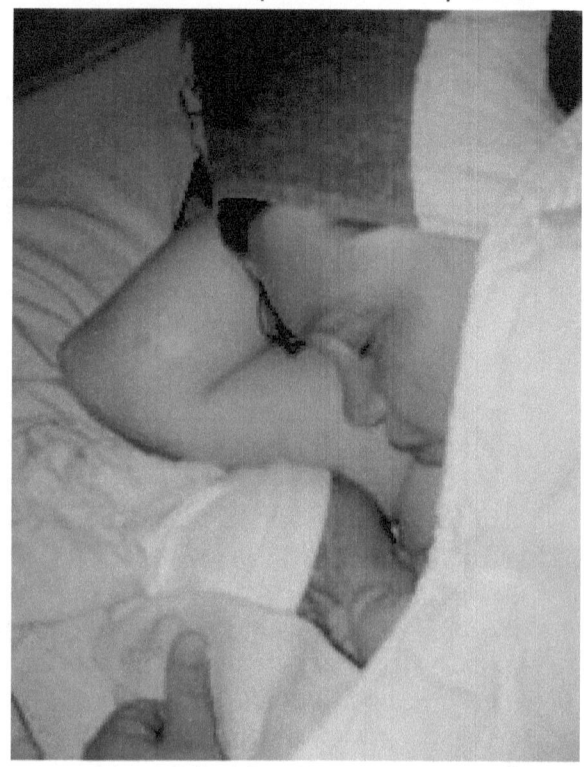

*"Munch"* – Photo: Anna Urbanski

## *The Early Daze with my 5th baby*

Today Myah is a week old. The week has passed in a hazy dazy blur of milk, rest, laughter, tears and amazement. We are adjusting to life as a family of seven and I am in a constant state of remembering to to be slow and patient. It is a time of intense mothering for me – I am breastfeeding 2 babies, my 22month old and my newborn. I have never done this before so it is a new challenge for me.

I struggled on the day Myah was born because I was awake pretty much all night the night before, and so was Sage, so sleep deprivation and an overtired toddler, plus 3 more overexcited children meant that we were all disrupting each other's space. No one could comfort each other and it was really difficult. Grace came over that evening with a box of goodies and a foot massage for me which helped calm me down. We all went to bed early and got an awesome night sleep. The next day I woke up fearful that we would have another overexcited/overtired day but the good nights' sleep we all had seemed to save our sanity. We all worked together and reminded ourselves that we need to be patient and slow. Lauren came over with her daughters and a big pie. We chatted and cuddled and ate fruit salad, drank tea and talked about the birth.

Myah's umbilical cord and placenta were still attached, as we were having a lotus birth. We believe the space that the lotus birth holds keeps us protected and still. We can immerse ourselves in each other and it creates a quiet space for our family. And it helps Myah transition into the world on her own, under her own terms. On Myah's second day earthside, after 60 hours, she let go of her placenta while she was being cradled in her older brother's arms. We buried it the following evening as a family ritual in the backyard under a passionfruit tree.

My milk came in at the end of the second day. I was so abundant in supply that when I fed my toddler, it was such a relief as she really helped with the engorgement! It settled down quite quickly – I felt like a really luscious and milky mother Goddess!

The whole first week has been spent gazing at Myah – she has so many cuddles from us all. When she is awake she is so alert and her

# The Wild Rainbow

little eyes gaze at you with so much intensity you almost feel like she can read right through you. The kids have been having plays at the park. We've had friends come over with food. We've been so well fed with lots of nourishing food. The meal tree is beautiful and a great way to keep us all supported – especially for me so that I don't have to think about what to cook. I can recover from the birth and spend my time getting to know Myah and also know that my family are being nourished.

On Saturday Lex came and took Caes out so he could have some boys' time with Ollie away from all us women, which was greatly appreciated by me, and also awesome for Caelan. Courtney's Mum made us a big tub of stirfry and dropped it around at our house. Steven and I have been resting as much as we can, taking time to have naps so that we can both parent our big tribe without being too tired.

It's so beautiful to see the world I am in and what I have created for myself. I really feel like I am in a community of conscious, aware and beautiful people who love and trust me as treat me as though I am a part of their family. We all look out for each other and each other's children, we help each other, we cry and laugh together, we understand each other. It is making this time of transitioning into a family of 7 much easier to cope with knowing that I have so many women to call on if I need it.

Myah's pregnancy and birth experience has been one that has taken me back to my roots. She is my baby who has reconnected me to my ancestors and to our ultimate mother, mother Earth. She has showed me that our bodies, like the Earth body, provide us with all that we need and if we listen and tend to her, nourish and water her, then she will work in perfection. We are all designed to perfection and we are all Goddesses. Thank You Myah for connecting me back to myself.

# Journeying as Mother

When I asked women what they wish they were told about for the early days (daze) of life with a newborn, this is what they said:

*I wish I knew how sacred and timeless the first days are with your newborn. I wish I knew the importance of skin to skin and of simple just holding your baby and staring at him. If I knew this, I would have restricted visitors and not let others pass him around. For the first few days, I would have kept him to myself and just stared at him, never putting him down from my arms.* - Whisp

*That I could take as long as I wanted to return to the world outside* – Melinda

*I wish I knew to rest more and cherish the time in the baby bliss bubble with just us. I wish I knew that two weeks was not long enough for my partner to be home. I wish I knew how normal it is to be teary when my milk came in. I couldn't stop crying and I felt bad about it.* - Hailey

*That babies peel. I was so freaked out when her hands and feet started peeling.* - Natasha

*I wish I listened when I was told all about the Birth Centre and how it would be perfect for me! Ha! No way, I needed my Ob and private room!*
*I do wish I was comforted more and had some real advice, encouragement and true support with breastfeeding. I caught thrush in hospital, but it was not diagnosed. 6 weeks of pure agony until it cleared itself, as thrush most often has a 6 week cycle.*
*Having someone diagnose and help me clear it would have helped so much.*

*I truly am so proud of myself and my stubbornness when I think back to getting through each feed for so long in such pain.*
*I loathe being told how lucky I was/am to feed. No!! It was bloody hard work, determination and guts to get it working.* - Clare Peterson-Morrissey

*I wish I was told how important it was to stay nourished. I felt so run down and kept getting colds. My immune system turned to shit once I had a baby. I felt like I just couldn't get enough nutrients in and I was so thirsty. It wasn't until ages later that I found out that breastfeeding requires more calories than pregnancy! No wonder I was always so hungry and thirsty. I thought there was something wrong with me* – Angelina

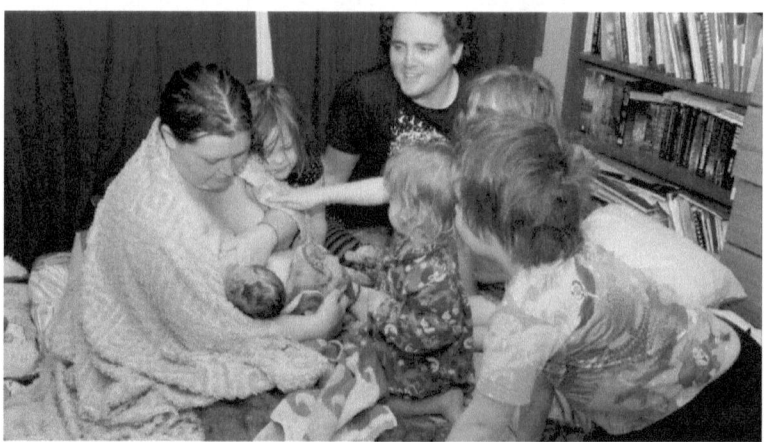

"Family" – Photo: Brooke Patel Photography

*I wish I was told I could stay in bed, that I didn't have to get out of my pj's and that one day I can return to the world. I returned to the world too quickly. I thought we were supposed to. I wish I knew I could take my time and go at a pace that worked for me and my baby* - Missy

## *Being Nourished*

It is essential to be nourished. To be nourished is to be 'filled up'. It is necessary for your growth and health in so many ways

Women are often nourishing others, and need to practice more self-nourishment. The nourishment starts on the inside. When we tell ourselves and others the truth and identify what we really want and need, we are nourishing ourselves.

How do you feel nourished?

By lazing in the sunshine with a good book?

By lying on the couch and watching a comedy that makes you laugh out loud?

Can you always have your favourite tea and chocolate on the shelf?

What about a warm bath filled with bubbles, salts and oils?

Do you feel nourished when you go for walks, have little (or big!) naps?

What about art? Does drawing/painting/sculpting nourish you?

Do you have a great circle of sisters that you can laugh and cry with? That you can tell them anything without knowing they won't judge you?

What about when someone cooks you breakfast?

Think of what makes you feel nourished. You will know when you feel warm and fuzzy inside when you think about these things.

Then go and do them.

## *Breastfeeding*

My breasts have nourished 10 children, 6 of those were my own, 2 were of babies whose mothers were close friends to me and 2 were donated breastmilk to sick babies whom I did not know initially know.

Breastfeeding my babies and them having access to breast milk are of extreme importance to me. Breastfeeding for me has been a whole journey of discovery of myself and my relationships to others. It has been both simple and challenging, blissful and painful, tiring and exhilarating. Feeding my first baby was difficult as I struggled with my body changes and breastfeeding as a first time mother. I didn't know what was normal, how breastfeeding worked, I just trusted that it did, and that I needed to persevere with it and seek support when needed.

At different times through my journey with breastfeeding, I've had blocked ducts, mastitis, cracked nipples and grazed nipples. I've had a baby with tongue tie, which made breastfeeding difficult and very painful and a baby that took the first 4 weeks to be able to latch properly which took incredible patience and love.

I've tandem fed for a whole year, which was a very intense (and hungry!) time of parenting was for me. I struggled as my hungry newborn seemed to constantly feeding, and my high needs toddler always coming over to my boob for a quick snack before she went off to play again.

But I've also had a breastfeeding journey of love and bliss. I have many fond memories (and still a reality for me at the time of writing this book) of sitting on the couch for hours at a time staring at my babies faces. I have had a journey of sitting in a sweet daze, where I could really feel the hormones of breastfeeding course through my body, feeling the mamatoto connection of my milk nourishing my baby and my baby's sweet content face nourishing me. Breastfeeding has bought me connection on deep levels with my babies and the other babies who are not biologically my own who have had my breastmilk.

I understand as a midwife and a mother, but most importantly, as a woman, the struggles, the breakthroughs, the highs and the lows when it comes to breastfeeding and the most crucial time for breastfeeding support is the first days after birth. To have support and assistance while you and your baby navigate this new journey of breastfeeding together makes an unbelievable amount of difference to whether or not you continue on with breastfeeding or not.

Optimal conditions and environments for the first feeds:

Skin to skin - skin to skin has incredible benefits for both mother and baby, this is nature's design. Bonding and attachment are enhanced; baby's temperature, heart rate and breathing are more stable and normal. Skin to skin contact immediately after birth allows the baby to be colonised by the same bacteria as the mother.

Once your baby is born, pay attention to the cues she makes, to show you that she is ready for a feed. Trust your intuition, be slow, be patient. You are both learning this together. Keep your baby skin to skin with you. One of them is the promotion of breastfeeding and enabling your baby's instinct to be used so she can crawl up your belly and self-latch.

For the first feeds having certain set ups will enhance the process of breastfeeding. A supportive environment, being as relaxed as possible and feeling private, peaceful and undisturbed are all a part of the recipe for a successful breastfeed.

Bathing and weighing the baby can wait, it is not important. In fact, bathing doesn't even need to be done until mother and baby are both ready. Babies are not born 'dirty'.

Learn to recognise feeding cues. Babies are in an alert state after birth (unless their mother had narcotics/other drugs during the labour) and they have hand/mouth activity, followed by rooting on the skin, then spontaneous crawling up the belly to the breast for self-attachment. If the mother had a natural birth and her contact with her baby is unlimited and unrestricted, then it's completely possible and preferable for the baby to crawl up the mother and attach to her breast.

In the first few days, you have colostrum, which is thicker, fattier milk, and more concentrated, which the perfect design for newborn babies, who have very tiny stomachs. Colostrum, amongst many things, contains antibodies that protects baby against infections of the throat, lungs and intestines. It also contains many antibodies and growth factors. The growth factors promote development of baby's digestive system and the antibodies promote the immune system.

Before your milk comes in, your baby may feed up to 12-14 times within 24 hours. Although this is tiring, it is normal and not something to worry about.

Keep your baby with you.

Seek support.

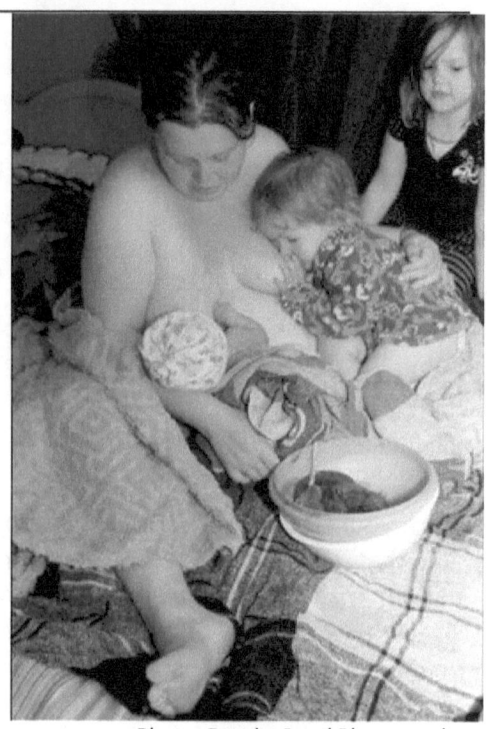

Photo: Brooke Patel Photography

The most common question that I have been asked as an experienced mother and as a midwife is 'how do I know my baby is getting enough milk?'.

- ➢ baby is generally settled between feeds
- ➢ wet nappies. Six or more cloth nappies or 5 disposable nappies in a 24 hour period. Sometimes in the first few days, 'urates' may be present. This is uric acid crystals from the kidney, it's not blood. It just means that your baby hasn't had a huge amount of milk and that it will disappear once baby has a higher intake of breastmilk.
- ➢ 2 or more bowel motions a day. During the first few days, your baby has meconium, which is black, sticky, tar like poo. As the colostrum changes to milk, the poo changes to a mustardy yellow colour. This is normal. After that time, passed the 4 week mark, breastfed babies may have less than this and may not poo for a week or more, but when they do, it is soft

# Journeying as Mother

- Gains weight. This may not be consistent and is definitely not the only indicator of a healthy baby. Her weight gain may slow down and plateau and then pick up again when she has a growth spurt. Breastfed babies generally gain weight more slowly than babies who are bottle-fed.
- She has awake times where she is reasonably alert, active and happy.

Use your intuition. If you feel something is not right, or you are feeling confused, talk to someone. Maternal and Child Health Nurses, Midwives, Lactation Consultants and The Australian Breastfeeding Association are all useful to know of.

When I asked women what they wish they knew about breastfeeding, this is what they said:

> *I wish I was told it wouldn't just be easy and you don't have milk straight away. I wasn't told how hungry and sleepy it makes you either but how wonderful it feels to feed your baby* – Donna

~*~

> *I wish I had of knew where to find more support and how to look after myself so I could produce lots of milk.* - Bonita

~*~

> *I wish I was told that I needed extra calories and that I would be endlessly hungry and thirsty and that is normal!* - Wisp

~*~

> *I wish I'd known that breastfeeding was different to the way the nurses at the hospital had said. I was yanked, stuffed, squeezed and jerked whilst being taught how to feed by professionals. I don't think it's meant to be like that. My second wasn't. But he was born at home and I re-learnt with him in such a gentle way. No stuffing or jerking.* - Beck

~*~

> *I wish I had joined the ABA sooner & got help from them sooner - in fact, going to one of their presentations about*

*breastfeeding while pregnant would have been excellent!*
*- Lisa*

~*~

*That it can be really hard and not always the magic experience some people have or that you hear about.* - Seri

~*~

*Those early days are so time consuming per feed* – Sonia

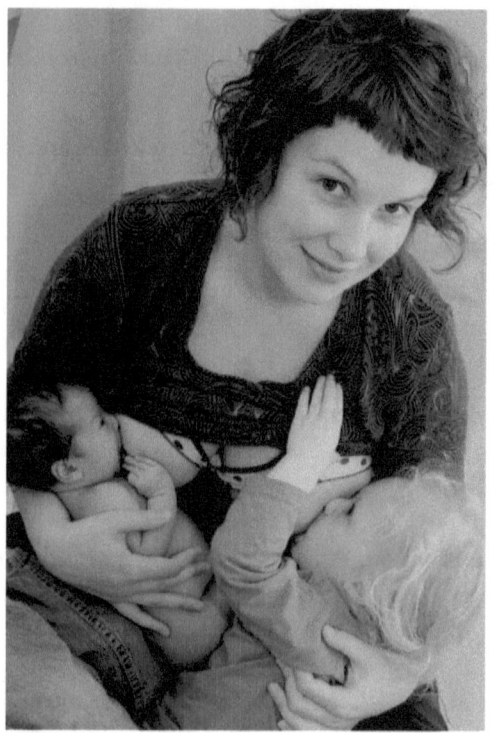

Photo: Brooke Patel Photography

Another crucial time is support for women who are breastfeeding their babies passed 1 year of age. In our western culture, only a very small percentage of women breastfeed passed their child's 1st birthday, which I find alarming as the health benefits alone of breastfeeding are so great that I feel mothers need support and encouragement in their efforts to breastfeed their child without shame, discrimination or alienation.

## *Breastfeeding, not special, just normal*

By Janet Fraser

I support a lot of women to find their way through personal and political gunk and reach a point where they can birth their babies in nice simple births. As the end of pregnancy draws near I encourage women to start thinking about how they're going to manage the early stages of the new breastfeeding relationship that's coming soon.

For some of us it's relatively simple because we've done it before, no particular drama, just boob till the kid starts high school or driving, whichever comes first.* Sadly for many women breastfeeding is complex, painful and difficult and this is largely due to the appalling lack of support, direct undermining of normal infant feeding and our obstetric birth culture which bears a huge responsibility for the lack of breastfeeding in Australia.

Recovering from previous breastfeeding experiences gone awry is vital to providing ourselves and our babies with the relationship we deserve. Many women also need to unpack their family's mythology around birth and breastfeeding in order to locate obstacles we all unknowingly carry within ourselves. First time breastfeeder's, or those with many children, can often benefit from working on this stuff.

Breastfeeding is far more than a delivery system for nutrition and antibodies. It is the way that babies relate to the world, and the security children carry with them. Every time my four year old breastfeeds to sleep she is doing what she has done since her first day earthside and that emotional connection cannot be sufficiently emphasised.

Breasts are the easiest parenting tool you will ever own so use liberally and wisely. They aid sleep because babies are meant to breastfeed to sleep. They bring calm to distressed, hurt or ill children. They bring relaxation to women who are infused with oxytocin for years on end. They provide free, instantly, constantly, ongoing medicinal, nutritional, emotional support to babies and children. You can't actually buy anything that even comes to close to that in any way.

While our society would have us believe that the number of women who can breastfeed is very small, the logical reality is that the vast majority of women and babies are perfectly suited to establishing and maintaining a breastfeeding relationship over a number of years. Humans have managed to feed their young for some thousands of years now and just as evolution has created some pretty clever bodily functions we unthinkingly accept like breathing and elimination, so too lactation is just another normal capability of women's bodies; nothing special just what is needed to feed human babies.

The following pages list some simple things I've observed as helpful to creating, sustaining and maintaining fullterm breastfeeding are easy to come by, and can make the world of difference to a motherbaby dyad in an anti-breastfeeding world:

***1. When you're pregnant, find yourself a breastfeeding support group.***

It is vital to make friends with women who breastfeed fullterm, who view breastfeeding as normal, can offer you support after your baby is born and won't be strangers since you already know them. Most of us never see breastfeeding, our families have lost our breastfeeding culture along with our birthing culture and we seriously believe that we come from mothers who were defective and unable to breastfeed us. This does not set up an environment where normal infant feeding can be nurtured and maintained. Seeing breastfeeding helps us learn how to breastfeed.

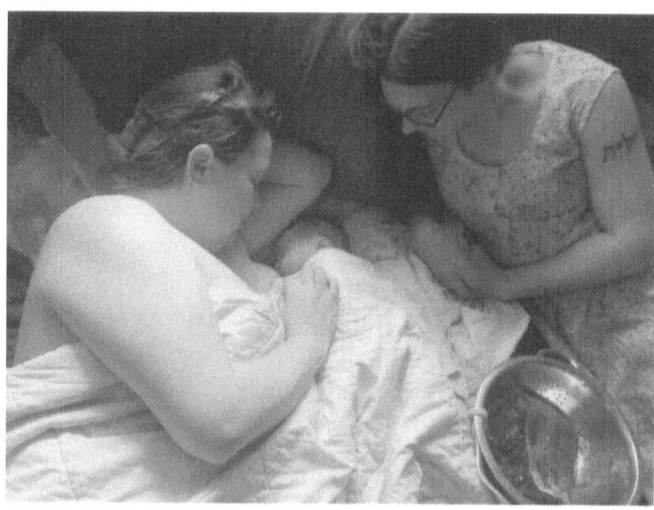

*"Center of attention"* – Photo: Steven Booth

Once upon a Nestle-free time, we would have grown up seeing breastfeeding, we might even have remembered breastfeeding as children ourselves. Most of us don't have that kind of memory but we can help ourselves along by seeing lots of women with differently shaped breasts breastfeeding babies and children whose styles of breastfeeding might vary immensely. If the breasts you see around you were unable to breastfeed, evolution would have bred them out of us millennia ago. Just like every woman here is a tribute to the birthing body her ancestors perfected so too are her breasts. Your breasts come from a long line of grandmothers who breastfed when that was what was normal and substitutes had not yet been invented. Large or small breasts, inverted nipples, flat nipples, large nipples, every breast can breastfeed. In rare cases insufficient breast tissue develops during puberty but even this is not a barrier to breastfeeding, it simply requires more planning, community and commitment.

Partners are also vital to breastfeeding and regular exposure to breastfeeding, unpacking belief systems around breasts, sexuality and parenting are going to be beneficial to the quality of support partners need to provide. We are all products of the anti-breastfeeding world, we have all imbibed myths and outright lies from marketing. Establishing breastfeeding needs both parents to be committed to it and the non-lactating partner needs to increase their level of responsibility around parenting other children and household maintenance when babies are born. Normal physiological birth makes this easier too since caring for women and babies after caesarean surgery is far more demanding than post birth support when a woman has had a beautiful and simple birth.

*2. Give birth at home.*

Hospitals aren't only the absolute opposite of everything needed for a normal physiological birth, they are also the exact opposite of what babies and women need to establish breastfeeding. Just as breastfeeding is the normal way to feed infants, normal physiological birth is the normal way for an infant (or two or more) to leave the mother's womb. Anything else puts up potential barriers to breastfeeding. The simple fact of shift change directly undermines breastfeeding as more and more staff come by with advice and suggestions few of which will be helpful to you coming from their obstetric paradigm.

Babies in hospitals are often induced and are thus premature which means they can struggle to breastfeed. To induce a baby means she is born a drugged baby from the syntocinon, pethidine and/or the epidural involved. The drugs all come with saline drips and major effects on women's bodies which lead to huge amounts of fluid being retained and breasts which are swollen and difficult for babies to latch onto. So not only is the baby drugged, but the breast is a beachball the kid can't latch onto.

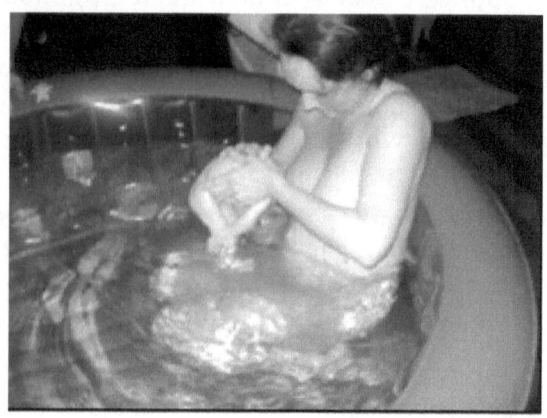

*"Talulah"* - Photo: Renee Adair

It is normal for mothers and babies to be separated after caesarean surgery (and many obstetric births which included vaginal involvement) and again this is a severe potential disruption to breastfeeding commencing. A baby who has then been drugged, taken from the womb prematurely and then separated from her mother at birth is most likely going to struggle to breastfeed. This is unsurprising and it's why birthing at home where your baby will be born to her own timetable, without drugs, trauma or separation is pretty obviously the way to really support the commencement of a breastfeeding relationship.

We can talk all that stuff about skin on skin after caesarean surgery, which is a popular discussion topic lately but in reality if you're having skin to skin after your surgery are you sure your surgery was warranted? Remember a minimum of one in three babies will experience caesarean surgery. Add to this that homebirthing families are generally families who support breastfeeding and could well be the best possible group to find for my number one tip, and you've got every base covered for creating the most likely environment for breastfeeding to kick off drama-free.

In the unlikely event of a woman or baby needing intervention you can mitigate the effects with these basic points anyway. Support for pumping, maintaining a supply and daily life will be forthcoming from that group you find to support you while pregnant.

Breastfeeding, like birth, is an odds game and there are no guarantees of anything. We do however know what works to directly oppose breastfeeding so removing that gives the motherbaby dyad the best possible chance!

**3. Debrief, unpack and understand your previous breastfeeding experiences as well as your family's beliefs around breastfeeding.**

Most babies in Australia are weaned very young and it's not because women don't want to breastfeed, it's because everything in our system is set up to thwart even determined women in their desire to simply feed their baby the normal way for humans to feed.

Most women whose breastfeeding relationships are ended prematurely have grief, anger and distress around it which is unsurprising. This is usually packaged up and given back to us as the "guilt myth" which is really about our society's discomfort with women's anger but also because it makes the "failure" to breastfeed solely about the woman, not the system which failed her and her baby.

Understanding how breastfeeding really works, the factors which influence our capacity to breastfeed, looking at our family history and culture around breastfeeding, honouring the grief we feel, working out what responsibility is ours and what responsibility should be held by the obstetric surgeon, MCHN, GP, hospital staff, local pharmacist or any other passing underminer, will all help work out what went wrong and thus what can be avoided in future. Very few medical people have any idea about breastfeeding and are best avoided. MCHNs are particularly attuned to promoting artificial baby milk and all the practices which undermine breastfeeding so don't go to any.

Examine your feelings about breasts, breastfeeding, the idea that your breasts will be more than decorative and sexual. This can be very challenging for some women and survivors of sexual assault or abuse can find they have complex feelings around intimacy and breasts and children. Support is always available but as above, best accessed before the baby is born. There will always be left field things like tongue tie, vasospasm, hypoplastic breasts or other stuff which is no one's fault and which we can only manage when presented with them.

Knowing what to avoid and what to embrace is key. Again that group you need to find while pregnant will be vital to this.

### 4. Accept no samples, do not purchase artificial baby milk, dummies, sterilisers.

If anyone gives you anything like this thinking they're being helpful, stow them safely in the garbage bin where they don't do too much harm. Worry about landfill another time. Anything readily available that denormalises breastfeeding as the way to feed a baby is undermining you from the get go. Don't do it to yourself. If you do struggle at some point with breastfeeding, people around you commonly try to alleviate their distress by offering you the chance to stop breastfeeding. This does not work in the long term.

The beautifully generous supply of milk when lactation begins can be easily managed with a hand pump or by learning to hand express. These can be borrowed from the women you know who are your breastfeeding support network and you only need to use them for the first week in most cases just to reduce the engorgement and let the babe latch on comfortably. The baby will regulate the supply she requires so long as you feed the babe when she needs feeding.

Establishing breastfeeding can take days, weeks or even months and it simply isn't helpful to have that kind of substandard caper in your home. A relationship of such importance to health and wellbeing for women and babies which can last up to seven years is worth spending some time developing even if it takes a few months to really get the hang of it. The effect of not breastfeeding is with us for life in all sorts of ways so committing to it means you never have to live with a lifetime of regret.

**5. Cosleep, babywear, feed the babe when she needs feeding, basically just parent the kid.**

Some modern experiments around baby care have failed parents and children dismally. They have however made very wealthy those who produce cots, baskets, artificial baby milk, dummies, nightlights, soothing music tapes, prams, rocking chairs, watches, clocks, video monitors, heart monitors, breathing monitors, stupid creepy hand things, psychotherapy, and so on and so forth. One of the fastest ways to make breastfeeding difficult is to put yourself in a different room from the baby to sleep. You wake up to a cry, stumble in, grab the kid, nod off in the expensive rocking chair then stand up and try to pat an unwilling baby back to sleep who cries as soon as you put them down because they're smarter than us and trying to tell us that we need them in our bed. Put the baby in the bed is the only parenting advice my mother ever gave me. It works! The baby snuffles, or latches themselves on, you feed, you both doze, you go back to sleep. You can learn to breastfeed lying down without too much trouble particularly if you ask those breastfeeding women in point one for some help. I've laid on many a floor to show many a woman how it's done.

It always irritates me that I have to spell this out since "feed the baby when she needs feeding" seems only logical. Basic baby care means human babies actually need to have nutrition readily available 24 hours a day from birth in the same manner they did in the womb. They don't leave the comfort of constant nutrition via the placenta and come into the world programmed to three meals and two snacks a day. They come out with little bodies which need the exact same nourishment and luckily, breasts provide it. So let the baby feed when she needs to feed, don't make a baby go hungry with the current fad for timing feeds. Do you know anyone who eats four hourly for 15 minutes per course? No, neither do I, least of all someone who weighs 4 kilos and has only just learnt to breathe and suckle. You can only feed a baby 24 hours a day if you sleep together, anything else is going to send you into a dribbling heap and ruin your breastfeeding relationship.

Wear your baby when she's not in bed with you. Nothing is more portable than a breastfed sling baby! Baby on the inside, becomes baby on the outside, no difference except the funky fabric wrap contains them instead of your womb. You become in tune with one another, you can breastfeed in most slings and that community you located while pregnancy will have a heap of women experienced in babywearing while breastfeeding, all eager to assist you.

You can't breastfeed a baby in a pram without unearthly flexibility and remarkably large breasts so it's more practical to bring the babe to the breast in a simple carrier of some kind. Cheaper and more convenient than a huge pram anyway. Babies facing away from parents in prams are going to feel abandoned so simply keeping them close in a carrier solves that kind of problem before it becomes a problem.

Expensive breastfeeding clothing has swept the market in recent years but honestly a shelf singlet is cheap, effective, keeps your tummy warm in winter, comes in many colours, and is just as effective. No need to spend money on that stuff, just make sure your tops have stretch in them so your breasts fit out the top of them easily. If you're going to be tandem feeding, make sure they're very stretchy so you can get both breasts out when needed.

This is by no means an exhaustive list of what enables breastfeeding nor have I tried to tackle some of the common problems which plague artificial baby milk-normalised cultures like our own. Back to basics understanding of breastfeeding however is that it really is at heart a remarkably simple system of providing so much to babies and women via so simple a method as suckling. Setting ourselves up to breastfeed rather than "see how it goes" "hoping" or feeling fearful can make the difference in both how we manage breastfeeding but also importantly, our ability to seek help should we need it.

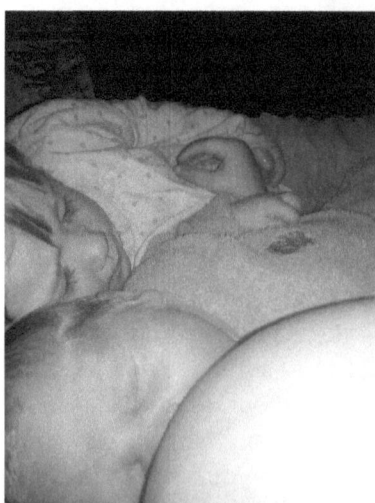

*"Booby Babes:* - Photo: Sheree Stewart

Remember you will be co-sleeping till at least university so this is no problem.

# Journeying as Mother

## *Traversing the Underworld.*

My spiral into darkness with postnatal depression

I never understood how women could get postnatal depression. I understood the baby blues, I understood how the changes that come are difficult, but I just couldn't grasp how you could spiral into depression after having a baby. With my first 3 babies, I had no support, except that of my husband. We had times of struggle and hardship, but I certainly didn't feel depressed.

When pregnant with my 4th baby, I employed the help of 2 sweet women to be my doula's and they supported my emotional needs all through pregnancy and the first month after my baby was born. They also helped to organise a meal tree, which is when a roster is organised and people are assigned to come and drop off a meal to your family, so the mother doesn't have to use her energy to cook for the first month, and so that she can regain her strength and concentrate on the life with the new child. I feel that this type of support set me up for the whole year. I felt confident, strong, in tune with my baby, I loved myself more and found raising 4 children beautiful and fun.

When I was pregnant with my very much wanted 5th child, my pregnancy was beautiful. People were so supportive, I felt like I had found a community. Women would gather around me, offer me support, ask what I needed and everything felt great. The birth of my 5th baby was incredible. It was a loving, instinctual, easy unassisted birth at home in the water. There was barely any labour pain!

I felt so blissed out and happy. However, my blissful state changed. And it changed fast. Little things were happening in my life, but to me they felt so huge. I remember the day after my baby was born, an acquaintance came over to visit. Her son came bursting in the door and loudly demanded to see my baby and sat next to me poking her. I asked him to move away and her mother also asked him to as well. As his mother sat beside me, she was explaining to her son about my baby's placenta, which was still attached and wrapped in a cloth, and preceded to unwrap the cloth. I covered my hand over it and told her that we aren't playing with the placenta. I felt that my space had been invaded and that she wasn't respectful of the journey of my baby and I. She apologised, but it was just the very beginning of things in my world starting to unnerve me. Day by day, life with 5 children felt to be a huge struggle. It was busy. It was more than busy. It was constant. If my husband wasn't around to assist me, I would fall into a heap, crying at everything and anything. I started yelling all the time. I felt like no one was listening, so all I did was yell. My baby hated the car, and 20 minute car trips turned into a time of torture that I couldn't bear. The baby just screamed, which made the toddler scream, which made the older 3 annoyed at the noise and then they would start bickering. My eldest 3 were often sent to their older brother's room where he had a TV, and were ordered to watch shows, just so I could cope with a crying baby and a very needy toddler. My husband also decided it was his calling to start uni, and begin a 4 year full time degree. I begged and cried for him to not go, I didn't feel I could do this on my own. I couldn't parent all these children. He said that he couldn't defer. He had to go. It was a calling. It was true that when I got into my midwifery course in 2004, he also got offered a place in uni. My course wouldn't allow me to defer and I didn't want to risk the chance of missing out, so I went to uni and Steven let his dream pass him by for now, and he was primary carer while I studied my bachelor. So, I saw where he was coming from, and felt it was wrong for me to refuse him his dream.

~*~*~*~

Some days were ok. Some days the kids played happily. Some days we had fun in the park, picnics in the sun, laughs with friends. I tried to keep my community going in this time. I figured that I didn't have to do it alone, so tried to create a community of mumma's and their young kids where we could talk and share. It seemed to be that people always cancelled on me at the last minute, or some would come, would bring her children that would absolutely trash my house, without picking up afterwards and then stay uninvited for dinner.

## Journeying as Mother

If Steven wasn't home, dinner would be baked beans on toast or toasted cheese sandwiches. I just couldn't cope. Days went by in a blur and they got worse and worse and worse.

~*~*~*~

At one point, I went with the kids to stay with my Mum for a week. I told her the extent of what was happening in my life. She said to me "well, you had all these kids. It's up to you to deal with". I felt so alone. And so unsupported.

Upon driving home that day from mums, which is a 4 hour drive, I almost killed my whole family. We were 70kms into the trip and my then 5 year old kept kicking my then 7 year old in the head with her big boots. She just wouldn't stop doing. The screaming from the girls woke up the baby, who is generally terrible in the car but managed to fall asleep, and she was scared of her sisters crying which made her scream. I felt so out of control that I stopped the car and just screamed. I then went and grabbed my 5 year old and put her in the front seat, and made my then 8 year old sit in the back seat. I fed the baby for a moment to calm her down, then put her back in her seat. Things seemed ok for about 20 minutes, when my 8 year old boy started fighting with the 7 year old in the back. This of course, scared the baby, who started crying again. I drove for about 10 more minutes, as I knew there was a town close by. We stopped there at a park. I told the kids to run around in the fresh air. I fed the baby again and got her to calm down. I rang my husband and he spoke to me calmly which made me settle down. We all hopped back in the car and all seemed calm. We put music music on, sang some songs and we were all ok. Until the fighting and the crying started again. It happened 3 more times on that car trip. All of a sudden, I could feel my mind going numb. Everything was starting to go black and I felt like something else had taken over me. I just couldn't do it anymore. I don't know what happened, but I rang Steven. I didn't say anything, but he must have known how bad I was, and he just started talking to me. Talking to me about the pies he is making for us, talking about how he had cleaned the house, talking about how much he loved me. I stayed on the phone until I could see the city in the distance. Then I knew I would be ok. I went home and went to sleep, wishing I would never wake up.

## The Wild Rainbow

~*~*~*~

I went to the doctors, and he told me that I am fine. I'm just tired, who wouldn't be with all those kids? I got told to rest. Meanwhile, the blankness in my mind came more and more and I started getting physical symptoms. My blood pressure, normally 110 / 70 was sitting at 160 / 100, I was getting numbness in my arms, having trouble speaking. All my blood tests came back normal. I was "healthy". Steven and I spoke of different options. Maybe I could go and do house sitting somewhere for a month. Just me and the baby, getting some fresh air in the country, with nothing to care for but ourselves. Building up my body, mind and soul. It seemed nice, and my heart smiled when I thought of it. And then Steven suggested I go to Cambodia. I have a friend there who has a volunteer organisation and she does work with birth centres, schools and orphanages. Something ticked over in my mind and it made me smile. It was the first time I smiled in months.

~*~*~*~

It seems drastic, I know. But it was a drastic solution to a drastic problem. Actually, to me, it seemed like the least drastic solution to me of anything else I could think of at the time.

~*~*~*~

When I told my Mum, she nodded her head and said 'go if you think it will help'. My husband's family hated it. His father didn't say anything except 'you chose an odd time to go, you should wait until the babies are older' and his Mother wrote long letters publicly to me on face book telling me how she knows I am going through a difficult time, but how dare I leave Steven and 4 young children when they need me. And what am I thinking taking a baby to an unsafe country like that. We stopped talking to each other for a while. I guess she didn't know the full extent of what was happening, and maybe if she knew the other option for me was suicide, then she wouldn't have said so much.

I don't know. All is forgiven any way and I followed my heart, and when I did it changed my life.

Life in Cambodia was amazing. It gave me strength, insight, perspective and hope. My physical symptoms vanished almost as soon as I landed in Phnom Penh. Sitting with Denise was like sitting with the Goddess. She had so much wisdom; we had many chats about many different things. I laughed so hard that sometimes I thought I was going to burst. And most of all, I missed my kids. After 3 weeks in Cambodia, I was itching to get home. I couldn't wait to see those faces, to cuddle those soft bodies and to laugh with them again.

My story isn't one for you to read and judge me. It also isn't a story for you to read and feel sorry for me. Severe post natal depression isn't an uncommon story. I believe we just don't talk about it because it is a deep wound, an unspeakable wound, one that we can't talk about because they are stories about the wounded mother and her wounded children. Society doesn't like looking at stories like that, and if they do, instead of supporting and giving compassion, we judge and isolate, which only breaks the wounded mother more.

~*~*~*~

It is for this reason that I hesitated for ages whether or not to include such a deep, heart wrenching personal story and felt as though I would stress over people's reactions to it. But then, eventually I realised that with my story, I am not alone. PND is, sadly, extremely common in our western culture. In fact, it seems that so many mothers are out their struggling alone or with not enough support networks and with less ability to cope that suicide is now the leading cause of death of mothers.

~*~*~*~

So with courage, I shared this story with you all to raise awareness. And I have the hope that if one mother with PND reads this story, and it enables her to see a way out of the dark place where she is, then I feel sharing this has been absolutely worth it. A glimmer of hope is all you need to start the journey back to wholeness.

*List of contacts*

Below I have put a list of contacts (for Australia) that you can connect in with. So please don't feel alone, there are places out there for you to reach out to.

Emergency – Police, Ambulance or Fire
000

PANDA (Post and Ante Natal Depression Association)
1300 726 306
www.panda.org.au

Beyond Blue
1300 224 636
www.beyondblue.org.au
An Australian not for profit, independent organisation, providing info for anxiety and depression and other related disorders

From The Heart (Western Australia)
08 9340 1622
http://www.fromtheheartwa.org.au/
From the Heart WA (formerly PNDSA) is a volunteer run consumer organisation providing support, understanding and information to women, partners and families who are affected by stress and depression related to pregnancy, childbirth, and the addition of a new child to the family.

Gidget Foundation
1300 726 306  Free call in Australia from 9am - 7pm
http://www.gidgetfoundation.com.au/
The Gidget Foundation exists to promote awareness of Perinatal Anxiety and Depression amongst women and their families, their health providers and the wider community to ensure that women in need receive timely, appropriate and supportive care

24 hr Maternal and Child Health Nurse Line  13 22 29
(for Victoria, Australia only)
Speak to a registered and qualified Maternal and Child Health Nurse. Available 24 hours a day, 7 days a week

Caroline Chisholm Society
(03) 9361 7000
(Country Victoria) 1800 134 863
http://www.carolinechisholmsociety.com.au/
The Caroline Chisholm Society is a charitable organisation, both privately and government funded, and is non-denominational. The Society offers support to pregnant women and parents with children up to school age. The Society provides a range of programs for families in need, including counselling, housing, material aid and in home family support. The families that the Caroline Chisholm Society works with are often bereft of wider social and family supports and are very grateful for the practical, emotional and financial supports the Society can offer.

LifeLine
13 11 14
www.lifeline.org.au
Lifeline provides access to crisis support, suicide prevention and mental health support services.

On Call Nurse
1300 60 60 24 for the cost of a local call from anywhere in Victoria. (Calls from mobile phones may be charged at a higher rate.)
http://www.health.vic.gov.au/nurseoncall/about.htm
NURSE-ON-CALL is a phone service that provides immediate, expert health advice from a registered nurse, 24 hours a day, 7 days a week

Psychologists
www.psychology.org.au
They have their Find A Psychologist link, and there is Medicare funding for pregnancy related issues (only for 3 x 30 min sessions) which can be added to the more commonly known Better Access scheme for up to ten sessions.

Birthtalk
http://birthtalk.org/
Birthtalk is a unique support and education organisation based in Brisbane, Australia, and run by a registered midwife, childbirth educator and mums

## *Create community*

Now that you have the numbers for some outreach programs, I have put together some simple ideas for you to remember in your life with your new baby around community. I wholeheartedly believe that PND can be significantly reduced if we have enough support systems in place. Creating and being a part of community helps to achieve this.

Create community and get in touch with other mothers!

You can do this by doing simple things:

1. Take your babies and children to the park. Say hi to the other parents there. Who knows, they could be the friend you haven't met yet.
2. Join in with already existing playgroups. You can be linked in with the mainstream playgroups from your maternal and child health nurse. Other playgroups are out there if you look for them! There are playgroups for teen mums, attachment parenting, unschoolers, older mothers, mothers groups for mothers who like to knit, who like to read, who like to bake... there are so many mothers groups out there, you are bound to find one that you fit into.
3. Join in an infant massage class or music class for babies. There you will find other mothers, who you may get along with. And if you don't, then you and your baby will have a fabulous time with massage or dancing that you can't lose.
4. Join a yoga class. There are many Mums and Bubs yoga classes out there. A yoga class for the 1st year after birth, where the women can take in their babies. A great way to stay healthy, stay with your bub and meet other mumma's.
5. Go to the library. They often have free story time for babies from 6 months to school age.
6. Start a mothers walking group. Put your baby in the sling or pram, catch up with other mothers and go for a walk in the sunshine.
7. Join a playgroup.

## *Playgroups*

Playgroups can be awesome or detrimental for your mental health. You need to find a playgroup that suits who you are. When I was 19 and just had my first child, the maternal and child health nurse linked me in with the local playgroup which didn't fit me at all. Most of the women were in their mid-30's, had been working corporate jobs and spent most of their time talking about their house renovations. I on the other hand, was a young 19 year old, living off Centrelink, studying for my VCE and renting a small flat with my then boyfriend and cat! The women all tried to be friendly, but we just didn't click and I felt like I didn't belong. I just ended up feeling more isolated. 10 years later, when my 5$^{th}$ baby was 10 months old, I came across a playgroup, partly run by the beautiful Mish, who I had known since highschool. The playgroup was called 'Rad Kids' and was open to parents of all persuasions! It didn't matter if you were single, alternative, queer; this playgroup was one where I didn't feel judged and was welcomed warmly and encouraged by the amazing people there.

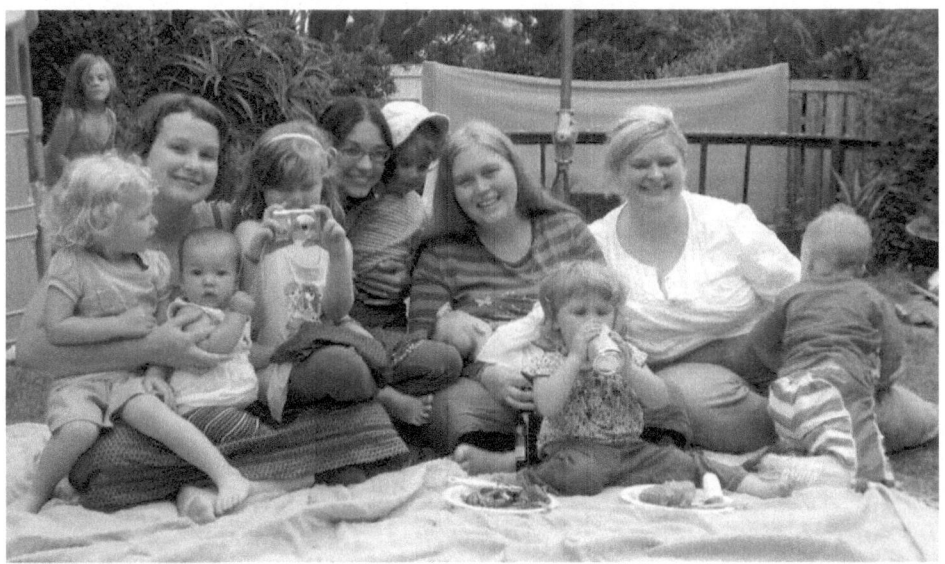

All you need to do is find the group that suits you. Here is a small list of playgroups that you can contact that may suit you and your children

Playgroup Australia
http://www.playgroupaustralia.com.au/
A great resource where you can look up any state or suburb and find a parenting group that suits you and your child.

:
Natural Parenting Playgroups
http://naturalparentingmelbourne.com.au/playgroups/
Playgroups in various locations around Melbourne, with the emphasis on natural parenting. They share the philosophy that all parents have an instinctive ability to care for their children in a responsive and respectful manner.

Melbourne Attachment Alternative Parenting
http://groups.yahoo.com/group/M_A_A_P/
A Melbourne group for parents interested in gentle, respectful and nurturing parenting to come and meet like-minded parents in a safe, friendly, and supportive environment.

Rad Kids
http://loopholecommunitycentre.org/node/2813
A group for parents of all persuasions: single parents, alternative, anarchist, queer...this is the "other" parent's group. Kids of course are welcome! Based in Preston, Melbourne.

Melbourne Babywearers
http://au.groups.yahoo.com/group/melb_babywearers/
The organisation has regular meet-ups in Melbourne so that we can enable, show, learn and discuss babywearing.

## *Stay calm, look after yourself, find some support*

Here is a little poem that was given to me by a midwife when I was pregnant with my first baby. She reminded me of what was important. I still have this poem stuck on my kitchen wall.

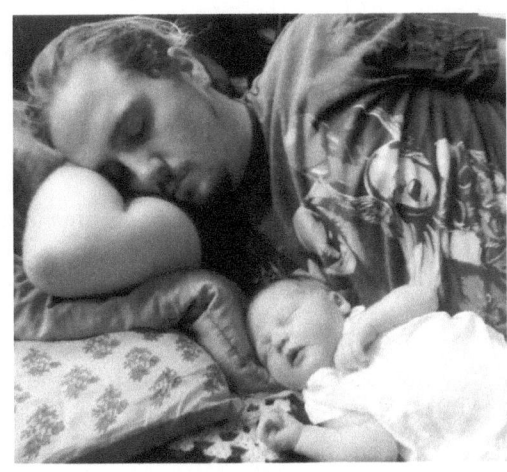

"Super Hero" - Photo: Sheree Stewart

<u>What Did I Do Today?</u>
Today I left some dishes dirty;
The bed got made around 3:30.
The diapers soaked a little longer,
The odour grew a little stronger.
The crumbs I spilled the day before,
Are staring at me from the floor.
The fingerprints there on the wall,
Will likely be there still next fall.
The dirty streaks on those windowpanes
Will still be there next time it rains.
Shame on you, you sit and say,
Just what did you do today?
    I held a baby till she slept,
    I held a toddler while he wept.
    I played a game of hide and seek;
    I squeezed a toy so it would squeak.
    I pulled a wagon, sang a song,
    Taught a child right from wrong.
    What did I do this whole day through?
    Not much that shows, I guess that's true.
    Unless you think that what I've done,
    Might be important to someone,
    With deep green eyes and soft brown hair,
    If that is true . . . I've done my share.
                  - Author Unknown

## *Journey of The Wild Rainbow*

*The big adventure of Rainbow Mumma and her Sweet Dragonboy*

After struggling on so many levels after the birth of my 5th baby, spiraling into dark, dark places where there were times I didn't think I would find my way out, I found a spark of light and managed to slowly and steadily be breathed back to life.

I was starting to come to a place of finding myself. Of finding who I was. I had already been on the road of 'mother'. Since I was 18, I had been either pregnant, birthing or breastfeeding. Once my 5th baby was 1, I started on a new journey to find myself as 'woman'. It felt relieving and freeing to know that my childbearing days were over. I started to think about where the rest of my life would take me and who I was as a woman, not a mother, and I started finding more power and purpose in where my life was heading. Who I actually was, who I was becoming. I saw my potential and it blew me away.

I had started doing a year-long Shamanic Midwife course and in this I learned more deeply about my innate body wisdom, my connection to spirit and world and my body's natural rhythm to the earth. I started charting my cycle (which had only returned a few months prior) and was reveling in knowledge and knowing of how much my body and the universe were connected. I was closely in tune with how my body was working. My body and the earth were of the same pulse.

It was one windy autumn morning that I stopped as I was charting my cycle when I realised that in one month I ovulated twice. And I had a moment of panic as I realised that I was quite possibly pregnant. The panic overcame me and I tried to brush the thought aside. This wasn't going to happen. I'm not having any more babies. I would never be able to go through what I had just been through the year before. I wouldn't survive it. I just wouldn't be able to. I'm too tired. I already have lots of children.

I went to the supermarket that same day and got a pregnancy test. I can't even remember doing the test, I just remember looking at the pregnancy stick and seeing it show up with 2 blue lines almost instantly. I was pregnant. I cried, and cried and cried and cried. I told Steven and then I cried some more. "I'm not keeping it" I said and I locked myself away in my room for a couple weeks.

I felt so devastated. I didn't want to know what was happening. I didn't want to face it. But there was a point in where I had obviously had to. Doing Jane's Shamanic Midwifery course meant I had to do a 3 day workshop on 'pregnancy – the inner journey'. I was so scared and I almost had decided to pretend that I wasn't pregnant during those 3 days. Of course, you can't pretend when you travel to the shamanic realms, so I wrote to Jane and told her that I was pregnant, that I don't want to be pregnant and that I don't want to tell anyone I'm pregnant. She replied to me with a 'congratulations and you are obviously going to have to share, just remember what is said in the circle stays in the circle'. She was so right, so I went along and listened to the women in the circle share their pregnancy stories. Their happiness, their love, their excitement. Fuck, I thought. They are all so happy about their babies. After listening to their stories, I decided to pretend that when it was my turn that I would talk about how happy I was too.

It got to my turn. I held the talking bowl in my hands and said "Hi, I'm Sheree and I'm pregnant with my 6th baby and I'm really not happy about that at all" and then I burst into tears. I cried and cried and cried. No one said anything; they just held the space for me. There was no judgement. I was held in love. I was honoured. I held the bowl for what seemed like eternity until the tears were gone. I said no more words. When the tears were gone, I passed the bowl to the woman next to me.

I felt so vulnerable. I felt like I wasn't ready for this. The devastation and the loss of the year before made me nervous. My marriage seemed to be all over the place, some family members had stopped talking to me, I lost some friends and a woman who I deeply loved had cut me completely out of her life. I didn't want to lose anything else. My mind was only just starting to get better. I was so scared that everything was going to turn to shit.

Over the 3 days of the workshop, I did many drum journeys where I travelled into my womb and met my baby. I looked at his face, I listened to his voice, we talked to each other. It was so vivid and powerful.

## The Wild Rainbow

There was one particular drum journey which shifted something deep inside me. It was actually the drum journey in which I decided I was going to keep my baby.

As I listened to the beating of the drum, my attention focused inwards. I entered in, I saw my baby straight away, in his embryo form, looking as though he was still dreaming and in a faraway place in the stars.

After that, the energy shifted and the embryo became a baby. He wasn't moving and looked really still. I started to worry and I called out to him.

> *"Where are you?" I cried out*
> *Baby replied "I'm here Mum"*
> *and I said "I couldn't see you move"*
> *Baby said "Why were you worried?"*
> *I paused and I said "Because I want you"*

This was the FIRST TIME EVER I wanted this baby! It was such a strong feeling and a massive shift for me. I couldn't stop crying. It was the first time in ages that I felt like everything might work out.

Coming home to Steven and talking to him about the reality of keeping this baby was surreal. It felt as though the words were coming out of my mouth but I wasn't actually talking them. I still felt so vulnerable that we decided to not share our news with anyone straight away. I was coming to terms with what was happening. I was being confronted by my own ideas about what was happening that I needed to deal with those first before I was able to deal with anyone elses. Whenever I would think about the reaction from friends, family or even strangers, I would find myself feeling overwhelmed. So, I stopped thinking about everyone else. And I went into my own space where I could be sovereign to myself, where I could see the issues coming up and deal with them on my own without the unwanted advice or opinions of others.

The first 20 weeks passed with me feeling a whole range of things, and often feeling all of these feelings in one day. I remember one time feeling ready to tell a few people really close to me about my baby dragon so I invited them over where we were going to celebrate one of the Sabbats and I was going to share my news with them then. They were all excited and as the day arrived, I got text messages from the 3 of them, all at separate times, telling me they were no longer able to come. It was so devastating to me. I felt so small and alone. The feelings of not being supported and not being able to cope crept back up. Needing to feel held and supported was the key to me being ok in this journey.

The little dragon baby growing in my womb had other plans though. He went and visited many people in their dreams (there were 11 people, and most of those were people who I wouldn't have considered in my close friends) who he went and visited. In a space of a month, I had received messages from people who had told me they had dreamed or seen me pregnant with an incredibly powerful baby and that he was going to make my family complete.

My pregnancy continued on and as I watched my body expand more and more to let this child in, I felt the excitement building. I was having a baby – or in Chinese astrology, a water dragon.

There were some times in the 2nd trimester where when I look back on, were actually quite beautiful. I held myself and protected myself until I was strong enough to emerge back in to the world. There was a gentle holding of my own space, the space of my husband and the space of my children. As the time passed, I felt more strong and capable. I no longer felt like a frazzled, scattered Mumma bird, but a strong, all knowing and protective Eagle – able to protect and nourish her young and all those around her in the animal kingdom know it. The time passed, and as it did, I felt stronger. The dragon baby was coming to me because I could cope with it. I was his Mumma. He chose me because I could do it. I was the only one who could mother this amazing child. He was mine and he was going to change my whole life.

Over the pregnancy, I transformed Steven's former shiatsu treatment room into a dragoncave. I got my favourite people to come and paint the wall – a huge labyrinth with a dragon at its mouth, and a spiraling, star splatted galaxy. It was incredible. It became such a colour cave, a magic place to be. I created altars that were full of gifts and items from nature that people gave us. There were handmade prayer flags, my handmade shamanic drum, seashells, feathers from peacocks, ravens and rainbow birds. There were rocks, crystals, bark and flowers. It was so beautiful. It was so magic.

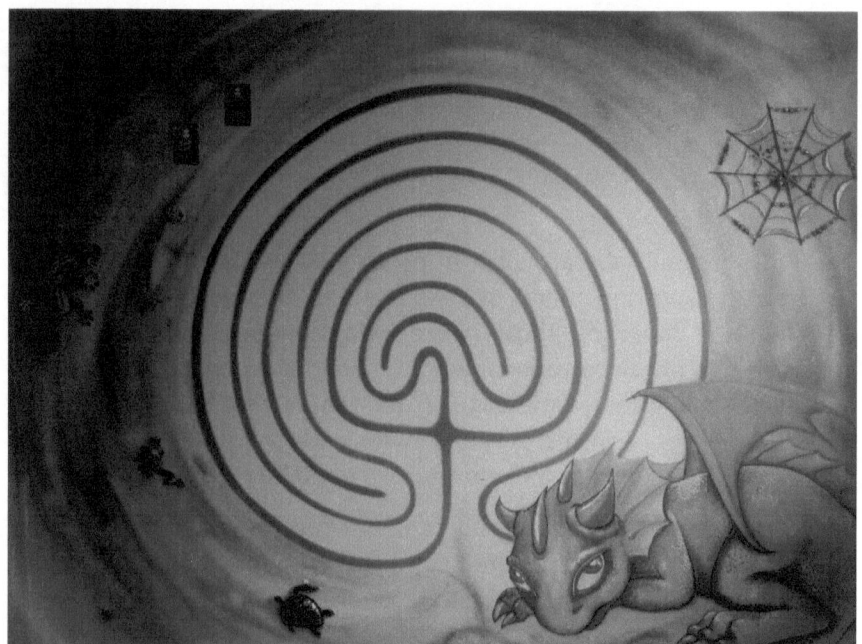

*"Dragoncave"* – Photo: Steven Booth

I did many drum journeys and I found what I needed to keep me sustained, nourished and held. It was imperative to my mental health that I felt loved. And I needed to find and keep deep connections with those who loved me as much as I loved them. For this pregnancy, birth and postpartum period to work harmoniously, I needed to find my tribe. Over the pregnancy, people came and went and those who were truly meant to be in my life have shown themselves. There were many hard lessons learnt and the pregnancy just kept giving me the opportunity to take another layer off, take off another mask until I was becoming closer and closer to my centre and my truth.

My dragonbaby was taking me through the labyrinth on so many levels. I didn't have to do anything but trust. I could close my eyes if I wanted to and just stay internal and I would still be walked to the centre of the labyrinth and back out again. The labyrinth begins and ends at the same point. It is not like a maze which has twists and turns that can lead to dead ends. With the labyrinth you start at the mouth and follow the convoluted path which although sometimes feel confusing, if you just keep following it, you will reach the centre.

The last few weeks of pregnancy were difficult as the baby grew more and more. My hips were incredibly painful as I had severe pubic symphysis diastasis and the baby with his head very engaged made a painful combination. I would sometimes get waves of feeling overwhelmed on how I could possibly look after so many children. Whenever I would get that way, I would contact a friend named Clare who has 7 children and just go 'bleerrrgghhh...this is happening' and she would always respond with the perfect words which would quieten down my mind and ease my heart.

One late evening, when I was 39 weeks and the world was getting ready for a solar eclipse, my womb started contracting. They were regular and 4 minutes apart from the beginning and I felt excited that I would soon meet my baby. I lit some candles on my altar and put some water in the pool. I knew it was still early, but I knew I would be able to rest in the water. After about 4 hours of these contractions, with them increasing in intensity, Steven came into the room and told me that Myah had woke up vomiting everywhere and is now in the bath. Then she vomited again and then again and then again. I decided to go and try and lie with her and breathe through the contractions. As I did, I fell asleep and woke up the next morning, still pregnant, just in time for the solar eclipse. I felt devastated that my baby hadn't come. Instead of holding a newborn in my arms, I was still holding him in my womb and had a sick toddler to care for. This really dampened my spirits and I asked Mish and Lucy if they could come over and be with me for a while. I remember as Lucy came and gave me a hug, I sighed and said 'I'm still pregnant'. She just looked at me and said 'that's ok'. That's all I needed. I just needed someone to tell that me that I'm ok. She came and massaged my feet and my neck and made me cups of tea. Mish snuggled with me all day and sung songs to the dragon. I felt so tired. But I felt so held that I knew I would be ok. I just needed to rest.

That week passed in a blur of sick children and of me feeling so pregnant and vulnerable. I decided I just needed to stay in the house, stay in my pj's and just wait for the baby dragon. I made sure people came to visit me every day and I made sure that I felt loved, supported and held – they were the key ingredients to my mind being ok.

# The Wild Rainbow

The day before Eli was born, I asked Mish to come over. It was such a nice quiet day. Even though there were 6 children in the house, it didn't seem chaotic and loud, it was kind of strangely quiet. Mish sang to my belly, calling the dragonbaby out, we talked about nothing, we laughed about nothing, we sat in both patience and eagerness as we waited, waited, waited for the baby.

That night after Mish had went home and Steven and I had got the munchkins to bed, we sat on the couch together and watched some shows. Monday night is always 'Mum and Dads movie night' in our house and we always watch some series together. At the moment it was 'Dexter' and 'The Walking Dead'. I laughed to Steven saying that if watching serial killers and zombies isn't going to bring out the baby, then nothing will. I had a little giggle as Mish sent me a text to say she was watching zombie shows too and we should synchronise our efforts and bring the dragon earthside. She had also given a crystal to Steven to rub on my belly that had been sitting out getting some lunar/solar eclipse lovemaking charges which I thought was awesome as I always sensed the baby's energy was tied in with an eclipse.

I went to bed late, tired but happy, with random contractions still happening, but not enough to bother me. My sleep bought me some wild dreaming for a few hours. When I got a contraction, it came into my dreaming, and it made for some wild adventures! I was falling off a horse, tripping over a large tree root in the jungle, feeling sick in the stomach after eating poisonous foods. One dreaming adventure came to a halt when a contraction was big enough to wake me. I woke up suddenly, wide eyed, staring at the roof and it took me a moment to centre myself and realise that I was at home in bed and was awoken by a contraction, and that I wasn't on a wild Incan jungle adventure. I checked my phone and saw it was just after 2am. I lay in bed for about half an hour in the silent, listening and feeling my contractions. A beautiful space, a moment in time where it was just the dragonbaby and I that were in on this secret that he was going to be born today.

Around 2:30 I got up out of bed and woke Steven. I wanted to go and sit in the pool, even though I knew it was early labour, I just wanted to rest in the water. I was so anxious about the noise of the pool being pumped up waking the younger girls, that I umm'ed and ahh'ed about it for a while until I got a contraction that made me go 'now, just go and pump it up, I want to sit in it!!'

Steven and I fiddled around like little birth faeries, him pumping up the pool, me getting the towels. I made a cup of tea and decided it tasted disgusting and found a ginger ale in the fridge which tasted far better!

We filled the pool only a bit as I was weary of running out of hot water, and because this was only the early stages, I didn't want to get overexcited and use all the hot water at once. The little bit of water that was in the pool was enough. It enabled me to relax and I could drift back off to sleep. I would wake for the contraction, breathe deeply through it, reminding myself to be calm, relaxed and open. When the contraction would start to go I would tell myself to let go of any tension and be soft, soft, soft, soft. As soon as the contraction was done, I would be back asleep.

I didn't know how far apart the contractions were at that point. They could have been 3 minutes or 20 minutes, but I felt so incredibly rested and rejuvenated by the sleeps I was having between them. Three hours of contractions like this and then the first rays of the sun were ever so slightly starting to show. This straight away bought up 2 issues for me – the first one was that it was going to be day time and I was going to be labouring! My homebirth babies were born early morning before the sun came out and I couldn't imagine labouring in the daylight! And the next issue was that I would be aware that my kids would be up soon. It was a school day and they would need help to get ready, pack their lunches and have someone drive them to school. I voiced all this to Steven and we decided to call some of our team to come and help with the kids. I needed Steven's attention to be with me completely so he called Mish and Lucy. By 7:15 they had both arrived. Mish arrived first; I felt her presence as soon as she came in the room. I couldn't look up at her, but I knew she was there. I was still feeling very present and aware but also very withdrawn and inward. I knew exactly what was going on, who was were, the happenings of the house, but I didn't engage with it. She started pouring water on my back, nice slow drizzles of hot water down my back. It made me feel calm. It made me feel quiet.

## The Wild Rainbow

Resting calmly and then sometimes falling asleep between contractions was helpful. I had a microsleep where I went straight to dreaming and I was suddenly in a forest. Back in the jungles I was visiting in my earlier dreaming. There were jaguars and colourful birds. I looked up and saw the jungle trees. They were so, so tall that I couldn't see the top of them. They were so ancient. And I could smell them. Mish was standing beside me and she was still pouring water on my back, but we were both naked. I looked at the jungle floor and I could smell the sweet and damp. Another contraction came and I woke up, back in my dragoncave – Mish still pouring water on my back, but she wasn't naked (well not that I know of, I didn't check!)

There was a space where something shifted in me and I knew I needed to move – as in, get out of the pool. I found it hard to do so and the couple times I tried, as soon as I stood up a contraction would come on strong. "Fuck" I would swear. "I knew that would happen."

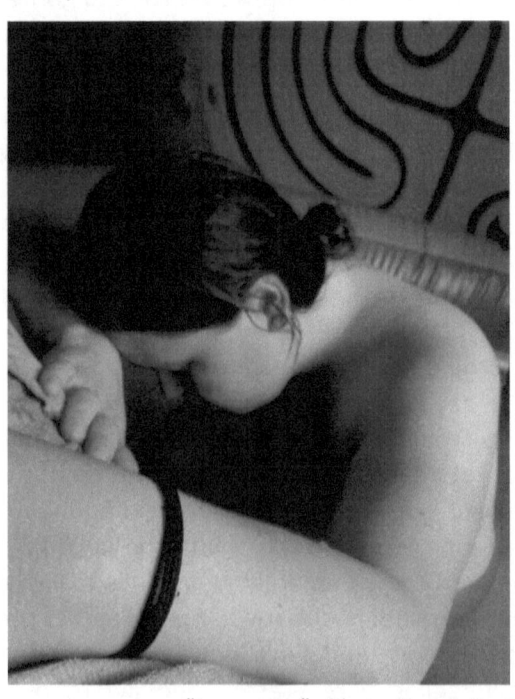

Eventually I realised that it was up to me to actually move, so I did. I went to the bathroom which seemed so bright and I stood up for some contractions. I knew they were going to hurt, so as they came on I reminded myself to stay soft and open, don't tighten up, don't tense, just stay soft. Melt into yourself.

*"Journeying"* - *Photo*: Steven Booth

I was in such a magnificent place. It was so surreal. Nothing else existed. I could hear a world outside of the bathroom door – it was my world of my children, my tribe of people, and my home. And still feeling connected to them, I was also in another world of my own. This strange amazing place was where the chrysalis transforms into a butterfly, where the rainbow serpent came out from the void and created the waters, the hills, the people and creatures. I was in the world where nothing but everything exists. I was bringing spirit into flesh; I was bringing my baby home to my arms.

I stayed in the bathroom for a short time. Standing up was good, well, it was painful, but it was good. It bought my baby's head down into my pelvis more which is exactly the perfect thing he needed to do. Going back in to the pool felt more comfortable, but I was getting to that point where no position was comfortable. I kept reminding myself to be soft.

In the world outside my dragoncave door, Lucy had taken 2 of our children to school and Mish took the other three kids to the park which is next to our house.

As soon as I knew everyone was taken care of, and everyone except Steven and I were off the property, I got a contraction that was so overwhelmingly big that it made my whole body tremble from its power and I got that overbearing urge to push. I tried to see if I could feel the baby's head, I couldn't feel anything. My waters still hadn't broken. Could I be fully dilated? I will just have to wait and see.

The next few contractions were the same. I felt that urge to push. I held face washers to my perineum and I could feel stretching, stretching, stretching from the inside, but on the outside there was nothing. There was no bulge, no baby's head that I could feel. A part of me started to wonder and think back to my last birth. When I had this urge to push with my last baby, she was born in 3 contractions. I had to pretty much hold my hand on my perineum and slow her from coming down so fast as I was afraid I was going to tear from her speediness!

This birth though, was different. It was different to all the 5 babies that I have birthed. I reminded myself that all my births have been different, none alike. One of my sisters words rang through my head as she reminded me just days before: 'this baby, this birth, this dance'.

The contractions were so big that I felt I had to push really, really hard with them. And sometimes there would be no progress at all. My whole body was shaking and sweating as I was overwhelmed by the next contraction – I kept looking at Steven's face, trying to find some strength. He held me close and gave me exactly what I needed. It was

## The Wild Rainbow

so good to have him there, just me and him, bringing our dragonbaby into our world together. As I was working hard, parts of my wedding vows to Steven came into my head:

> *... Let's live like Dragonling, in our garden on our time on Earth, to look after the Baby Dragons that have been put into our care...*
> *I feel like this spiralling path has led us here, to this cleared, opened space...*
> *Let's create Heaven together and live it every single day with our Baby Dragons.*

I worked so hard to get this baby out. Time wise, it wasn't long, it was around 45 minutes (which is the longest I have taken to push out ANY of my 6 babies!) but effort wise, it took so much from me. I wondered if he was in a wonky position. Was he oblique or directly posterior? Was I going to feel a little shoulder through my cervix, was I going to have to transfer to hospital now? I decided it didn't matter. I decided that although it hurts and it is hard work, I needed to keep working with this little one to get him out. The chrysalis and the butterfly came into my mind – the struggle and strength it takes to transform into something so spectacular and freeing. I was both the chrysalis and the butterfly. As was my baby.

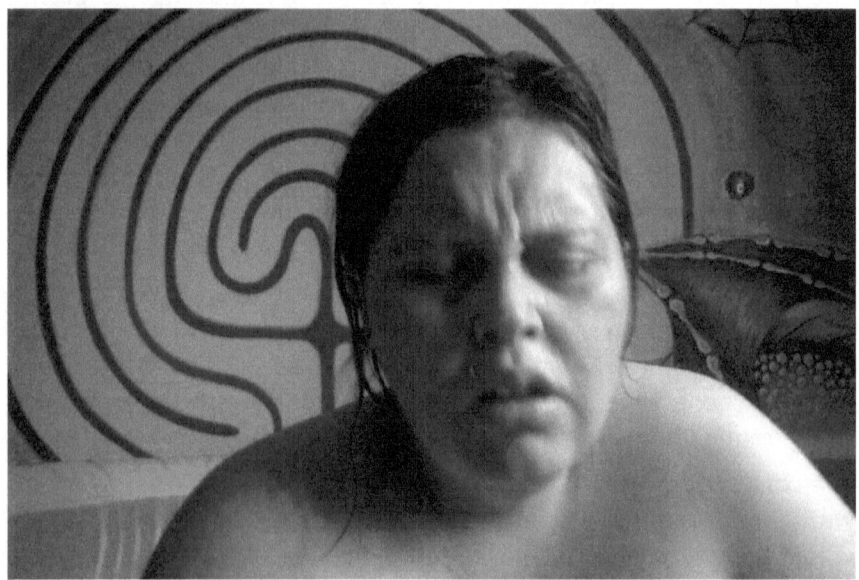

"In the Labyrinth" - Photo: Steven Booth

The contractions kept coming and instead of backing away, I said yes to the challenge. I felt his head come a little more, then a little more, then a little more. The waters broke, not a huge gush, but a noticeable one and it reminded me that I was nearly there. I eventually felt that familiar bulge of a baby's head behind the perineum and as I reached down to feel, I touched his head which was full of soft hair. It felt like seaweed dancing in the water. I was so excited to be seeing him soon, all I could focus on was getting him out. His head felt so big and I had moments of thinking 'far out, that's a big head, how am I going to get that out?'

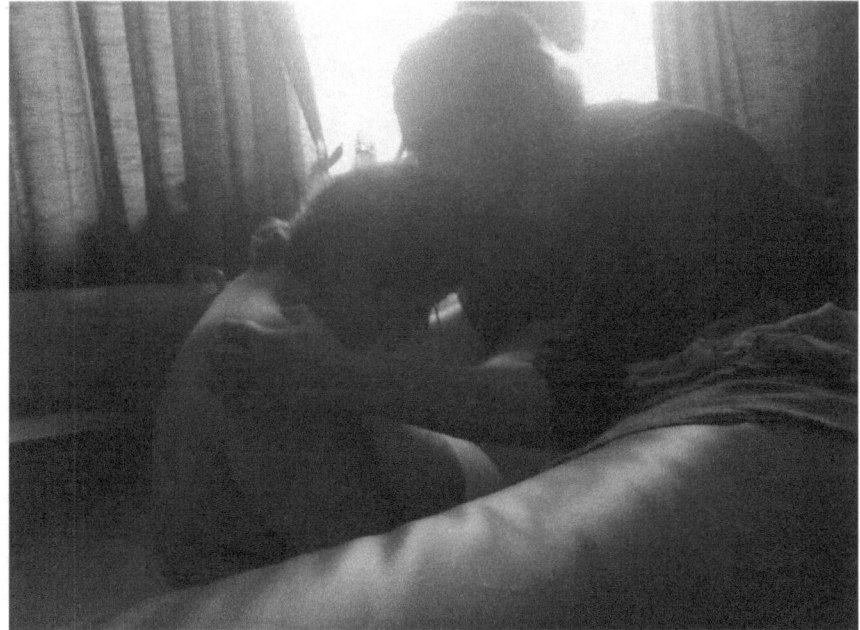

Photo: Lucy Johnston

I remember that contraction which slowly bought the last of his face and head out into the birth pool. I was squatting holding onto Steven and as his head was out, I reached down to him. In that time, Lucy had just walked in the front door and Steven asked me if I want her in the room. I nodded yes, he told her to come in and I was in this surreal world of a baby half in my body, half in the world. I wanted someone to go and get Mish and the girls from the park (especially as my daughter really wanted to be at the birth, she was present at the birth of her littlest sister) but I didn't have any words to do so, so I let that

## The Wild Rainbow

idea go and reminded myself that all is perfect. This is perfect. This is the birth I am having.

The next contraction came and I awaited the sweet release of his shoulders into my hands in the water. I always loved that feeling of that last contraction when the shoulders come and the whole body emerges, slippery and wet. Instead, I was met with nothing but an overwhelming contraction. It was building up and the shoulders didn't come. It was getting towards the peak of the contraction and his shoulders were still inside where I had a moment of 'oh, fuck'.

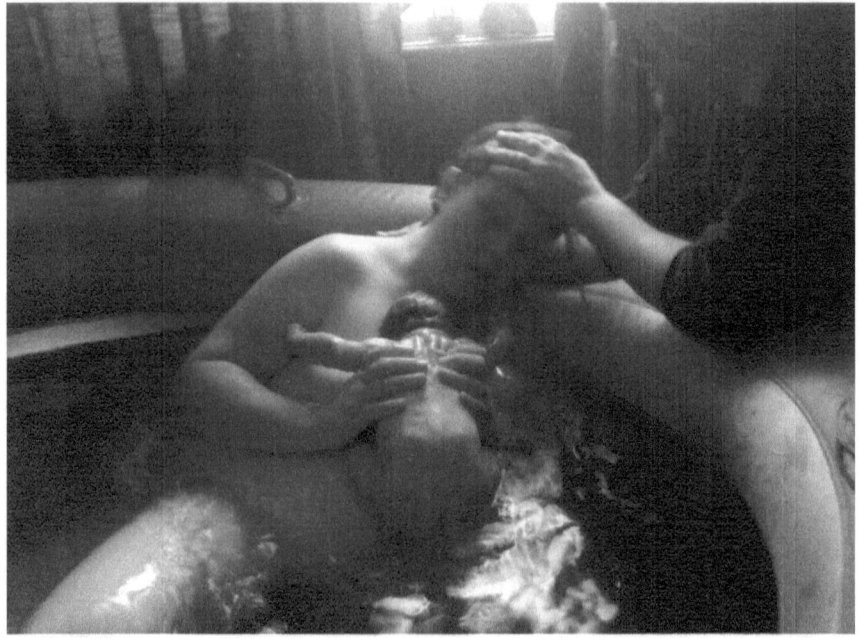

Photo: Lucy Johnston

Instead of panicking, I was met a clear voice that reminded me visions that I had had during my pregnancy. During my pregnancy, I would do shamanic drum journeys to meet my baby, and I would always ask him about the birth. Every time I would get shown his birth which would be me birthing in a position I would never think I would birth in (standing up with one leg kind of held up by someone) and I would get told over and over that the last contraction I need to change position to get him out.

With that in mind, I decided I was going to stand up out of the water. I went from a squatting position, let go of his head, held onto the pool and then kinked one leg out to the side. As soon as I did this, before I had the chance to stand up, he came spiralling out of my body into the pool. I reached my arms down to scoop him up and bought him to my chest.

He cried within seconds. A big, long, long dragoncry. I felt so relieved. I looked down to see that he indeed was a he! A beautiful boy. A big, built, strong boy, with a head of soft hair and a divine, perfect face.

Someone went out to the park to call in Mish and the girls, and they scurried inside to see the dragonboy in my arms. Beautiful and chubby, crying, calling himself home.

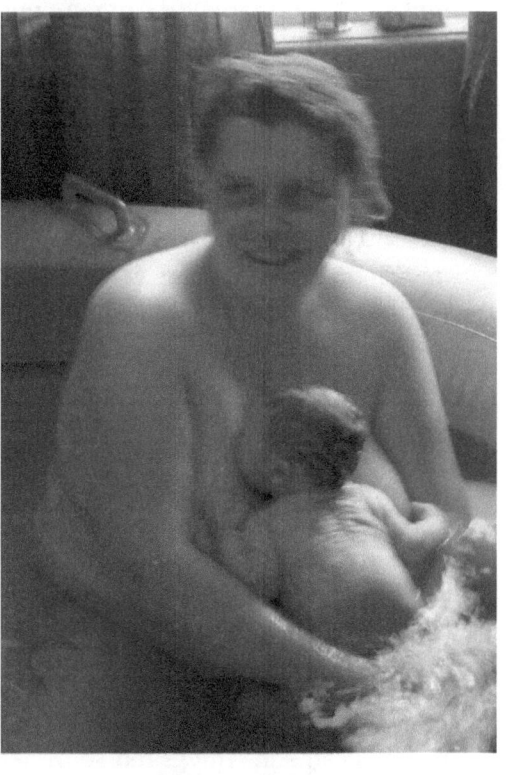

"Lionheart" – Photo: Lucy Johnston

When everyone was in the room, I felt so supported and held. Steven, Mish and Lucy were incredible. They all knew what I needed and they gave me everything, 100%. They honoured my space, they loved me when I needed love, and they gave me what I needed so that I could bring my dragonboy into the world.

His placenta came away easily and quickly. I remember feeling nauseous and then asking for a colander to catch the placenta in. Dragonboy was having a lotus birth, so he was still connected to the placenta via the umbilical cord (which was pretty short). It felt big and the membranes felt tough. I could feel the placenta just sitting there but needed to stand whilst holding Dragonboy so that the last final bodily release could happen. Steven was a brilliant placenta catcher, and caught the placenta in the colander. Sitting back in the pool, I

# The Wild Rainbow

marvelled at how big it was and how strong it looked. I have named all of my babies placenta's. I consider them to be the baby's womb twin. I looked at the marvellous organ, which kept my baby alive. It had big thick membranes, sitting over the cotyledons, overshadowing them; it reminded me of an eclipse. Eli was also born right in the middle of both a solar and lunar eclipse. It felt right to name his placenta Eclipse.

I went to bed all snuggled with my boy, who was beautifully pink and chubby, with his placenta in a colander beside him and we were looked after all day long. My Birth Faeries took my children to the park and out for babycino's. At times I was alone with my baby, soaking up his lusciousness, just me and him and no one else in the entire world existed. Other times, my bedroom was full of my children, my husband and women I deeply loved. We did placenta prints and gave them as gifts to our loved ones. We marvelled at his placenta that had the thickest, toughest membranes I had ever seen. They were so tough and they looked like dragonfly wings. Eclipse was perfectly round, with big, fat healthy cotyledons, with the exception of one cotyledon which has grown off to the side. I felt like this was a medicine gift to me from my dragonboy, so after he was lotus born, I took this cotyledon and made it into medicine.

He let go of his placenta after only 2 days and around that same time my milk came in. Things felt so perfect. I lay and look at him for hours, still not fully believing he is here. I didn't think my life could feel this beautiful and complete.

I look at my boy, who is born right in the middle of both a lunar and a solar eclipse, and I think of how special he is. For a baby that wasn't planned, who came by surprise and took us all on a huge ride, I feel the intensity of him as he is supposed to be here.

Our boy, Eli Zen, is both wild and calm, chaos and order. He is my moonfaced dragon who came to me bearing many gifts. He knows everything there is to know in the entire world.

His birth wasn't the sensual, blissful, orgasmic experience I was planning for. Instead, it was something way more magic and powerful. It was hard and confusing, it was confronting. It made me question myself, my beliefs, my intuition, my body, my baby. But I gave in to it. I was stretched to my limits (in all senses of the word!) but in being so, such a gift was given to me.

I am feeling amazing. My moonfaced dragon is amazing. My family of stars is just incredible. My community of rainbow warriors are beautiful. I totally just can't believe my life right now.

Welcome home dragonboy. We've been waiting for you.

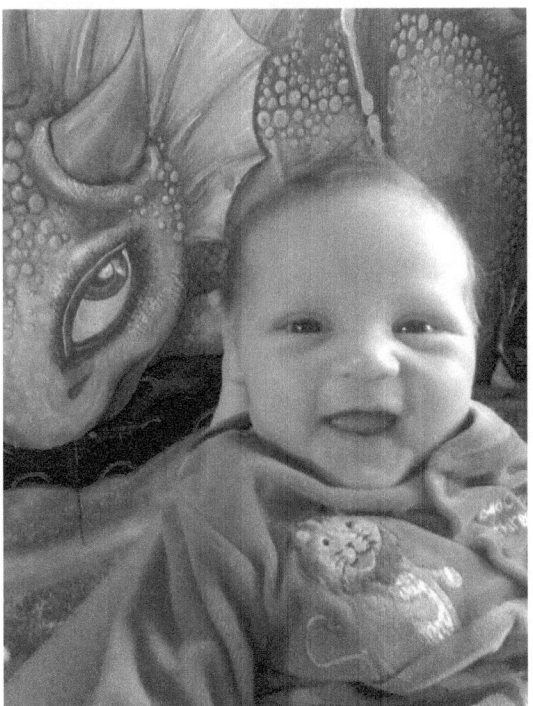

Photo: Sheree Stewart

*"I don't want to miss the world around me or inside me*
*Golden Child of the Galactic Centre*
*When are you coming home to me?"*

May 2007

# *Journey as Sage Femme*

A woman in harmony with her spirit is like a river flowing.
She goes where she will without pretense
and arrives at her destination,
prepared to be herself
and only herself.
~Maya Angelou

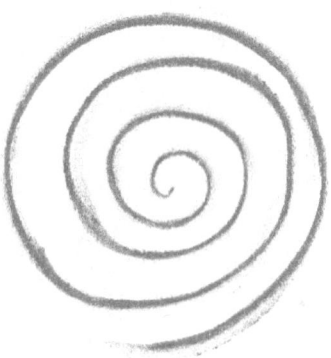

## *Finding the Magic*

### **The Priestess**

> *As part of a Transpersonal Art Therapy course I was undertaking, one of our exercises we were to do was create a fairytale type story using myths about an event in our life that started off as trauma in some way and ended up being a significant life affirming event. I had just finished my 3 year Bachelor of Midwifery and was struggling to work in the system. This is the story I wrote about my journey.*

Once upon a time there was a Priestess, with honey coloured hair and emerald green eyes. She was one of the very few chosen ones who was picked by the Goddesses to learn and train to become the embodiment of empowerment and to empower women and help them to connect to their femininity, sacred sexuality and their role as creatrix.

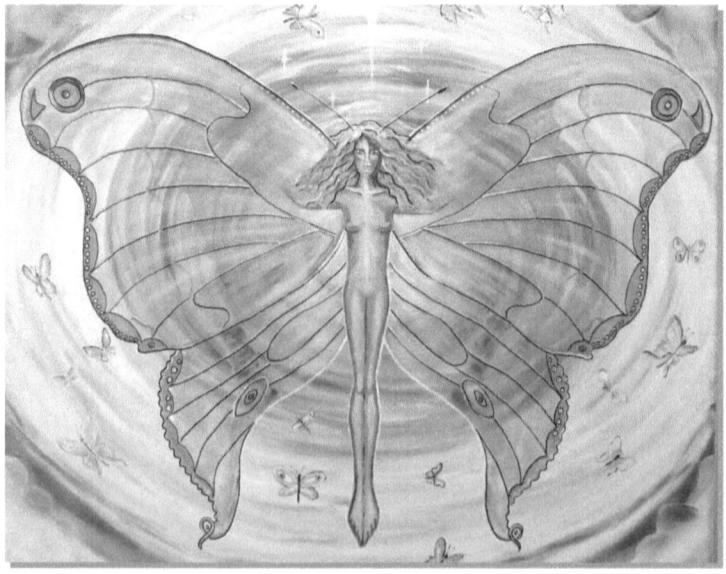

*"Transformation"* - Artist: Annie Joy

# Journeying as Sage Femme

The Priestess marvelled at this opportunity and she moved into the temple, along with the other chosen ones, to start the intensive training. Years passed and as they did, the priestess grew more passionate, courageous and loving. She could see her path with clear eyes and she understood her teachings deeply. They touched her to her core; they gave her purpose and meaning.

She understood the importance of being with women. She understood the very essence of honouring women in such an authentic way that the woman felt sovereign to themselves, autonomous in their own right. She supported them in a way that the women recognised themselves as courageous beings, as wild lioness women and as all powerful as they intuitively connected with their babies, their birthing bodies, their families. The Priestess had trained for years for this, that is, to be witness and loving support for women through all stages of their lives, to allow women the freedom to reclaim their inherent power and bliss. The time finally arrived when it was time for her to leave the temple. Her training was complete and her call to be out in the world to serve the women had begun. She was released from the temple to be of service in the wider world.

The Priestess was assigned to work in a birthing house of a special kind. It was a large building by the edge of the woods. It sat as a grey, dull, concrete square, in a strangely cleared space. Women would leave the confines of their warm homes and messy haired sweet children to come to the dull building to birth their babies. The Priestess found this most confusing. As she arrived and entered the building, the door was locked behind her. The doors were big heavy steel. The doors could not be opened. The Priestess shuddered, but she kept walking.

She knew something was not quite right. All of these people here claimed that they were the same as her – chosen ones, specially trained and marked, who studied the Law of Women through the great temples. But how could they be? There was just something about them that didn't seem right. She just couldn't shake that feeling and went to bed that night unnerved. Months passed, and as it did, the Priestess was growing weary. Her heart was heavy and she knew she had to go. She collected the little belongings that she had with her and walked to the big steels doors. She tried to work out how to open them, but all efforts led to more frustration. She was unable to pass through the doors. They were shut with bolts and magic and the more she struggled to leave, the tighter the doors closed in on her.

When she turned around she recoiled in horror as she saw that all the people who had claimed to be of the same clan as her own, had been fooling her. Her so called people had all been wearing masks of Goddesses and Priestesses, and once they knew she was barricaded in their birth house, they removed their masks to reveal their true faces. She was petrified. She felt her bones tremble as these unknown, cruel faces stared upon her. They were ugly and green with long rough hands. Their faces looked like demons with hollow uncaring eyes and dark hearts. They were not supposed to be here. They do not represent the ones who studied The Law of Women. These creatures took her by her arms and dragged her through the rooms of the buildings. The Priestess screamed as she was revealed with clear eyes and heart of the horror that was happening in the place that was supposed to be there for honouring woman as goddess / creatrix / starwoman.

Women and their babies were being tortured. Mothers bodies were being cut up against their will, babies were being injected with poisons. Families were being torn apart. The Mothers had blank, drugged faces. Their babies cried and refused to feed and the partners stood around lost, not knowing what to do.

Where was the empowerment? Where was the honour? The celebration? The wellness, the sisterhood, the initiation that these women were now mothers? To watch and witness this was killing the Priestess. She couldn't do it. She had to find another way. But for now, she couldn't. She was trapped.

Years passed. She fell more into alienation, depression and emptiness. The witness of abuse and torture of the world's most important beings sent her mind into darkness. At times she felt like cursing the Goddess for lying to her. She even began to slightly change like them, in small ways, but it was the only way she felt like she could cope without being abused and tortured herself. And without losing her sanity...

One day in the future, the Priestess noticed that she could see light from underneath the big steel door. She had never seen that before. It intrigued her and for the first time in a very long time, she went up to the big steel door. She touched it, just to feel it's coldness, but as she did, the big steel door opened. It opened! She couldn't believe it!

She left everything behind, and without turning back, she walked through those doors that kept her trapped there for so long. The Priestess looked out passed the strange clearing, into the woods and could make out some beings, hiding up in the trees. She couldn't see their faces but she could see their hearts. They were like her! She could tell easily because the Priestesses have golden hearts, full of light, and it shines through their chest like a luminous light. It is heart fire of the most magnificent kind. She squealed in delight when she realised that she had been rescued by other Priestesses whom she has never met.

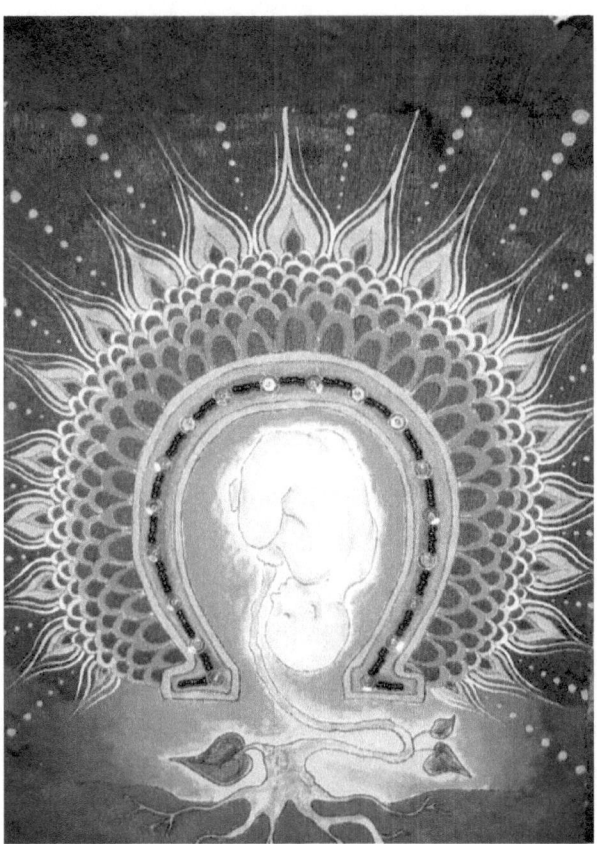

Artist: Michelle Guest

## The Wild Rainbow

They came out from the trees, tangled in spider webs, and armed with bows and arrows. There were 5 of them and they were all beautiful. They wrapped her in silk and carried her away from that big grey concrete place and took her into the cosmos. There she rested in the light. There she reflected. There she sat for what felt like blissful eternity in deep conversation and love with other Priestesses. Slowly she began to trust again. Slowly she remembered what her calling was. Soon enough, her inner strength returned. Her lioness fire heart ignited and she remembered how knowledgeable, empowered and passionate she really was. Being with other Priestesses made her whole again. She was ready to return to her calling, to her urge, to serve women and their babies.

And that is exactly what the Priestess did. Like a Phoenix rising from the ashes, the Priestess emerged transformed and regenerated, with a new found enthusiasm and passion for the work she does. And even better was that she had found herself a Rainbowtribe whose firehearts burn the same as her own. Together they created a new world, a new way of honouring and journeying with women and their babies. It was a new place of love, compassion, sisterhood, courage and truth. Everyone was honoured and everyone was able to grow fully into their potential to fully heal and fully love. All the beings in this place lived happily ever after.

*I embrace my desire to*
*feel the rhythm,*
*to feel connected enough to step aside*
*and weep like a widow,*
*to feel inspired,*
*to fathom the power,*
*to witness the beauty,*
*to bathe in the fountain,*
*to swing on the spiral of our divinity*
*and still be a human.*

-Lateralus by Tool

## *Alchemy of Midwifery and Women's Initiation*

*A talk given by Shivam Rachana*

The traditional midwife inherited the temple teachings of the high priestess - the one who walked the path into the essence of the women's mysteries. In birthing, the midwife again walks the path with the mother-to-be reliving and regaining her own knowing, as nature initiates the birthing woman into her own knowing that is, at once, individual and communal. This knowing, woman's knowing, is seldom written, for it is passed as living presence from one who knows to one who is ready to receive.

In its timeless ritual of incarnation/birth/rebirth, in the space between the silence and activity, the alchemy of midwifery occurs. In the surroundings of home, with those whom we love and trust, women's knowledge can be reclaimed and birth can be restored as the continuing pathway of women into the mysteries.

Let's look at the steps involved in restoring birth as a women's initiatory mystery. This heritage of women, can be recovered as her future path of power and wisdom.

The role/art of the traditional midwife included knowledge of the process of becoming a woman and the role played by a woman's sexuality. Menstruation, love making, pregnancy, birth, breastfeeding, mothering and menopause are all involved in a woman's sexual expression. These aspects of her sexuality can be understood by other women who have travelled the path.

The midwife is one who is able to be with-woman during those times of growth and unfolding. She understands the underlying forces at work during these times and can facilitate their expression so that the woman passes through the experience gathering the wisdom and insightfulness that are available to her via these processes.

Common female difficulties such as P.M.T., conditions of pregnancy such as toxaemia, high blood pressure, morning sickness, backache, birth complications, forceps deliveries, caesarean delivery, retained placenta, haemorrhage, post natal depression and breast feeding all stem from the incomplete expression of these experiences of living in a woman's body, either by the woman herself or by her ancestors.

The traditional midwife understands life in a unique and organic way. Her understandings come from the evolutionary expression of herself as a woman. Her embracing of her woman-ness in its many aspects equips her to be able to voyage with her sisters through their own deeper un-foldings.

Her training crosses the millennia. She reaches into dimensions beyond the physical to enable the physical embodiment of the processes. Her understanding of the natural order unfolding during these key times in a woman's life enables people to re-access their experiences and heal old wounds.

Few women in our culture have experienced totally, that is, completely naturally, their baby's birth. Most have, locked inside them, these unexpressed and unexperienced forces. The release of these frees her psyche and her body to live more fully and happily in the present.

Traditional midwives see the process of giving birth as an initiation. An initiation takes a person into a new situation after which they have new knowledge and understanding about their reality. They are different afterwards. There is a period of preparation that involves self-exploration, completing in-completions from the past so that the person in fully present. There needs to be a willingness to let go of the past and their perceptions of self if they are to be fully initiated. They are accompanied by a guide - one who has gone before - during the preparatory phase and then accompanied by a guide to a doorway - but only the initiate can enter the doorway, alone.

In other times, in other cultures, it was the practice for the young woman to spend time in the women's temples. Here she would be instructed in certain practices such as exercises, chants, dance to direct her awareness to certain parts of her body and bring her into conscious communion with her inner mysteries. These teachings were given gradually as she grew and developed. She was introduced to practices that were time-honoured by her people and known to enhance happiness and health.

These people recognised the body as a temple in which the being lived and, just as we live in a house and are able to function in different rooms for different purposes, so too it was with the body. We have become alienated from our bodies. We have become full of judgements and fears about them.

When the midwife sees birth as a natural function of the woman's body and knows that with the right support most women have their babies naturally, then this is what happens. If, on the other hand, the midwife/obstetrician is focused on the foetal heart monitors, urine analyses, times and duration of contractions, complications, there is not space for the tuning in to what is actually happening. There is no trust in, or tuning into, the amazing capabilities of the human body.

Whereas a medically trained midwife may see that a uterus is not contracting efficiently, a traditional midwife may see that the woman is feeling unsafe, or is anxious about this baby she is carrying. She may be wanting somebody who is in the room to not be there, or she may be wanting somebody else to be there. The birthing woman's total being is the primary event.

Most midwifery practice looks at secondary events that are expressions of the primary event. The primary thing that is happening is available to the midwife if she is receptive to it. It is transmitted by a wavelength or vibration that she will "feel" or "see" or "intuit". To do this she must be able to let the information in, know how to understand it and how to respond appropriately. This we can see as the requirement for responsible practice - an ability to respond.

How is it then that some midwives can do this more easily than others? I think it is related to the degree to which she is in touch with, or tuned into, her own reality. Her reality is her own truth, a part inside her that she actually is, not something that she has had imposed on her from others, be they parents, schools, peers or society. We all have an inner knowing part that lives always inside us to which we have access in varying degrees. It is the development of this crucial part of a human being that leads to living in harmony with the natural order of things and enables manifestation of that order. Birth is an event where the natural order displays itself strongly and majestically and reminds us of what we are all a part of. It is crucial, in my view, that this happens as often as possible and it is the office of the midwife to facilitate this.

With the barrage of Western technological development which, in its own right is quite magnificent, the natural process of birthing the next generation has been undermined. The homebirth movement, to which we are committed, has been the guardian and keeper of the truth. Between us we have a vast store of knowledge and it is, I think, our task to teach this. We need many colleges of midwifery being established and open to all women who want to honour the midwife who dwells within. We need to remember that mid-wife means with-woman and it will be women themselves who claim their heritage and support each other and bring into their everyday lives the strength, power, wisdom and compassion of the midwife.

If this is to happen, women need to focus on this and put aside dissension towards each other. Solidarity and loving cheerfulness will bring about change more quickly than anything else. When we work together to support women giving birth, the power of creation lives vitally within us and there is nothing we cannot do.

A person who has birthed her own baby is a woman liberated from the constrictions of a society that says you must rely on things and people outside yourself. A baby born naturally knows that the natural order works for him/her and that it is his/her attunement to it that brings about his/her success.

As this planet heals herself and awakens us to our role as co-creators of our future, each of us becomes a midwife at the birth of the new.

*Shivam Rachana*

(Edited from International Homebirth Conference, Sydney University)

*"A bird doesn't sing because it has an answer, it sings because it has a song."*

Maya Angelou

## Midwife- Mother- Woman

> *Drugs, machinery, and medical personnel are no match for a woman's own intellect and intuition. Birth is sexual and spiritual, magical and miraculous—but not when it is managed, controlled, and manipulated by the medical establishment, or hindered by the mother's own mind.*
>
> —LAURA SHANLEY

As with all the roads I take, the journey to becoming a midwife was not an easy one. The road was full of alienation and powerlessness. My ideas of what midwifery is seemed to be very different one to what midwifery actually is in our culture. Midwife means 'with woman' and I felt like anything but 'with woman' when I was thrown into the system. Rather, I was 'with institution', 'with policy and procedure', 'with fear-mongers'.

I was distressed at the thought that most of my colleagues thought of childbirth as a dangerous medical condition, a disaster waiting to happen. Interventions were rife and most of them were unnecessary. And then the ones that were necessary were only necessary because of trouble that was stirred from a different intervention earlier on in the labour.

In the system, midwifery seemed to be a shift of paperwork, charts, dilation, reporting to doctors and medication. Supporting the woman seemed to be of less importance. As long as the I's were dotted and the T's were crossed, and you didn't deviate from hospital policy, then you did well on your shift. I know that sounds harsh, and I know it isn't the case with all midwives, but working in the system, no matter how gentle, trusting or compassionate you are, you are still working in a system that is run on policy, protocol and guidelines, not women's wants. As compassionate woman, and as birthing mother, I felt wounded as I both witnessed and participated in this system.

In some hospitals, during handover, jokes were made about the women. In one small public hospital, if a woman had a lot of interventions during her birth, she was referred to as 'a hamburger with the lot'. If she had a birth plan she was 'a hippy' and if she refused intervention she was 'one of those people'. The word 'empowerment' was laughed at. At another hospital, the staff referred to their workplace as 'the sausage factory' – so many women coming in, almost on a conveyer belt, labeled and tagged, timed, poked and prodded, washed and cleaned then shipped off to the next ward. The more efficient the midwife was, the more she was praised for her 'good work'.

Something else I noticed was the lack of power that the women had in themselves. I noticed so many women, hundreds who I have supported, were unable to recognize their own innate authority. Even when some of the midwives I worked alongside in the hospital, sung the same heart song as my own and encouraged the birthing woman to find her birth power and trust in herself, many times, we went unnoticed and the women had no belief in their own abilities. Our culture has come to rely on technology and we have handed over a part of ourselves and our babies to the system. This makes us lose trust in ourselves, then we feel powerless and start to think we need saving. It has been so sad to witness.

Working in the world of birth, I witnessed violence against women by both doctors and midwives. I experienced horizontal violence from midwives. It seems that horizontal violence amongst midwives is extremely common, which is such a shame as midwives need to be in sisterhood, standing alongside and encouraging one another. In my student years, I noticed how some midwives were more close-knit than others. Some hospitals, there was an obvious hierarchy among themselves on who ruled the roost. Another hospital had midwives with philosophies around birth that were so extreme to each other that they often referred to each other in cruel and unkind ways. I have come to notice that midwives are people with a strong belief in birth - for some midwives, it is the belief that birth is dangerous and a disaster waiting to happen and for others, it is the belief that birth is as safe as life gets. These polarities in the midwives beliefs made it very hard for me to be able to practice in the way I wanted to, even though I have always practiced in evidence based, informed choice, culturally sensitive and women centered way. Not only this, but I really felt uncomfortable having conversations with many of the midwives, because I knew that they would completely disagree with the way that I birth and parent my children and I just didn't want my personal life to become a big debate in the tea room at work.

As a student Midwife, I was like a sponge - absorbing all this information around women, birth, life, and babies. I did have my philosophies and ideals around birth, but I never forced them on to anyone. My belief in my role as midwife is to give women information – all the information - and then the woman decides what to do with that information and then you support her and honour her through that journey. As a mother of 6 children where I experienced 2 hospital births, 1 birth centre birth and 3 unassisted home births, I can honestly say that just because I have chosen to birth in the way that I have, that those choices are definitely not for everyone. It is not that my choice might be better than your choice; it is that my choice might be different to your choice. And different is ok. What I did hate seeing in the system however, was that women were often given very little or no choice, they were often coerced or pressured and then were still led to believe that it was them that made all the decisions in their care. The times where woman were given information, it was often only a half-truth or information that wasn't evidence based or woman centered. A lot of the time, it was that the woman just wasn't given enough information for her to make an informed choice. I remember reading somewhere that you cannot make an informed choice if you don't know what your choices actually are.

## The Wild Rainbow

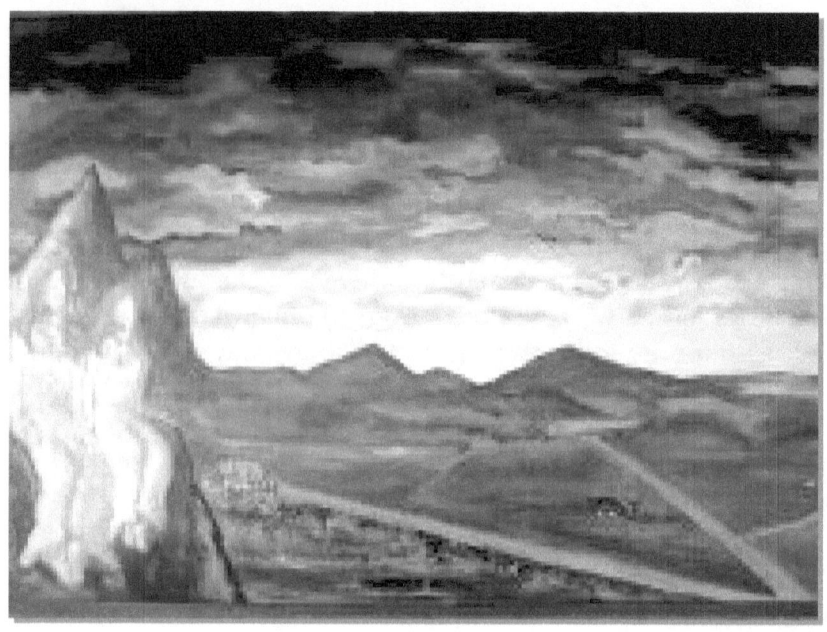

*"Dreams"* –Artist: Annie Joy

Being a student midwife was always a tough gig. It was always hard to know when to speak up, when to stand back, when to actively participate or when to just shut off and hold your tears back until you get 5 minutes to go and cry in the bathroom all on your own. If it wasn't hard enough dealing with all the horizontal violence from the midwives, many of the doctors I met as a student were simply revolting. In my ideas and ideals around birth, where I feel that birth is considered an initiation and a rite of passage that is sacred, to be met with midwives and doctors who thought of birth as something undignifying and dangerous was really traumatic for me to experience. To see such health care professionals come from such a fear based placed was scary. And it was also dangerous. Women need to be held, supported and trusted in childbirth. This brings them to a place of empowerment. Going into the hospital system as a student, I was shattered to see that women as mothers were not honoured as they should be. I felt like they were lied to, deceived and not properly cared for. So many times I felt as though I was out of my depths, in a foreign place, in the wrong place - a place that was wearing my heart out. I didn't think I was going to be able to finish.

## *Rose Between The Thorns*

One night, on my 2nd year of midwifery, I was assigned to look after 'Bed 8'. 'Bed 8' was actually a woman, and her name was Leah. I hate when they call the women by their room number. It is disturbing to see women reduced to numbers like that. Anyway, I went in to introduce myself to Leah, who was in good established labour. As I walked in the room, she had a beautiful, strong contraction that would bring her to her knees. When it started to fade, she would rise and breathe calmly and sip some juice. She was coping well. She had her husband in the room, massaging her on her demand. She had juice and barley sugars to keep up her energy and her body was changing positions, moving in a way that brought relief for her. Leah was a part of a public hospital system that was privately owned. So it meant if she wanted to birth her baby in that particular hospital she would need to 'be delivered' by one of the obstetricians.

The obstetrician she chose was the one whom I clashed most with. It was as though we were from completely different planets, our views were so extreme from one another and we found each other most challenging to work with. He had a piece of paper at the midwives desk which outlined what times he wanted to be called, what drugs women were to have, and what position he wanted the woman to be in while he 'delivered her'. All 'his women' were to be in lithotomy by the time he walked in the door. If you called him too late or too soon, all hell would break loose. The midwives were all scared of him.

Leah's labour progressed steadily and powerfully. It wasn't long before she was starting to feel pressure in her bowel. Everything was going perfectly and naturally. She was on all fours as it was helping her cope with the pressure and internal stretching. Her eyes were closed and she was concentrating. The lights were dim. The midwife I was working with shuffled a little nervously and said 'it's time to call the Doctor' and she scurried out of the room. For the next 20 minutes, Leah was involuntary pushing with her contractions. Her body was working as nature had intended it. I put wet, hot face washers on her sacrum and cold ones on her forehead. Her eyes remained closed as she focused on the incredible and intense work she was doing.

# The Wild Rainbow

And then the Doctor came in. He switched the lights on which broke our dim, dark and quietly held space. He looked at me, then looked at Leah who was still on all fours. Then looked back at me.

"Are you supposed to be looking after her?" he grumbled.

I answered him yes and he roared at me like a monster, which made me feel shaky and nervous. I felt like a little child who had done something wrong.

"Get her on her back; I am not a bloody vet. How am I supposed to get this child out?" I stood there stunned. The Midwife looked at me nervously and said 'why didn't you get her on her back?', then quietly scurried over to the Doctor and Leah and told her to change positions.

Once Leah was lying flat on her back, the Doctor took the vacuum off the trolley. There was no indication what so ever other than the Doctor's impatience and love of control that warranted the use of the vacuum. He told the midwife to set it up for him while he started to do a vaginal examination without even asking Leah. Then he reached over to the delivery trolley (which I name 'the torture trolley'. It is there for episiotomies, clamping and cutting cords, and generally just for hurting women and babies) and then proceeded to cut an episiotomy. This again, was without consent. He actually did all of this without even telling her what was happening. All he said to her was, "I'm just getting your baby out now. You have to stop yelling."

He grunted and mumbled a lot, and generally looked tired and grumpy. He put the vacuum cup on her baby's head and pulled and pulled. It hurt my heart – I felt so wounded to be witness to such violence. After many hard, violent pulls of the vacuum on the baby's head, she was finally born, a little blue baby yanked out unnecessarily and brutally from her mother's body. She was thoroughly rubbed with a rough towel, despite her vigorous crying. Cord cut, baby dried and then finally given to Leah.

"You need a couple stitches, not many" he lied, still not even looking her Leah's face.

"Thank you" she said to him. I cringed inside and felt nauseous when I heard her thank him.

I asked Leah what her babies name was. "Rose" she said. I looked at the midwife who was anxious and flustered, and scurrying around to the orders of the Doctor. I looked at the doctor, with his bloodied hands and his old, uncaring face.

"That's beautiful" I said to Leah. "I like that name".

And although my thoughts were wandering to the trauma I had witnessed, I held my heart in my hands as I showed her gentleness and compassion whilst acknowledging the journey she had just been on to bring her child earthside.

May we all be held in gentleness and peace, I thought. And I went into the bathroom and cried.

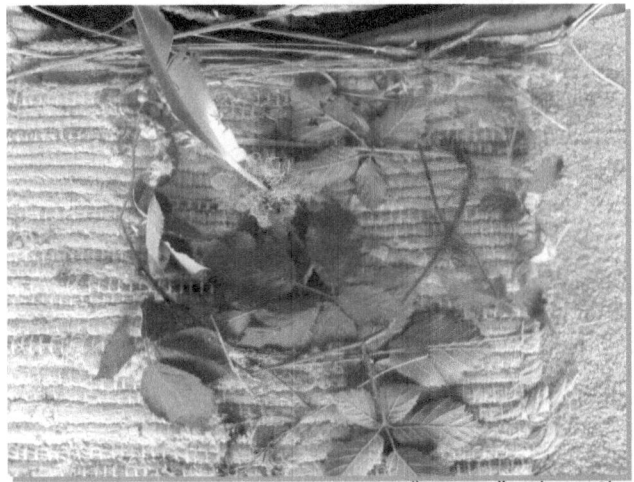

*"Autumn"* – Photo: Sheree Stewar

## *Big Dreamings - finishing my degree, finding my feet, holding my heart.*

Even with the mountain of stress that came with completing my course, I still managed to do it.

Love, awe and an overwhelming passion for supporting women during birth is why I continued on to finish my degree with the hope that I could one day be the one advocating and being with women as they traverse the world of birth and motherhood.

Through the many struggles and wounds to my heart to finish my bachelor of midwifery, I remember the day when my piece of paper came in the mail to remind me that following my heart is all worthwhile. Event through the hard times, I feel as though my calling to be this, to be a midwife, is what I am supposed to do. A part of my nature is that I dream big and I believe in the impossible, so once I set my mind to what I am going to achieve, I go out and achieve it, no matter how difficult or impossible it seems. I refuse to place limits on myself. I refuse to live a life half lived.

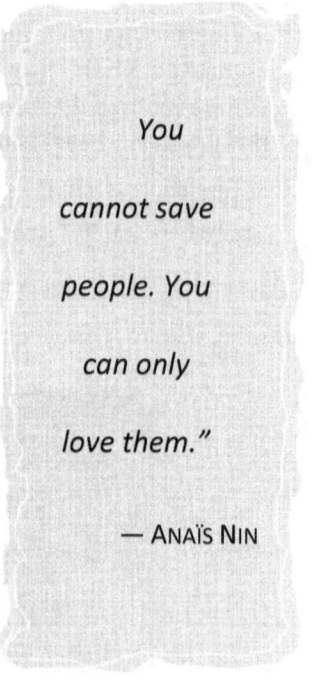

*You cannot save people. You can only love them."*

— ANAÏS NIN

I've had people ask me how I have gotten so far in my life. Was I bought up with luck, money and a positive nurturing support network and family? Was I encouraged to go out there and live my life to my potential? As a part aboriginal young woman who grew up as the only aboriginal family in the small redneck, racist town, I can tell you that I have lived my life and gotten this far not because of privilege. As the daughter of a working class family who lived around alcoholics, drug addicts, violence and pedophiles, I can tell you that I got where I am now not by being privileged. Nothing has ever been handed to me on silver platter. I got where I am from working really fucking hard and because I believed I could. I believe it to be possible to live authentically and to your potential without selling your soul to the system, even when you only have the bare essentials. The choices I make have more to do with my view of the world and making do with what I have. It's about working towards my dreams in a real, honest way. I would hate to look back on my life in regret that I didn't live with heart and soul. And I also want my children to be proud of me. I want them to look at their mother and feel proud that I got to where I am today with passion and integrity.

My big dreaming was that I was going to get out there in the world and make a difference. I was not going to live and work and hate what I do, or even feel 'just ok' with it. I was not going to live and work in anger, pity, sympathy, disgust or judgement, like I see so many others doing. I was going to live and work from my heart, in integrity, kindness and compassion, just as my Nan always taught me. And I was going to do all this in my own way.

I didn't need to go out and change the world with loudspeakers, yelling to the world what is wrong with it, what we are all doing wrong that is creating the demise of our planet. I didn't need to hold up big signs and yell at the system from outside its big, ugly grey walls on how it rapes women and steals their baby's spirits. And at times, there isn't anything wrong with that. In fact, we need that. But just not from me.

I was determined to play my part in the world in my own quiet way. In tenderness, in stillness, in the fleeting moments that people will remember forever. Completing my degree was my stepping stone to make a difference and change the world we live in for the better in my own way. One gentle word at a time. One act of kindness at a time. There were many reminders to me during my course of how I work with quiet integrity, compassion and non-judgment.

Sharing a tear as a grieving woman tells me how her husband isn't with her in the labour ward because he died just a month ago. Giving my hand to a woman to hold as she stares and cuddles the baby she gave birth to 3 days prior for the very last time before she went to her adoptive family. Sharing laughter with a big Greek family as they celebrate loudly and joyously the birth of their daughter and first grandchild from both sides of the family. Telling a woman and meaning it with my heart whose face was disfigured in the middle of the night by 'the devil men' on their horses in Southern Sudan that she is beautiful. Reminding women when they are in the throes of labour that they are strong and powerful and they can absolutely birth their babies with their strength and determination. Holding a woman close to me as she births her baby alone, with no other support in her life at all. Cuddling a heroin addicted baby and singing her songs in a darkened room, with a gentle voice. Telling the police officers who had to be present during the labour and birth of a prisoner that she does not have to be shackled to the bed while she laboured. Shedding a tear of awe at every single earthside arrival of a baby I am witness to.

I worked so hard through my course with the dream that I could one day be she who is advocating and being with women as they traverse the world of birth and motherhood. I wanted women to feel like Goddesses when they birthed, like they were honoured and supported for being the vessel that brings forth human life. I wanted them to feel that their needs were met, that their dreams and fears were listened to. I wanted them to feel as though they were the only thing in the world that mattered, for they are indeed a whole world, creating and bringing forth the next generation.

I want my work life and home life to come together in some way. I want the women who pay for my services to not be thought of and treated as clients. I want us to all be equal and loving and true to each other. I could envision myself as Old Grandmother Midwife, still answering the call of her heart, attending births where the birthing mother was once a wee babe who I caught in my own hands many years before. I want the babies, as they grow up, to come over and pick fruit off the trees and collect eggs from the chooks and have cold lemonade with me as their mothers and I chat about life and children and the simplicity and complexity of being human.

I would be a part of their lives in some small way forever. I don't believe it to be healthy, or even possible (even if you never see the person again physically but it is on an energetic level) that you can be a part of something so intimate with someone and then just disconnect yourself from them, unless you do a lot ritual work or cleansing work with the intention of disconnecting any energetic link that has come from the interactions you have had with them. It brings to my mind the idea of the ancient Chinese proverb of the red thread. *The invisible red thread connects those who are destined to meet regardless of time, place or circumstance. The thread may stretch or tangle, but it will never break.*

And I wholeheartedly agree with that. And although I understand that it doesn't mean that everyone who I am connected to through the red thread will be friendly or understanding or a good person. But it gives me a reminder that for what I want to do with my life, who I want to become, what I want to work with, that by working in a field where I am an advocate and a support for women, children, families and communities, the energetic ties that I do have via the red thread are, from my end, ones of integrity, kindness, compassion, honesty and an open heart.

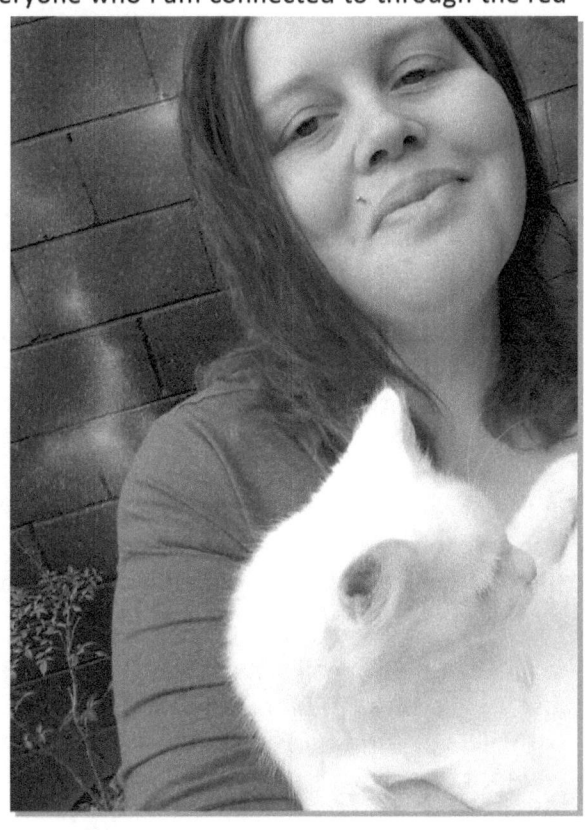

*"Selfshot"* – Photo: Sheree Stewart

These are all the reasons why I continued on with the struggle of getting the piece of paper, of becoming a midwife. I could see where my heart was. I could see how I could change the world in my own quiet way, in my own sweet time. I continued even though I struggled because I never lost sight of what I wanted to be, who I wanted to be. I could see the path of my future and this is what I saw. It was challenging at times, but it was beautiful. And it was incredibly fulfilling. And this, I know, was my contribution this Earth.

## *Ruby with a Red Bow - A Tale of Adoption*

During my life as a student midwife, I was assigned to do some work at a special care nursery. It was a level 2 nursery, not a NICU (neonatal intensive care unit), so we didn't have any very premature or sick babies. It was mostly the babies transferred from NICU after they were stable so they could 'fatten up'. There was often NASS babies (babies with addictions, mostly narcotics); a few sets of twins and 1 set of triplets, a baby under triple light photo therapy and a hypoglycaemic baby on I.V glucose.

On this particular day, I saw a big, beautiful baby who was obviously full term. I wondered why she was in the nursery when she looked obviously healthy and vigorous. The nurse I was working with must have seen me looking at her and came over and said that the baby was being adopted. The 'new parents' were waiting in the tea room, filling out paperwork. As she said that, a couple walked through the heavy nursery door and came towards us. "They are the birth parents; they've come to give her a bath. Do you want to help them?"

I said yes, but I did feel nervous. Actually, I had butterflies in my stomach. I didn't really know what to say. The usual 'congratulations' just wasn't going to work. So I just said 'are you going to give her a bath? I'll get some towels'. I felt silly that I was so anxious, so when I went to the linen cupboard, I made a conscious effort with my breathing and my mind. It immediately made a difference to my state of mind and I was able to return to them calmly and lovingly and with compassion.

Whilst we were setting up for the bath, they casually explained that they were going home after they gave Ruby a bath because her new parents are here waiting for her. Outwardly, they didn't seem overly emotional or distressed, which is how I had imagined it would be like for someone adopting out their baby. I didn't ask any questions and I never found out why they weren't keeping her, although I was curious and had often wondered since then. Ruby was in the bath, relaxing deeply into the arms of the woman who had just birthed her. She enjoyed it thoroughly and didn't cry, just a quick yelp once she was lifted out of the warm bath, and into the cool air.

She was dressed slowly and gently with carefully chosen clothes that Ruby's birth parent would meet her in. Her little white cotton dress and a white knitted cardigan fit perfectly over her soft skin. She had thick, wavy black hair and a fringe so long and thick that it that fell over her eyes. Her birth mother got a sparkly red ribbon which she tied on to her hair. She looked so beautiful but my heart twisted in sadness. I knew that these were the last moments that Ruby was going to be in the presence of her birth parents before she was to be handed over to her adoptive parents.

Her mother started to have tears well up in her eyes as she was gazing into the eyes of this sweet baby. I sat next to her unobtrusively, and she leaned over and grabbed on to my hand. I didn't resist, I held back on to her hand and gripped it firmly so she could feel supported. After a minute, when she released her hand from mine, I left the husband and wife together to have their last moment with Ruby.

I often thought of Ruby after that day. Hoping that she would grow up happy and that her adoptive parents gave her what she needed. I will always remember her sweet little face with the sparkly red bow tied to her hair. I thought about Ruby's birth mother, and how her life unfolded for her.

A week later, on the 2nd last day of my placement, the special care nursery received a thank you card from the birth mother. It read 'Thanks to the nurses and midwives who showed us kindness'. And under it, it had the names of the staff that showed her kindness. And one of them was mine.

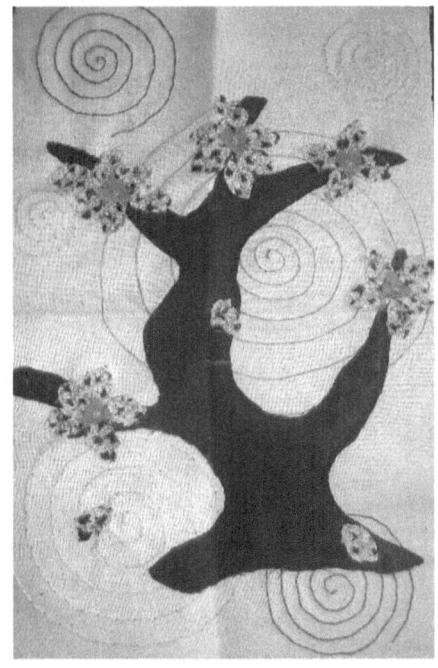

*"Birth Flag"* - Brooke Patel

## *Baby Lavender - the life and death of.*

Amel had been in the antenatal ward for a week or so with high blood pressure, which eventually turned into Pre-Eclampsia. She was pregnant with her 1st baby. I met her when she came to the birth suite, and I was the Midwife on duty.

As soon as she was wheeled into the birth suite, my heart started to ache. I knew this was going to be a hard day for her. She had started bleeding, it was painless, but she was bleeding nonetheless. Her blood pressure was abnormally high and she had all the signs of Pre-Eclampsia. I introduced myself to her and asked her how many weeks pregnant she was. "23 weeks and 6 days" she said, sobbing. Her husband was standing in the corner with dark circles under eyes, he had been having sleepless nights, I could see.

The room was full of people - Doctors, Consultants, Midwives and a Paediatrician. I felt so overwhelmed for Amel. She had choices to make and they had to be quick. I listened to the baby's heart rate. 164 beats per minute. Great, perfect.

The Paediatrician stepped in front of the cavalry and asked what she wanted to happen with the baby. The baby would still be very small, 24 weeks old. The baby could survive with months and months of intensive care. Did she want her baby resuscitated? She had to make the decision fast. The Doctor stepped in. Was she aware she would be going to a High Dependency Unit or Intensive Care Unit after the baby was born by caesarean? She had to think quickly. She was bleeding more heavily now.

I asked Amel if there was anything I could do for her. "Don't leave me" she said. So I stayed.

The events blurred passed. It all went quickly but it was all so emotionally charged it also seemed to take forever. The placenta was tearing itself off the wall of the uterus - placental abruption is its medical name. The caesarean was done at an extraordinary fast rate. Jay, her husband was not allowed to come into the operating theatre as Amel was going to be under general anaesthetic (G.A)and hospital policy is no one but medical staff allowed in theatre when there is a GA.

> Beauty is life when life unveils her holy face. But you are life and you are the veil. Beauty is eternity gazing at itself in a mirror. But you are eternity and you are the mirror.
>
> — Kahlil Gibran

Once the GA had taken effect, Amel had sticky tape put over her eyes and a tube down her throat so that it could do her breathing for her.

The surgeon started cutting, and then pulling Amel's abdomen and uterus. I prayed silently.

Baby was born. It's a boy! A beautiful perfect boy. He was so small, he reminded me of one of my Rainbow Brite dolls I had as a child.

He wasn't crying. I listened to his heart. He had a faint heart beat and it was slowing.

He was dying right in front of me.

My heart was breaking. This little man was dying and his mother was anaesthetised and unconscious. His Father wasn't allowed to be in the theatre. So it was just me. I wrapped him in a blanket with patterns of blue flowers and lavender and held him to my chest until his heart stopped beating.

I carried him to his Father so that they could meet. "I'm sorry Jay". He didn't want to hold his son at this moment so I told him I would take him down stairs with me, back to the ward.

I had a special task to do. My shift had just finished and the Midwife who was assigned to take over from me came and greeted me and said 'I'll take it from here, you go home'. But how could I? I spent the whole of this child's life with him. I witnessed his birth and his death. I couldn't just leave until I felt it was completed. The midwife mumbled something about me not getting overtime and walked out of the room as I prepared myself for the next part.

## The Wild Rainbow

I made a memory folder for his Mother and Father who would never get to hold him, who would never get to experience his expression and life pulse. I dressed Baby Lavender in a golden yellow nightgown, and re-wrapped him in his blue flower and lavender blanket. I took photos of him and put the photos of him in the memory folder. I pressed his fragile, perfect hands and feet in ink and made prints of them in his memory folder. The memory folder that was for Amel and Jay to celebrate the too short but extraordinary life of Baby Lavender.

I felt an overwhelming sense of gratitude. I felt enormous love in my heart for this baby who I felt chose me to be his carer. I was there for his birth. I was there for his death. I was there to celebrate his life and mourn his death. Amel went to the Intensive Care Unit and I never saw her or her husband again, but I sent them their memory folder and a letter which expressed my immense thankfulness for allowing me be a part of their intense journey. And I went home that day with the song of baby Lavender in my heart.

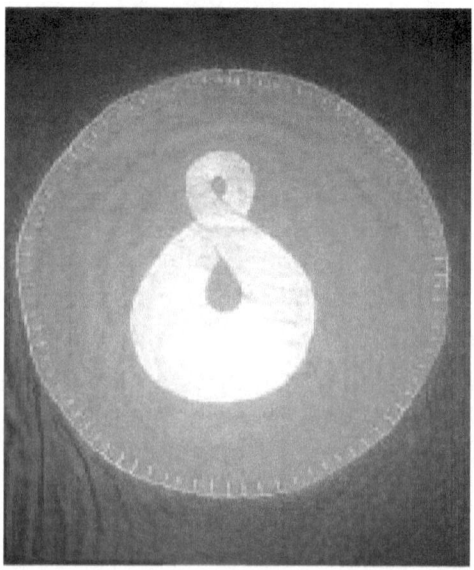

*"Birth Flag"* – Melinda Whyman

## *Standing Together – a natural birth in a high risk ward*

This was my first shift back on the ward since I resigned and I felt nervous.

I didn't want to go up to the high risk ward, but they changed my allocation and so I had to venture up there, alone. I entered through the big double doors, and they shut slowly and heavily behind me. The Midwife was sitting on her wheelie chair at the front desk, chewing on a pen, her face looking anxious and tired. There was a buzz of bright lights, doctors in their blues and overworked midwives. We were understaffed again.

The chaos and stress was evident and the sickly red walls of the midwives desk made the chaos and the buzz even louder. Someone was shouting out if the anaesthetist was ready in theatre for the twins and another woman was being wheeled passed me on her bed, apparently going to a ceaserean as well – her baby had no stomach and one kidney. Her husband was walking alongside her, his face twisted with helplessness. I felt overwhelmed about what I had just walked into. I felt scared. I could never imagine how a labouring woman would have felt safe walking through those heavy doors.

Putting my bag away, and then awaiting handover at the midwives desk, I spotted a familiar face of a Midwife who I worked with many times as a graduate. We worked well together and had a great trusting relationship with one another. When she came through the doors, I almost went running up to her to hug her I was so glad to see her. She came to the desk with the noise and the buzz and the chaos and told everyone to stop panicking. She was quickly approached by one of the afternoon staff who was concerned that 'the primip in room 7 only dilated 2 cms in 4 hours'. The midwife told her to just leave her alone and stop worrying about everything and she quickly allocated her to me and said 'people in this place don't know what midwifery led care is. You must show them. And I'll keep the doctors away'. Then she was swamped with chaos and concern and scurried off to deal with the mess.

## The Wild Rainbow

I went in the room to meet Tracy. She was doing fantastic. She was labouring well, contracting 4-5 minutes and they were strong and all consuming. I was not concerned at all about her 'slow progress'. It wasn't even slow. It was perfect. She had a dose of pethidine before my shift and was a bit sleepy. Not being able to get comfortable, I suggested a change of scenery so we wondered off together to the bathroom. She went and sat on the toilet and ended staying there for 2 hours. We kept the smallest light on so the room was dim and quiet. She alternated between the toilet and the shower, when she eventually said she was getting an urge to push.

The midwife in charge was updated with what was happening and she wanted to get Tracy up into the room seeing as though there was no birth stools in the whole ward for Tracy to sit on. She stood up and a contraction overwhelmed her body. She made a roar, primal growl and once that contraction passed, she said in a definite voice that she will not be sitting down.

I could see her body needed to stay upright to birth this baby, so I put a dry towel under her feet so that the tiled floor in the bathroom wouldn't get slippery from the wetness of birth.

The midwife in charge had a slightly panicked look on her face when she realised that Tracy was going to birth in the bathroom, in the dark, but my reassurance to her that Tracy's birth was normal and that I was confident in supporting her to birth her baby in the bathroom was enough for her to back away and leave us alone. I promised her I would tell her when I need her. Tracy pushed well, and each contraction gradually bought her baby closer and closer earthside. Her perineum stretched beautifully, a little at a time and each contraction I could see more and more of babies head emerge, I realised just how strong Tracy was. Her baby was big, with a large and not very moulded head!

The next contraction enabled her baby's body to be completely born. I caught this beautiful baby girl, plump, blue and slippery into my arms and passed her to her mother, who was ecstatic and in awe, both of her baby and of herself. Her baby was born quite quickly for a first baby and although we were interested in how much her baby weighed; we all let our curiosity subside whilst skin to sin and milky cuddles reigned. A few hours later we found out that her beautiful baby daughter was 4.7 kg and Tracy had only a small first 1st degree tear that didn't need stitches.

Speaking to her the following day, she spoke about how in awe she was of herself of birthing her baby. She spoke of how when she felt safe and supported, that her body changed somehow and she responded to her contractions in a different way. Her body's innate wisdom was telling and showing her positions to be in to birth her big baby with most ease and comfort.

I felt so inspired by her, and how once she was out of the 'labour room' and into the dimmed, private, bathroom, she opened up on all levels and was able to birth her baby undisturbed. It was one of those times when I left the hospital after working on the labour ward and actually feeling like a midwife - I was actually working in partnership 'with woman'. I went home smiling.

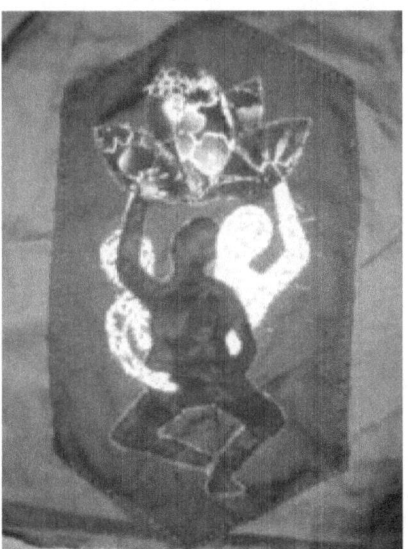

*"Birth Flag"* – Courtney Gale

> *Birth is not only about making babies. Birth is about making mothers-strong, competent, capable mothers who trust themselves and know their inner strength.*
>
> BARBARA KATZ ROTHMAN

## *The Bright-Eyed Baby and Me*

Abeba came to the hospital as soon as her waters broke at home. This was her fourth baby, and her longest labour in her previous births was 3 hours. She felt confident birthing and she wanted a homebirth with her three sisters helping her, but as she had newly arrived in Australia from Ethiopia, funds were very tight and she could not afford an independent midwife.

As her Midwife at the hospital, I listened to her babies galloping heart beat and watched unobtrusively for a moment. I felt that at that point of time there was nothing I could do for her. She was very connected to her birthing body and was deep inside herself. I dared not break her space. I did not speak after that initial introduction until she called for me to be with her, right near her baby's birth.

She laboured well, and powerfully. With each contraction she would swerve her hips and stamp her feet. She would roar loud Ethiopian words and turn and face her face to the sky, eyes closed.

She stood for her entire labour, which lasted about 1 ½ to 2 hours.

The Midwife-in-charge came storming in at one point 'just to check if everything is ok', and 'is she going to deliver soon?' I told her she was not needed at this time and I reassured her I would get her if need be. She looked at me as I was squatting on the floor behind Abeba while her body started to push.

"You will get a sore back if all of your deliveries are like this" she said as she scurried out of the door before I could reply. Abeba's husband looked at me and said 'is that a problem? Her standing? All her babies are born this way'. "No problem" I smiled. The next wave pulsated through her body and her babies beautiful head emerged at once. Lush, thick, wavy black hair and eyes that opened, wide and awake, staring at me, upside down. It was an incredible sight!

"Welcome" I whispered

I felt Abeba push and her amazing baby slid into my arms. "Abeba, bebe" I said softly as I passed her to her mother. She kissed her baby and held her, still standing. About 10 minutes later she said ever so softly 'I'm finished', as her shiny, nourishing placenta was out, no longer needed for Abeba. She wanted to lie down to breastfeed. I didn't interfere, I just let baby attach herself to her mother's breast as I went to get Abeba a warm blanket and a hot cup of tea.

I felt empowered by Abeba's confidence and trust in her birthing. I loved the simplicity of her birth and the trust that everyone in the room had for her birth to be simple and easy. I will carry the story of Abeba and her bright eyed baby with me forever.

~*~*~*~

*Birth is rolling, rumbling*
*A sacred passage way*
*No time, nor age will wipe the memory of*
*birth from a woman*
*Birth imprints*
*Empowers*
*Birth is woman*
*A wild sea of chaos, calm and lust*

- Lucy Johnston

## *Healing the Mother Wound*

### Working with birth, working with earth

My Mum's side held our aboriginal ancestry. One strand of our family coming together after the white fellas came in was as a result of my Great-Great-Granny forced into Albacutya, Antwerp Mission, which at some point travelled to Lake Boga Mission. It was there that my Great-Great-Granny met my Great-Great-Grandfather (also an aboriginal coerced into the mission). My tribes are Wergaiia and Wamba-gourmanjunyuk tribe (the thunder tribe) and my totem animals are the pelican and the black cockatoo. So much is lost from my culture. Most of what remains to my knowledge is cassette tapes that my Mumma made of interviews she had with some of our family when she was researching our ancestry. Other than that, it is just my dreaming that tells of my ancestors tales. Of what living in harmony with the Earth and living in tribal community was about.

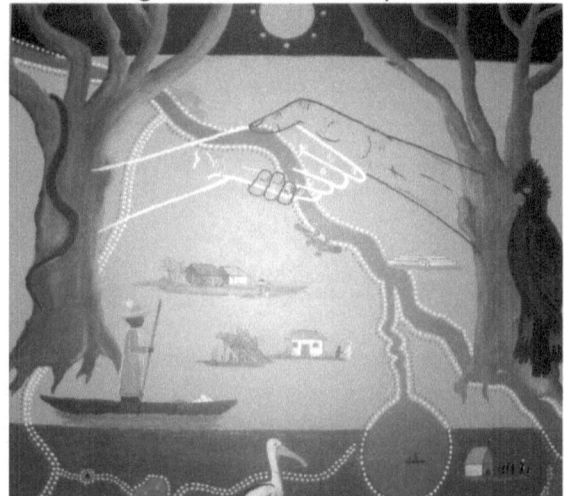

*"Together"* - Artist: Annie Joy

Spirit and heart has been viciously wiped from aboriginals in Australia. In such a short time, aboriginals were forced to assimilate into white culture. Their children were stolen, the women used as slaves while the men were left standing there hopeless and helpless as their women and children were taken from them, right before their eyes. There were many slaughters of my ancestors. Many cruel and unkind things were placed upon them.

Is it any wonder that when white man put the 'white fellas venom' in the hands of the black man, that he drank from it? Bleary eyed and a clouded drunken mind must have seemed far more tolerable than standing there in helplessness as you can do nothing but witness the obliteration of their women, their children, their land, their culture, their spirit.

With this knowledge of my family's history, it gives me insight as to why I have always felt like I am searching for meaning, why I am always so intent to connect, to plug in, to communicate, to feel a part of something that is bigger than myself. Being disconnected to my world on all levels is the biggest detriment to who I am as woman, mother, human. When I am not in harmony, I am in chaos. I am lost. And I lose sight of what I need to keep me living. I lose sight of the mother pulse, the pulse that keeps my heart beating, the beat that keeps who I am connected to the Earth Mother.

As some years passed and I journeyed further into the realm of birthwork, I started seeing the connection between our Earth and birth – how they are both linked and connected in the way earth and women are cared for, how they are treated and respected, how they are perceived to be. I started seeing 'coincidences' – seeing glimpses of 'mother' in both woman and earth and their startling similarities.

I saw the connection of when we neglect our earth mother, when we use her, rape her, destroy her, violate her; when we cut her down, drain her and take everything she has without giving back, we are left with a soulless place. A place where spirit is gone, a place that was once fertile, rich and lush is now barren and parched. And even after we take everything from Her, we still expect her to continue to give us a place to live, a place to keep us warm and safe, to feed us and grow us. If the Earth Mother isn't nourished or left to thrive in the healthy environment, then we are left with a land that can't sustain life. We are left with the Earth Mother who doesn't have the support structure, energy, essence or right environment to thrive. When we take and take, and don't give back, then eventually she dies. And when this happens, it means that those that live upon her will also die.

This is the same as our physical mother. If she isn't nourished, honoured and supported to thrive to her full potential, then she will become shriveled and sad, desolate and blank, and she won't be able to provide an adequate, nourishing, sustainable environment for her children. We need to keep mothers healthy. We need to keep them happy. We need them to know how much we love and cherish them for it is them that are the Creatrix, the world within a world.

Women as Mothers are so undervalued in our society. We are so caught up in the whole 'at least you have a healthy baby' mantra, we don't realise when we say that, we are actually just sweeping her trauma and experience under the carpet. By not validating and hearing the story that women so often try to share about their birth, then we are forgetting that woman are human beings with feelings, emotions and values that have the right to express themselves. I actually find it degrading and insulting to reduce a woman's birth experience, a huge transformative event of her life, to 'at least your baby is healthy'. The story so often happens that she leaves the hospital, usually with her broken and cut body, to her home with little support and a crying baby. She is often required to go back to work way before she is ready and she is often required to parent her children either on her own with basic support from her partner and with no other outside help. There are not many parenting in communities in the western world, except for some families living on the fringe. It is a very isolating parenting culture and this is very dangerous. If no support structures are in place and if we continue, as a culture, to undermine the important, huge work that woman as mother does, then we are going to sit back and watch our society crumble. Our Mothers will crumble under the pressure. If we take and take from our Mothers and not give anything back in return, then the future is bleak. No wonder postpartum depression is at an all time high in our culture. Although mothers are incredible, they are still mortal and just like the Earth Mother, she still needs the right conditions in order to grow and thrive if she is able to take care of the rest of us. If we continue to put so much pressure on the mother and we undermine and undervalue her, continuously taking, then it is all downhill from here. If our mothers 'die', then as her children, we all do too. Even if this isn't a physical death, it certainly is as a community, as well as emotionally and spiritually.

What can we do to heal this?

If we heal birth, we can heal the Earth..

Journeying as Sage Femme

## *Healing Birth, Healing the Earth*

@ Dr Sarah J. Buckley MD 2005 www.sarahbuckley.com
Previously published in Living Now, Winter 2002, supplement Women Now and reprinted in Living Now in May 2009.
An updated version is published in Gentle Birth, Gentle Mothering: A Doctor's Guide to Natural Childbirth and Gentle Early Parenting Choices (Sarah J Buckley MD, Celestial Arts, 2009).
Thankyou to Sarah and her publishers for permission to include this.

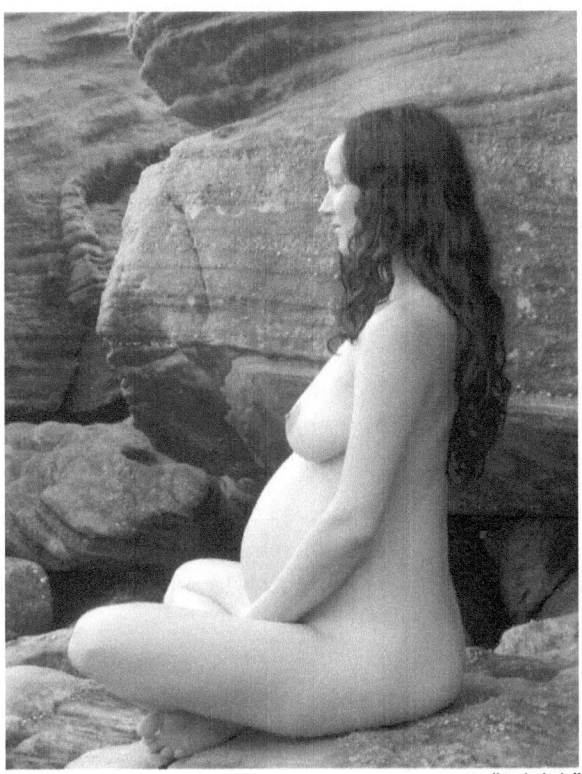

*"Talulah"* - Renee Adair

## *Birth, she is dying.*

This primal and unspeakably powerful initiation, the only road to motherhood for our ancestors, has been stripped of her dignity and purpose in our times. Birth has become a dangerous medical disease to be treated with escalating levels, and types, of technological interventions.

What is worse perhaps is that the ecstasy of Birth- her capacity to take us outside (ec) our usual state (stasis)- has been forgotten, and we are entering the sacred domain of motherhood post-operatively, even post-traumatically, rather than transformationally.

These deviations from the natural order, whose lore is genetically encoded in our bodies, have enormous repercussions.

We live in a society where new mothers have unprecedented levels of distress and depression, and where our babies, with their colic, reflux, and sleep problems, are also having their distress medically treated. We live in a society where depression and anxiety are among the largest burdens of disease worldwide, according to the World Health Organisation, and children as young as four are being diagnosed with these conditions; and where young people, at the prime of their lives, are choosing in large numbers to opt out, with mind-altering drugs, or to opt out permanently through suicide.

More than this we have set ourselves as a species on the road to self-destruction through our despoiling of our collective mother, the Earth. The havoc that we wreak through waste and greed has many parallels with our treatment of mothers and babies, and of our primal environment — our mother's womb.

And just as we have pitted ourselves against the Earth, forgetting that we are interdependent, so too have we begun to pit the rights of the baby against the rights of the mother; imagining a separation, a competition that does not and cannot exist.

The wounds of Birth and of the Earth are severe but, as the Goddess Hygieia tells us, "The wound reveals the cure".[1] My belief is that we are suffering in birth from lack of passion; of love; of surrender; and from a misunderstanding of our own power, and I believe that these qualities can provide us with a way of healing birth and, at the same time, healing the earth.

## *Passion*

We all began our lives in a passionate act. Our human bodies crave the intensity and pleasure that sex brings and many cultures have recognised the capacity for healing that is inherent in the sexual act.

Why is sex so powerful? As well as giving us the potential to create new life — the ultimate power — sex involves peak experiences, and peak hormone levels, of love; pleasure; excitement; and tenderness. These hormones (our bodies' chemical messengers) and their actions are exactly the same as those of birth.

In other words giving birth is, inherently and hormonally, a passionate and sexual act. From the perspective of hormone levels in both mother and baby, we could say that birth is the most passionate experience that we will ever have.

Oxytocin, the hormone of love, builds up during labour reaching peak levels at the moment of birth and creating loving, altruistic feelings between mother and baby. Endorphins, hormones of pleasure and transcendence, also peak at birth, as well as the fight-or-flight hormones adrenaline and noradrenaline (epinephrine and norepinephrine). These fight-or-flight hormones protect the baby from lack of oxygen in the final stages of birth and ensure that mother and baby are both wide-eyed and excited at first contact. Prolactin, the mothering hormone, helps us to surrender to our babies, giving us the most tender of maternal feelings as our reward.

But these passionate hormones are not just feel-good add-ons. They actually orchestrate the physical processes of birth (and sexual activity) and enhance efficiency, safety and ease for both mother and baby. This hormonal cocktail also rewards birthing mothers with the experience of ecstasy and fulfillments, making us want to give birth again and again. All mammals share virtually the same hormonal crescendo at birth, and this is a necessary pre-requisite for mothering in most species, switching on instinctive maternal behaviour.

Birthing passionately does not necessarily mean birthing painlessly (although this may happen for some women). Giving birth is a huge event, emotionally and physically, and will make demands on the body equivalent to, for example, running a marathon. But when a woman feels confident in her body, well supported, and able to express herself without inhibition, the pain that she may feel can become easily bearable and just one part of the process. She can then respond instinctively with her own resources, including her most basic and accessible tools: breath, sound and movement.

The problem in our times is that the passion of birth is neither recognised nor accommodated. Birth has become a dispassionate medical event, usually occurring in a setting that discourages emotional expression. If we are to reclaim our birthing passion, we must give ourselves permission to birth passionately and we must choose our birth setting and birth attendants with this in mind. It is likely that birth in these circumstances will be easier, helping us to step into new motherhood gently and gracefully. Passion is, to my mind, an opposite and an antidote for despair and depression. This is clear physiologically and hormonally.

If we give birth, and are born, in passion, how different would our primal emotional imprint be? And what about our brain chemistry, which is being set even as we are born? Some studies have linked exposure to drugs and procedures at birth with an increased risk of drug addiction, suicide and anti-social behaviour in later life, and other commentators have suggested that contemporary problems such as learning disorders and ADHD may also be linked to drugs and interventions at birth.

As a birthing mother I have both witnessed and experienced the enormous passion that can be unleashed at birth, and that can fuel both passionate motherhood and a lifetime's work on behalf of mothers, babies and the earth, and I ask: "Can we afford, as a species, to be born, and to give birth dispassionately?"

## *Love*

Passion and love are as powerful a combination at birth as they are in sexual activity. And in birth, as in sex, we release oxytocin, the hormone of love, in huge quantities. Here again, our hormones are directing us toward optimal and ecstatic experiences yet this system is also extremely vulnerable to interference.

For example a labouring woman's production of oxytocin is drastically reduced by the use of epidural pain relief — this is the reason why epidurals prolong labour. And even when an epidural has worn off her oxytocin peak, which causes the powerful final contractions that are designed to birth her baby quickly and easily, will still be significantly lessened and she is more likely to have her baby pulled out with forceps as a result.

The drug syntocinon (pitocin), which has been called the most abused drug in obstetrics, is also implicated. It is a synthetic form of the hormone oxytocin, and is used for induction and for augmentation (or acceleration) of labour. Large numbers of women giving birth in developed countries receive large doses of this drug in labour for one of these reasons. For example, in Australia this figure approaches 50 percent.

When a labouring woman has syntocinon administered by drip, for induction or augmentation, her body's oxytocin receptors may lose their sensitivity and ability to respond to this hormone. We know that women in this situation are vulnerable to haemorrhage after birth, and even more syntocinon becomes necessary to counter that risk.

We do not know, however, what the long-tern consequences of interference with the oxytocin system may be for mothers and babies, and for their ongoing relationship.

I had a very powerful experience of oxytocin as the hormone of love while labouring with my fourth baby, Maia Rose. As the waves of labour strengthened I found myself looking into the eyes of my beloved, telling him 'I love you, I love you, I love you...' as each wave of labour washed over me. This ecstatic experience has created more love in my heart, in our relationship, and in our family, and has taught me, in a very physical way, that giving birth is also making love.

## *Surrender*

Surrender is not a popular virtue. In fact, surrender is often seen as a weakness in our culture, where we are instead encouraged to be active and in control of our lives. This very yang, masculine attitude may serve us in some circumstances but we cannot birth our babies through sheer force of will. We need to learn the more subtle — yet equally powerful — path of surrender.

I sense that, for modern women, difficulty with surrender can reflect a lack of confidence in our bodies. This is not surprising when our society is distrustful of the natural order in general, and women's bodies in particular. This view is further reinforced by the obstetric model, with its long lists of all that can possibly go wrong with our birthing bodies, and its myriad of technological fixes, designed to rescue us from these exaggerated dangers.

Along with this forgetting of the awesome but natural power of our female bodies, we have also lost our birthing patrons: the goddesses and saints who have, for millennia, guided women through this transition, where the veil between life and death is at its thinnest. Today, this guidance is available to us, when and if we need it, in the living form of a midwife: a woman who has pledged to be with (mid) women (wyfe) in birth. A good midwife can remind us by her presence that we carry genetically the birthing successes of all our foremothers and that we know already how to give birth.

As midwife and author Jeannine Parvati Baker reminds us, giving birth is women's spiritual practice, requiring "...purity in strength, flexibility, health, concentration, surrender and faith."2 It has also been said that to be consciously present at birth is equivalent to seven years of meditation. When we birth consciously, putting our great rational mind on hold, and allowing our instinctive nature to dominate, we can access the wisdom that all spiritual traditions teach: that the ego is our servant, not our mistress, and that our path to ecstasy and enlightenment involves surrendering our egoic notions of control. This level of surrender will also serve us well through our many years of motherhood.

When we surrender conscious control, we also allow our deeper innate rhythms to surface: this can be a profound experience for a birthing woman. In allowing her labour to go at its own pace, without hurry or interference, a woman learns to trust her own, and her baby's, natural rhythms. Such trust is another gift; another way that Mother Nature ensures optimal mothering and maximum survival for our young.

In surrendering to birth, we also learn about our role on the earth: we are neither the rulers nor the architects of creation. Life comes through us, simply and gracefully, when we allow it.

## *Power*

It is easy to say that our problems in birth stem from the excessive power of the medical system and its agents, and a lack of power for the birthing woman. However a deeper analysis is necessary, I believe, because the time has come to dispel this idea of a power imbalance and to assert our innate authority in birthing.

We live in a culture that prizes, and puts its faith in, technology. We reward those, such as doctors, who are masters of technology and indeed we are fortunate to have their skills available to us when we need them. And even though we may want less technology in birth, we are witnessing more and more litigation against obstetricians, almost all of which blames them for not using enough technology.

Along with technology, we also prize information. In pregnancy and birth, becoming informed is equated with being responsible, both of which are strongly encouraged culturally; yet there is also a price to pay. We may have all of the information in the world, but we cannot predict our experiences in birth. And we diminish our own authority in birthing and in mothering — we disempower ourselves — when we put more faith in information from the outside (tests, scans, others' opinions) than our own internal knowing of our bodies and our babies.

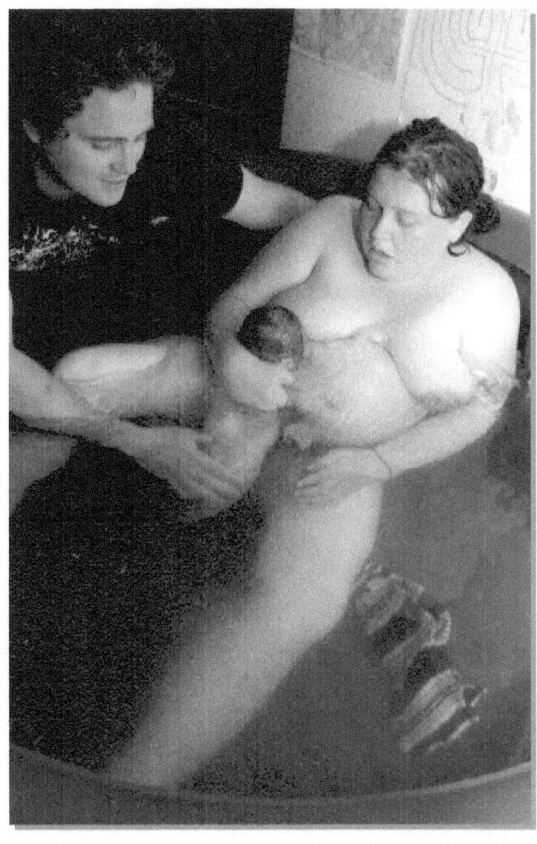

"Myah's Birth" – Photo: Brooke Patel Photography

The truth is that our babies are constantly informing us of their needs and desires, and how we can best care for them. This is a physiological reality — the baby's placenta is in constant communication with our bodies, transferring blood and nutrients and generating the placental hormones, which organise our bodies and our psyches for the optimal and specific mothering that this baby requires. In the same way, our cravings, yearnings, dreams, and inclinations in pregnancy can be communications from our babies, showing us the deeper ways of knowing that are richer and more true, even if less numerical or detailed, than information from the outside, such as medical tests.

In fact from the very beginning, when we first suspect that we are creating new life in our womb, we can use this ancient system and allow our bodies, rather than a pregnancy test, to inform us. Often the truth will unfold gradually, allowing us the space to learn and adapt at our own pace, and giving us opportunities for reflection and dreaming.

When we choose this traditional women's path, the path of all our foremothers, we can both discover and reinforce an inalienable trust and power in ourselves and in our female bodies. This deep faith is the best preparation possible for birth and is also, to my mind, the basis of true responsibility; we are able to respond with our own truth. We also become able to use the medical system, if we choose, without giving away our power.

Beyond this, when we tap into women's ways of knowing we can open channels of communication with our babies, enhancing the psychic powers of communication that Mother Nature intends for mothers of all species. Mothering can become a meditation; a deep mindfulness that is satisfying spiritually as well as physically and emotionally. Again I believe that this is nature's intent and a possibility for all of us.

How would it be to live in a society where we are all, through giving birth or being born, in possession of our own power and our own deep knowing? Where science and technology are our tools, rather than our masters? How differently would we treat our babies? How differently would we treat each other? How differently would we treat the earth?

Birth is dying, but, like cells in her body, we each have the power to enliven her and to resurrect her in all Her glory. What is needed, I believe, is the collective passion, love, surrender, and power that we pour into the ether as we birth our babies.

And in healing birth, we are healing ourselves, our babies and the Earth.

~*~*~*~

Many people inspired this article. Jeannine Parvati Baker contributed some core ideas and phrases; ecstasy in birth, 'healing the earth, healing birth': 'giving birth is women's spiritual practice' and 'the wound reveals the cure', which is the canon of her Mystery school, Hygieia College. www.birthkeeper.com

Thanks also, for inspiration and ideas, to Leilah McCracken (www.birthlove.com) Michel Odent, and especially to my teacher Shivam Rachana and the women's circle that we share in the International College of Spiritual Midwifery. www.womenofspirit.asn.au

This article is also based on my research, presented in "Undisturbed Birth: Mother Nature's Blueprint for Safety, Ease and Ecstasy", and all other references will be found in that article. Both this article and Undisturbed Birth feature in my book, Gentle Birth, Gentle Mothering: The Best Articles on Gentle Choices in Pregnancy, Birth and Parenting.

~*~*~*~

References

1. Baker JP. Hygieia College Mystery School. www.birthkeeper.com.

2. Baker JP. Prenatal Yoga and Natural Childbirth. 3rd ed. Berkeley CA: North Atlantic Books, 2001.

## *Myah's birth – welcoming my baby tiger.*

> *"There is power that comes to women when they give birth. They don't ask for it, it simply invades them. Accumulates like clouds on the horizon and passes through, carrying the child with it."*
>
> *Sheryl Feldman*

I felt restless and irritated in the 2 days leading up to Myah's birth.

Nothing could take that feeling away. I was irritated that I was irritated. Felt so restless. Steven took me on drives in the car because that seemed to help. When I sat with what I was feeling I understood that those feelings were my babies more than my own. Preparing for labour must bring up those feelings in a baby. Waiting for the stars to align, for the baby to make the signals to her mother's brain to start releasing the hormones needed to bring her earthside.

On the night before she was born one of my friends suggested we go for a late night swim together. She is pregnant with her 3rd baby and we were both feeling like uncomfortable whales! I decided to just stay in. I didn't really want to leave my home.

That night I went to bed with restless legs, a restless mind and a restless baby in my womb. I barely got any sleep. I just couldn't settle. The Braxton-Hicks contractions were irritating. They had been coming since 34 weeks and I was so tired of them. I lay on the couch, I meditated, I had a shower, I wandered up and down the house. I noticed after some hours that they seemed to have a 'bite' to them and not wanting to use all the hot water for a bath in case I actually was going into labour, I woke up Steven and asked him to fill up the birth pool. We sat together while the pool was filling and he lit some of my candles that I was given on my Blessingway. We talked about how it was so exciting that we will get to meet our new baby today. What would s/he look like? What would his/her voice sound like? What will be his/her favourite things be?

Sage awoke while we were filling up the pool and she was obviously really tired but wouldn't go back to sleep for Steven. She came in the pool with me, which she loved. She paddled around, put the hose with the warm water running onto my belly. I had an empty ice cream container near me because I felt nauseous and whenever I said 'oh I feel yuck', Sage would hold the bucket up to my face, in case I needed to use it and would say to me 'Mum, yuck, yuck'. We played together in the pool for a while. She was so comfortable in there – she was back in her birth space as she was born in the same pool just 22months earlier. At some point I asked for Sage to hop out of the pool and she snuggled up with her Dad on the couch. Although I sure that I was still in the early-ish stages of my labour, I started thinking about calling on women to help with Sage as they all live 45 – 60 minutes away from me. It is always impossible to tell just how quickly or slowly birth will progress so it was all done intuitively and instinctively.

There was music playing in the background. It was very calming and it held an awesome space because it kept me calm, focused, present. When contractions came, I would close my eyes and lean against the side of the pool. Sometimes I would count when the peak of the contraction came, or I would envision myself walking through a labyrinth. When your body surrenders to the power of labour, it is easier to be in. I remember once reading in 'Ocean of Stars' by Lesley Crossingham that we all go around the medicine wheel, whether we want to or not. You can choose to go freely or you will be dragged around it with you kicking and screaming.' Remembering this, I chose to go freely. On my own. With my own instinct.

I felt really present throughout the whole labour which was unusual for me. There were still times of being swept away but even in those times, I was still aware of when there were people around, what my body was doing. Steven was doing shiatsu on my back, it was beautiful and helped me drop down further into labour. When Lauren arrived, I was deep in labour and I remember her hands were cold on mine as they touched me and she kissed my hand and my head. Brooke and Courtney and Courtney's baby arrived in song. I remember spiralling and shifting through some contractions. They were short but they were intense. I remember hearing Taioma (5months old) singing my birth song. I opened my eyes to look at her and she was looking at me, wide awake and upside down, very alert and happy and singing. It felt so right in my space. Hearing the song and being with my women and Steven there, I didn't feel I needed to make the call to anyone else at that time. I felt that when labour progressed more in the morning and the kids were awake I would call on others to come in with me.

I was starting to feel restless and irritated again. I felt that the contractions were good – they were strong and intense but they just weren't lasting long enough. When Steven and I talked about it post birth, we thought that at that point they were 4 minutes apart and only lasting 30 – 40 seconds. I felt as though I needed to get out of the pool and move around and try and shake the baby down into my pelvis a bit more as she still felt high. I got up restlessly and held onto Lauren. I didn't want to let her go, I felt safe in her arms. But the restlessness of labour swept me away and I wandered into the end bathroom. Then I wandered down to get some grapes to eat but had a strong contraction so stopped what I was doing. I went into the other bathroom and had another contraction whilst standing. Courtney came in and gave me a cuddle and told me I was beautiful and amazing. She asked if I wanted anything and I asked her to wash me some grapes. I came out of the bathroom in time to have a grape (which tasted so, so sweet!) and had another strong contraction. I leaned on the desk and Courtney massaged my sacrum – it was so heavenly, I could feel the baby descending – she was no longer high up. I managed to eat a couple more grapes and decided to go back to the birth pool.

It was when I got back into the pool that the contractions I was having were really intense. I tried to see how much I was dilated, and couldn't feel anything – nothing at all. Couldn't feel a head, a cervix, nothing, which really didn't help! I was at a point where I wanted to know how far dilated I was so I could prepare in my mind approximately how far I had to go. I faced towards Steven and said 'what if this takes 10 more hours?'. He reminded me I was doing so well and that it won't take 10 more hours, it will be before lunchtime. I was feeling so frustrated by that point. Just wanting to know how long it would take. Were the contractions going to get worse? How will I go for 10 more hours? Should I call someone else to come over now? What if the kids wake up soon and annoy me?

Around this same time, a cellular / ancestry knowing of birthing came to me. Birth takes as long as birth takes.

I felt a shift in my body. I faced towards Steven and feeling really frustrated as another contraction was coming I felt the familiar feeling of a baby travelling the last steps of the journey. It is like a tsunami wave that pushes the baby far away from where it has just been. It is a movement of travelling from one world to another.

It was at this point that Rhiannon, my 6 year old half woke up and walked out of her room, right passed where we were and Steven grabbed her in his arms and I heard him say 'Look Rhiannon, Mum is about to have a baby'. I was aware that Lauren wasn't in the room and was trying to say her name in words so her and Sage could come and the see the baby born swimming. They came out of the room in the final pushes of my labour. My baby was born into my hands and we were surrounded in complete love, awe and wonder by my husband, 2 of my daughters and 3 of my best friends. We all swelled with pride and burst with love as my 5th baby, my 4th daughter made her journey to Earth in such a peaceful, yet powerful way. It was such a beautiful, instinctive birth.

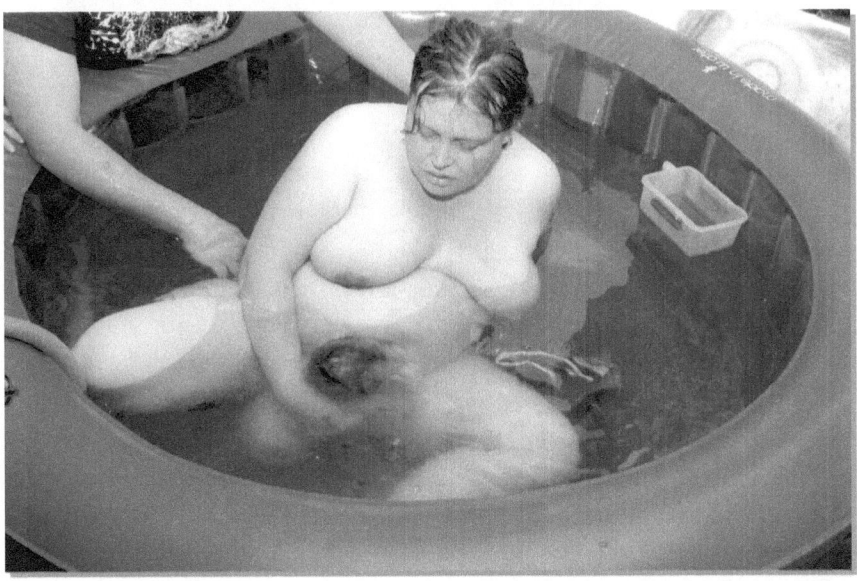

*"Baby Myah"* – Photo: Brooke Patel Photography

## *Taioma's birth – welcoming baby bear.*

told by Courtney Gale

Labor first started with a slight, steady tightening in my uterus, only enough to get my attention. This was around 11.30am.

As my labor with Simi (first born) was 16 hours long, I imagined I would be at this for a long time to come so tried not to get too excited. I was a little surprised, as I had imagined labor starting during the night and waking up with contractions as I had with Simi. I had heard so many stories about mothers going into labor when their other children were asleep or absent, so I wasn't expecting things to start in the middle of the morning. I went about my day, trying to predict what I might want to eat for dinner, so began cooking.

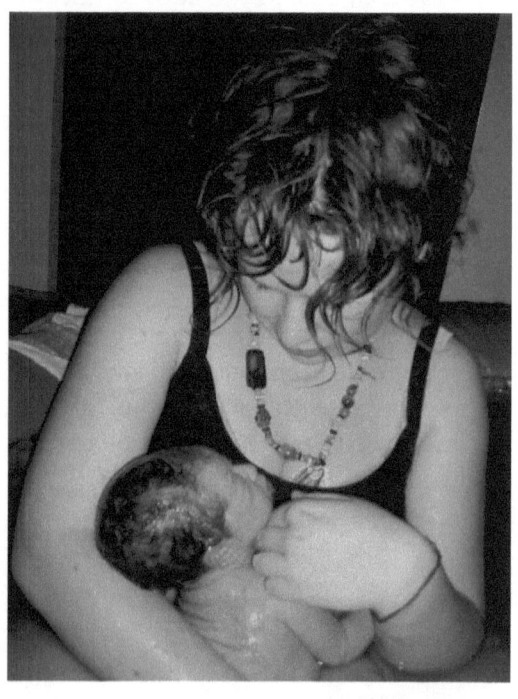

*"Courtney and Taioma"* – Photo: Sheree Stewart

At one point, I made a conscious decision to open and expand, so as each contraction came, I paused for a moment, expanded my vagina and imagined my cervix softening. It was around 12.30pm that I called my mum to tell her I thought things were starting and she reminded me not to get too excited – how could I not though?

Simi was showing signs of being tired, so I put her on the breast to fall asleep, looking forward to some time alone. Her suckling brought on the contractions more, which worried me as I was only in very early hours of this... How full on was this labor going to get!?!

Around 2pm I contacted my doulas via SMS to prepare them that they might be attending a birth very soon. Sheree replied immediately saying that if my little bear was to come on her birthday (also that day) that my cub would have to hurry up! I also rang Leo at work, letting him know I would like him home as soon as possible, as contractions were starting to take much of my attention. When Leo got home he put up my birth flags. These flags were so wonderful! I felt so loved and supported receiving each one from women in my community. Looking around the room at them even months after giving birth reminded me that I was not alone, my feelings were normal and many other women experience the same thoughts – to their lovers, children, society. Every piece of the flag unique, as each woman is. Some had writing; others had beads, spirals, feathers or handprints. One I particularly remember was a transfer of a Tarot card which had fallen out of the deck, picking itself for me – 'Trust', which had been my journey through this pregnancy. Trusting myself to become a mother of two and of having enough love. Trusting my body to free birth. Trusting that if something did happen, there would be time to transfer to a hospital. Trusting my baby's ability to form herself to her perfection, without observing or checking on her progress through ultrasound waves.

It was early afternoon that we contacted Leo's parents to let them know they would soon be grandparents again! Leo's mum Fane had been at our first birth, a gorgeous, concerned, furrow browed Fijian woman, who was ready to jump up and help at every given moment. She was the opposite of my mum who had also been there and was grinning the entire way through (though also keen to support). Fane was keen to attend this birth, but I didn't feel the want or need to have her there – as this birth was a completely new journey for me. I saw myself being surrounded and supported by my woman tribe, my friends and sisters.

Sheree was amazing at keeping in contact with me... asking me if I needed anything and when she should come. My answer was always "I think I'm still in early stages and I'll be at this for hours!" She told me she would come around anyway, just to hang out. On her way she let Lex know her plans, so she followed suit.

By the time Sheree arrived I was sitting against an electronic shiatsu massager and was starting to drift inwards, still opening and expanding. She got straight to work setting up the birth pool with Simi,

# The Wild Rainbow

2 years 9 months old assisting her. Between contracts I snuck peeks at this process, loving seeing one of my best friends support my first daughter in this transition to becoming a big sister. Simi's squeals of delight were beautiful to hear, as she played naked in the pool with the water level rising around her. Her curly blonde hair looking angelic through my endorphin influenced gaze.

When Lex arrived she travelled straight to the kitchen, did dishes and cleaned – this is where she found herself during my blessingway, as well as on later visits. Bless her. She also made me a plate of food, which I barely nibbled. Grace was the last to arrive around 6pm. By this point I was hitting transition, but in utter denial about it, as in my mind I was still in early stages and had ages to go still – I noticed I was shaking, but I thought they must have been for other reasons!

Sheree reminded me that the pool was ready, but I stayed where I was because things were working and I didn't want to wear out the pool experience too early. I eventually jumped in anyway. I took my skirt, leggings and undies off and left my bra and top on, not wanting to give the idea or tempt Simi into breastfeeding. Simi had stayed in the pool, so she was in there until she started to bug me, responding to my small noises and movements, wanting to be in my arms to feel secure herself.

Lex took Simi into the other room and watched Dora the Explorer on the computer. I felt guilt over bringing another child along while Simi still needed me so much – but as this was one of the issues I had worked on so much during my pregnancy that I was able to observe this thought and let it go.

I sank in to Sheree's arms, who was behind me giving my shoulders a massage and I swear she put some kind of spell on me, as labor hit hard! I was uncomfortable during contractions. Only 2 had hurt prior to this, when I hadn't concentrated on expanding, but the energy of these contractions were suddenly intense! Nothing I did helped me feel comfortable. I tried 314spiralling my hips, which is what had been recommended over and over again to me. "Spirals are shit!" I thought angrily.

I felt noise wanting to come out, so I started playing with noise and pitch. I found the right note for me, which then I felt the energy move up from my base and sacral chakras, up through my body and out my crown chakra. This was the only way I could cope with this amount of energy running through me – it was intense! I later found out that the pitch was connected to my sacral chakra, which is associated with childbirth. My body knew exactly what it needed.

When Sheree had told me weeks before that she saw my birth involving lots of noise I replied "I am happy for my doulas to sing or chat if that is what happens". She responded with "No, you will be making lots of noise." I thought that was a ridiculous concept as my first birth I was quiet and within the whole way.

Between some contractions I blurted out "I am scared", which I think was a surprise because there was a pause, then Grace asked me "What are you scared of?" I pondered this thought a moment, but nothing more came so I responded with a quick shake of my head. I didn't need to go any further; here I was surrendering to birth.

My roar started to disturb Simi, so after her shifting in Lex's lap for a while, she brought her in to my birth space. My whole team, including Leo, was around me now. Lex mentioned something about cutting up some fruit and I roughly growled to her to stay. I momentarily felt bad talking to her that way – she later told me it was great feedback and she liked knowing what I needed.

I finally let myself feel up inside my vagina. I hadn't wanted to do it any earlier, thinking that I was still going to be only 2cm dilated, but instead I felt a head there! It seemed kind of squishy (the fact that my waters hadn't broken didn't come to mind). I was so excited I blurted out the news and everyone gave little cheers!

I was on my knees leaning forward against the birth pool between contractions and upright roaring, feeling the energy rush through the contractions. Grace was behind me pressing wonderful pressure points in my pelvis, but during the contractions I only wanted her to place her hands on my lower back, which surprised me because I wasn't feeling pressure in my pelvis and sacrum, but wanting to be held in my "support" spot – which shouldn't have surprised me at all, really!

Simi wanted to get in the pool with me, she was getting quite uncomfortable by the noise I was making and other people's comforting wasn't working. She just wanted to feel safe in my arms. I knew I couldn't have her in the pool with me, as she would be climbing

# The Wild Rainbow

all over me. I let my fingers slip up my vagina again and the head that was previously there had disappeared! Fuck! I didn't know how much longer I could keep doing it! I cracked it and told Leo to take her away, which in my head meant to another room, but he whisked her off, naked and all, into the car and to his parent's house, a suburb away. I stood up in the pool and the gravity felt amazing on my body! My legs felt solid and strong, my body and pelvis heavy, "It feels so good to stand!" I exclaimed. I had only been in there about 90 minutes, but too much for my Earth constitution body!

I got out and started towards the bathroom and went to the toilet. Sheree bought me a towel possibly to wrap around myself – I just held on to it. I had a contraction on the toilet, which was so incredibly uncomfortable! I squirmed on the spot, trying hard not to fight it. Next couple of contractions I was holding myself semi suspended between the sink and washing machine, loving gravity's pull. I was fully bearing down and my waters broke. Sheree grabbed my towel and placed it on the floor under me – thinking the baby would come right there and then. Thinking the same thing, I looked her in the eyes and said "If I'm going to have my baby in the water, I better get in the water" and got back to the pool quick!

Lex tried calling Leo and left a message on his answering machine telling him to get back urgently! The next contractions baring down, still concentrating on stretching and expanding, I felt my body pushing and this overwhelming grunt coming up my body and through my throat and mouth. My body pushing on its own!

There were less than 10 contractions after getting back in the water, then I felt Taioma's head descend through my vagina and I instinctually brought one leg up (as I was on my knees). I reached down and touched her head. "What a lot of hair" I thought. Between these contractions I could feel Taioma's body moving in my vagina. As Simi had come out all at once, I had never felt the sensations of having a baby with only its head out. It felt disgusting! I wanted to shout at her to stop moving!

Next contraction she slipped out into my hands at 8.45pm! I caught my baby! I gazed at her under the water, still curled up like she was in a cocoon and my first thought was "whose baby is this?" Seriously, where had this black Fijian baby come from? Where was the little blonde baby I was expecting? This thought faded, followed by me noticing how short her umbilical cord was. Feeling concerned about lotus birthing, I was questioning how I was going to breastfeed to assist the placenta's separation from the uterus. But as I pulled her up to my left breast I realised the cord was loosely around her neck. Sheree had seen this at the same time and said "Just give her a little somersault". I looked at Sheree as if to say "Somersault? My logical brain is switched off!" So she gently took my babe and did this for me.

A moment later Taioma cried out. No-one was worried, as she was a wonderfully vibrant colour and the cord wasn't tight. It was also quite long, contrary to my earlier thought. Holding my baby was so amazing! Words cannot express the love I had for her and the triumph I felt – having birthed her the way I wanted, the way she wanted! I could sense the women around me, loving me, proud of me, holding me, but my gaze was glued to my gorgeous second daughter.

Thoughts came and went of Tom – the blonde, blue eyed boy me and other holistic practitioners had envisioned in my womb. I was so confused and wanted to cry, but chose to stay present to the endorphins and the beautiful, perfect baby in my arms.

Leo returned and Simi, still naked, jumped back in the pool with me, which was being topped up with hot water. The love I had for my family at this moment was profound! Seeing Simi for the first time as a big sister, no longer my baby – she was beautiful. I felt guilty that Leo hadn't been there to see Taioma enter the world, but knew in my heart that I needed Simi out of my birth space and my carers to be fully present to me and the birth. I have since confirmed with Leo that there are no negative feelings. He completely understood my desire to birth with my women around me, they journey I was on and he knew his role as Simi's care giver.

After breastfeeding a while, I felt the desire to push my placenta out. I half squatted over a bowl on the floor and was amazed at the ease it was to push it out. I then took my baby, her placenta, my daughter and my man to bed, where I tandem fed for the first time. Simi getting so much needed and deserved comfort from me. This tandem relationship would continue for almost a year, with me finally making the decision to stop, as the whole experience became too demanding on me, physically and emotionally.

## The Wild Rainbow

A whole lot of blood gushed out of me as I stood and I panicked. Sheree confirmed that the amount of blood loss was a normal amount and started me on some Chinese herbs straight away to encourage and assist my fundus returning to a normal size. I don't remember any after pains following Simi's birth – I wonder if my body was making up for it second time around! Every time I breastfed my toes were curling as my womb felt like it had a dagger in it! Where's my epidural for this pain?

Once Taioma was settled and asleep I left her with Leo and got up with Simi – cuddled her and finally ate my dinner I had prepared hours earlier – I was ravished! Giving Simi that one-on-one time straight away was so important to me, to honour her transition from only child to big sister. In my mind I just wanted to cuddle my squishy new babe, but in my heart I knew the importance of this time with Simi.

Before my doulas left, they collected the candles they had gifted me at my blessing way and left them in sight. They also took a photo of themselves, grins from ear to ear! My beloved priestesses of awesomeness!

The morning after Taioma's birth, so many hours after her umbilical cord stopped pulsing, as it was beginning to dry, we rinsed her placenta, getting to inspect it as Sheree showed us through the medical things to look for. After gaining Taioma's permission Leo started pouring cold water over it. She screamed and writhed in agony, as if it was being poured over her! If I had any doubt about the lotus birth process, seeing the way she reacted to her energy field being attacked by such a sensation would prove the importance of letting the baby slowly transition into the world and pulling all her resources and energy to her body, before finishing her own birth process. Taioma let go of her placenta 58 hours later, the shortest lotus birth I have heard of – she was very ready to be here! When this transition happened, it was amazing to see the change from her internal womb space, where we didn't even know the colour of her eyes, they were closed so much, and a quiet, not sluggish, but internal persona – to an awake, observant, wide eyed cub!

For 2 weeks I had friends and family visit every second day, bringing me food, company, compliments and love. I felt so incredibly nourished!

## *Travelling Sage Femme*

## *Ethiopia*

### *There She Goes Again...*

I needed to do something else. My graduate year was difficult and I felt like I was losing myself, not finding who I was as a midwife. I was getting so lost in working in the system, following protocol and learning the ins and outs of working in such a large place that I was starting to feel like I wasn't learning anything. I definitely didn't feel as though I was making a difference in womens' lives. In my graduate year, we grads had 2 mentors over the year, who would help us along if we had questions, needed help as well as just to support us in our journey. One of them was a gorgeous midwife named Fiona who ended up leaving the system to go into homebirth as well as other important women's work and our other mentor, an enthusiastic, knowledgeable, young woman tragically and suddenly died. With our support structure gone, and in such circumstances, it was even more difficult for me to be able to try and find my feet, find my heart and practice how I wanted to. Some of the midwives were fantastic. Some of them took me under their wing; some of them trusted me and left me to work how I wanted to. When we got a new team leader, she was an incredible woman with a lot of enthusiasm and passion for working with woman. She was caring and considerate to not only the ward full of women and babies she was responsible for, but to all her staff. She was empathetic to my needs as a mother to 3 young children and she always listened to my concerns. Despite this, I still felt overwhelmed and desperate for a change but I didn't even know where to begin.

# The Wild Rainbow

One day, when I was browsing on the computer, getting lost in stories and pictures around birth, I came across a website for a UK based charity called Maternity Worldwide. At this time, it was a small charity founded in 2002 by two extraordinary men, Adrian and Shane. This organisation grew out of the frustrations of a small group of public health professionals at the needless deaths in childbirth of so many women in developing countries. They were a secular organisation with no religious affiliations. There projects and services were open to all members of local communities regardless of their faith or background. Their work was also mainly in poor rural areas where some health services are often provided by faith based organisations as well as by the government. They maintain the standard that their partnerships with organisations are that which share the same vision and values as their own.

Reading through their information, I found some information on a bike ride challenge they were hosting in order to raise funds for a hospital they were working with in the remote highlands of Ethiopia. The event was a bike ride that spanned over 5 days, was 350kms and started at the capital Addis Abeba and finished at the hospital they were raising funds for in the remote highlands. This hospital was at the end of the road, it was just kind of there, in the middle of nothing but trees on a mountainous terrain. I was so fascinated by this and I was surprise when I actually found myself thinking of the logistics of it and if it was going to be something that I could actually do.

I laughed at the notion of it for a bit. It obviously wouldn't work. I was in my graduate year, we didn't have much money and I had 3 small children to look after. I also had not been on a bike ride for about 6 years at the point, was overweight and not very fit! Also, I had never travelled overseas before. So it kind of seemed ridiculous that travelling to remote highlands of a third world country where there is no means to communicate with family back home seemed like a not very sensible thing to do.

I tried to let it go.

But sometimes my heart screams louder than my logical brain and the noise eventually becomes so loud that I can't ignore it. I just have to listen to it. I just have to give in to it. And then the noise quietens. And this is what happened. I started dreaming of it in both my sleep and waking consciousness. The idea of it just kept coming into my head and it got to the point where I couldn't let it go.

Fear of travelling to Africa on my own, I decided to send an email to the group to ask if anyone from Australia was going. I was thinking that if anyone was going, even if they were interstate, I would travel to them and then we could fly together to Africa so I wasn't alone. Within 10 minutes, an email was returned and I was told that yes, 2 sisters from Australia were actually going, and I was given their email information. I promptly wrote an email, asking them where they were and if I was able to fly with them. The eldest sister replied to me first and told me where she lived. I was so astounded and almost couldn't believe it. She lived about 4 blocks away from me. That was my sign from the universe. I was going to Africa.

## *Leaving Comfort, Meeting Despair*

Boarding the plane was emotional. As I kissed my husband and 3 small children behind and walked through those doors that separated me and my family, the reality of what I was doing hit me. I had silent tears as I walked through the airport lounge. As I looked around, I saw that others had their own silent tears as well. Tear of leaving a world behind to go to a new one, even if it is just for a little while. The plane trip took ages, it was so long to be in the sky, in a world above the clouds where there is nothing to see but your thoughts. My mind reeled. What am I doing? Am I doing the right thing? What if I get kidnapped while I am there? What if I get lost somewhere in the highlands and no one ever finds me again? What if someone shoots me? What if I lose my passport? What if, what if, what if? Well, whatever happens, there's no point in freaking out about it now. I just let it all go. And waited to see what lies in front of me once I touch the ground onto this new world.

As I flew past Yemen, over the Red Sea to Ethiopia, my heart fire became alive. I was surprised at how green and lush Ethiopia looked from the skies. From up here, you couldn't tell that the land I was flying above was poverty stricken. You couldn't tell that this was a country full of orphaned children, dying babies and starving families.

# The Wild Rainbow

You couldn't tell that this was a country where people die from not having access to basic needs of survival such as clean water and food. I could barely believe it, until of course, the plane landed and my feet touched the soil of this ageless, broken country.

Coming through the gates of the airport, my eyes were met with 30 men in green uniform, holding guns. And even though I know they were standing there in peace, I felt so unnerved at that sight. I had never seen anything like that. All I was thinking was that I am so glad that I didn't travel to Africa alone. We were picked up by one of the crew and taken to the small motel, a few doors down from a shanty town. As we pulled up, people came knocking on the windows asking for money. I was told to lock my door, which I promptly did, but this didn't stop the begging. About 12 kids tried to pile in and ask for money. When they realised they couldn't, they started climbing on the bonnet of the car, up onto the windscreen, their faces caked with dirt and dried up snot pressed up against the glass as they pleaded for money. Their eyes looked so sad. Their bodies looked so skinny and dirty. I didn't want to look anymore, so I looked out the back window where I knew the kids couldn't climb up. As I did this, I saw man with no legs, using his arms, with thongs on his hands, to scoot across the big road to the grassy medium strip that separates the 2 roads. On that strip there was a plastic bag full of something, I wasn't sure what, and a dirty child sized blanket. Oh. I sighed. I realised that that is where that man lives. That was his home. I was in the country for one hour and I already could feel the heaviness. So, this is what despair looks like. It was looking at me right in the eye.

## *What a ride!*

The bike ride itself was physically challenging to me. The state of my physical fitness definitely showed! I felt embarrassed as poverty stricken old women with bare feet and a large load of wood on their backs would overtake me as they walked up the hill when I struggled to ride my bike. I felt embarrassed at my large body. I knew I was overweight but nothing made me feel more uncomfortable about it as much as being overweight in Africa. It seemed so unfair that I

# Journeying as Sage Femme

obviously have an abundance of food, when they have nothing. It made me feel selfish and wasteful.

For the 5 days where we were riding, we were looked after by an awesome support crew. Two jeeps followed us, one in front and one at the back and we would stop for food that was made for us. There were lots of mangoes, avocadoes and paw paw, eggs, vegetables with spice and lots and lots of injera. Every time we would stop for a break, countless people would seem to appear from nowhere and come right into your space. This made me feel so nervous to begin with but after a few days, I realised they were coming from a place in interest and intrigue. Most of the places we went to were not tourist destinations, they were just villages we passed through with nothing in them, so we must have been quite a sight to them! Some of them had never seen white people before, or pushbikes! I became used to the attention and at the times where I wasn't too fatigued, I kind of enjoyed it. The interaction was great, even if most of the time, we didn't understand a word the other was saying.

Kids would run behind you while you rode and they would hold onto your bike, making a difficult ride more difficult by them pulling you back with their weight. They would laugh and point at you, try and steal your water bottle and they would clap their hands and wave.

Adult men would run alongside you and the one who could speak some English would yell out "where you go?"

I would yell back "Gimbie!"

"Why?"

"To the hospital!"

"Oh!" they would yell and then give me an approving smile and clap their hands and let me go on my way.

If I took photos of the kids, I would show them their selves on the screen of the camera and they would laugh and squeal in delight. That was something that I always liked. No matter what the language was, we all laugh the same in the same language.

On one of the nights, there was no particularly safe place to stay. No compound, churchground or motel like we had been privileged with

# The Wild Rainbow

the nights previous. We ended up setting our tents beside a cornfield and paid some men to be our guards for the night. With their white shawls and their big guns in their hands, they looked really scary, but they made me feel safe. At night, when I was lying in my tent, I heard one of the guards do a massive, long, incredibly loud fart. Then the other 2 men laughed out loud. Then a different guard farted which made them giggle even more. They started laughing harder and talking. Then they continued to fart and laugh, fart and laugh, fart and laugh. It made me realise that no matter where we are in the world, and who we are in the world, we are all just people who think, dream, cry and laugh. No matter how difficult our life is, no matter what we are dealt, we all have moments where we laugh and feel joy. Even if it is about farts. I went to sleep smiling.

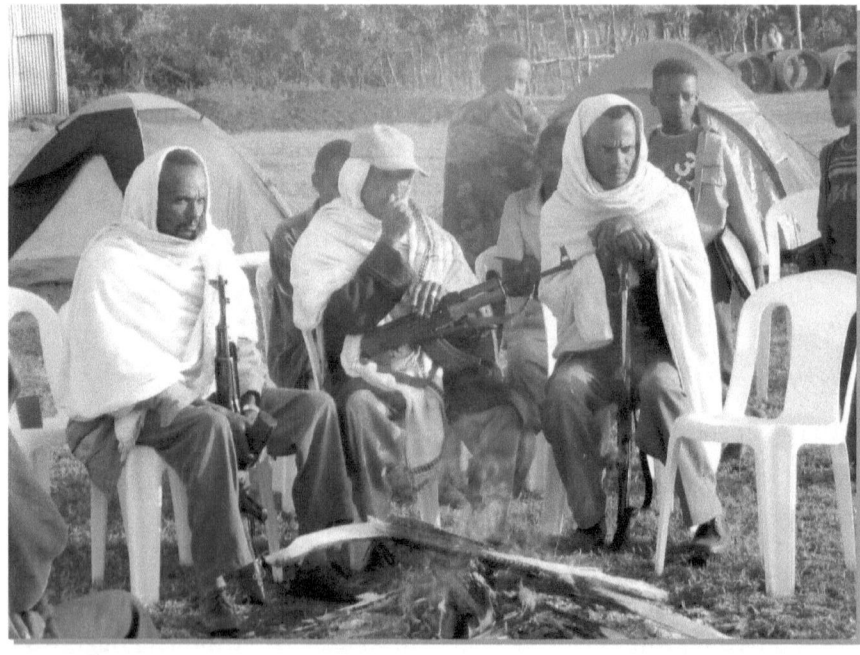

Photo: Sheree Stewart

## *The End Of The Road*

The hospital is at the end of the road. Passed the hospital is more villages, but there is no roads to or from them. They are the remote Ethiopia.

Arriving at the hospital, I was full of tears. I had tears of awe that I had made it. I had tears that I did the challenge, that I rode my bike that far after many times of doubting myself. I had tears as I looked at the man riding beside me who was the one who had the vision of coming here and helping these people. It seemed the whole village was standing waiting for us, watching us. They were clapping and smiling. They were cheering that people had come to them.

We went through a back way to the hospital so that the whole village didn't come into the compound and we put all our bikes and belongings away. I was shown the house where I was going to stay and met some of the volunteers who were working there.

I instantly fell in love with 2 fifty something year old volunteers who were nuns from Ecuador. These women had no fear. Their hearts were as big as the sun. Together they would do daily bike rides down to the remote villages where there were no roads. They would take food, water, medicine, and kindness. They would laugh with the women and sing songs with the children. They would weigh the babies and make sure they were breastfeeding without any issues. They would teach the children how to count. Their smiles were infectious and you couldn't help but be uplifted by them. I asked them how they were able to stay so positive when they are surrounded by despair and poverty every day. One of them replied 'It is because we see hope in them and we want that hope to never go away'. And the other replied 'this is my work and my calling to be with these people and be kind'. Their attitude to support others in the capacity that they do really did bring home the idea of not only supporting people through physical means such as providing basic needs such as clean water, food and access to free healthcare, but that showing compassion and kindness play a massive part in rebuilding a broken poverty stricken community as well. Although kindness doesn't make the poverty go away or feed the belly, it feeds the heart and brings hope. And we cannot underestimate the power that that has.

The day we arrived felt long, and even though my heart felt tired, I was full of gratitude. The long day ended with us sitting on the porch of a gorgeous house full of inspirational volunteers who had left the comfort of their homes and families behind to come and be a part of something bigger than themselves. I was drinking a beer and the sky was full of our laughter. There were 3 monkeys swinging in the trees just meters away from me and there were fireflies glowing and buzzing in the grass below me. Even though it was dark, I was able to see the silhouette of the trees – the lush, vast treescape that seemed to dance on forever below me. I just watched everything, with childlike eyes and wonder.

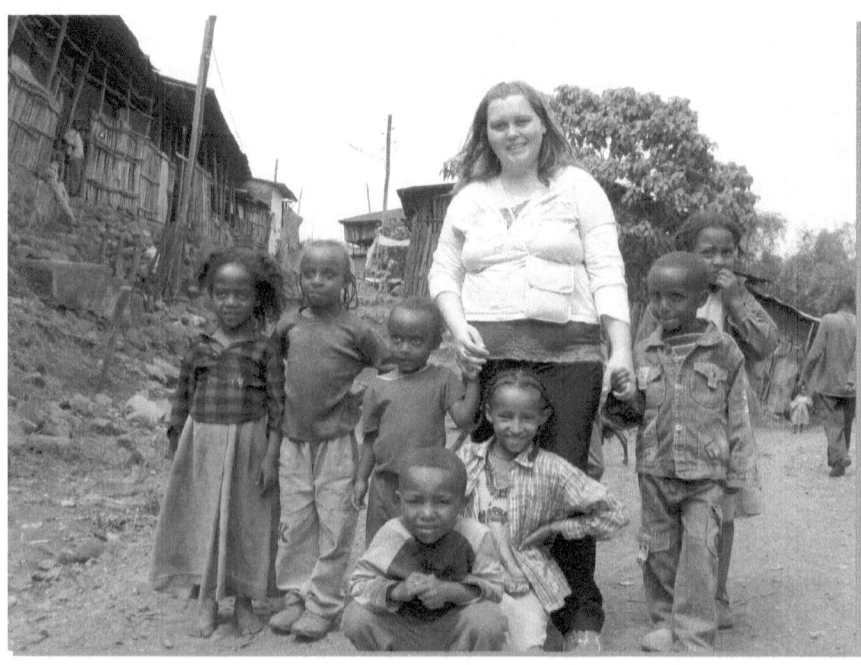

*"Gimbie"* – Photo:

## The Hospital

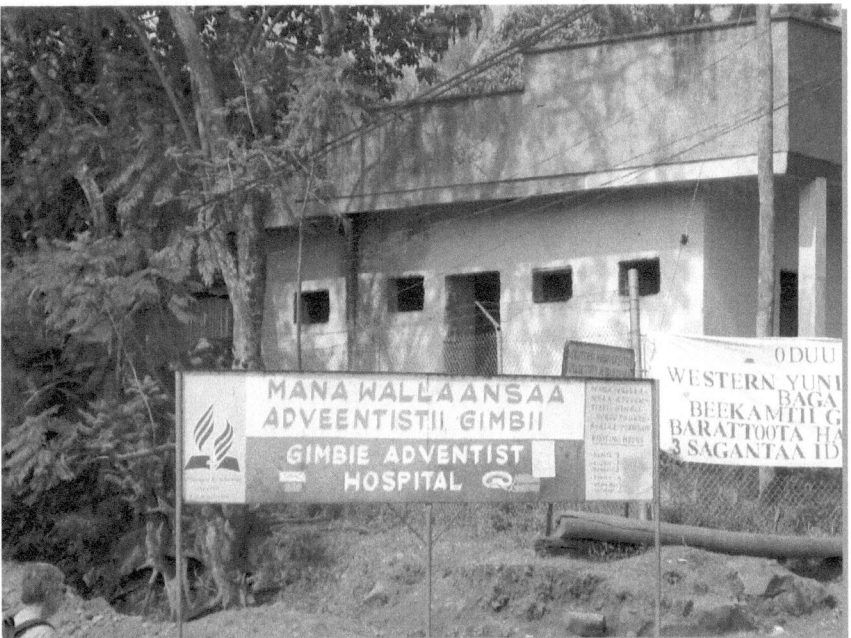

*"Gimbie Adventist Hospital "*– Photo: Sheree Stewart

The next day I had a tour of the hospital. I got to see how it worked and what was there. Everyone was so friendly. Everywhere I went, there was a sea of smiling faces.

I saw the Pathology clinic, which was a gorgeous man standing around in a white coat in a small room, testing blood and urine samples that were collected in empty glass bottles. He was so proud of the work he was doing. He told me how he cannot even describe what it is like to help his own people. As a part aboriginal woman, knowing what it is like for my own people back home, all I could do is nod in agreement.

We walked past the laundry, which was a room outside, separate to the hospital which had several large drums full of water sitting over a woodfire. This is where everything was washed, cleaned and sterilsed, including the sheets for the operating room. They would wash them in a drum of hot water, then hang them on a line in the sun and beat them dry with a large stick. The sheets were full of holes from all the stick beating, and they were still far from anything considered sterile, but at least they had sheets for the operating room, even if they were full of holes. At least they were kind of clean.

The general ward was full of people there for both short and long term stays. There was a child around 4 years old there who had broken his leg. He was there for 2 weeks, without his mother as she had to go back to the villages to look after her other 6 children, 2 cows and crop. There was no father, he had died, but the fathers' brother came and helped with the animals, property and finances. The little boy didn't seem bothered that he was away from his family for that long. He seemed to love the attention that he was receiving from the staff and the other patients on the ward.

The Intensive Care Unit was another small room, which had 2 beds in it and a broken, useless machine. I asked how does this room qualify as an Intensive Care Unit when there was nothing in there and was told that it is because it is the room that is closest to the Nurses' station, so that if anything happened to the patient, then the staff would be able to see. Not that they could really do much to save them anyway. I didn't know whether to laugh or cry.

There was an antenatal clinic with full attending classes for women and their families to come and learn basic health and safety during pregnancy. They were taught what things to look for in pregnancy and birth that could be potentially dangerous and what to do if those situations arose. Everyone benefited from this and the women went home feeling more empowered and the men went home feeling more knowledgeable and confident in what to do for their women if they noticed certain sign, symptoms and behaviours.

The birth room was a tiny little room that was big enough for one bed and the midwife attending the birth. The woman would labour and birth on her back and have her legs in stirrups for the second stage of labour, the birth of the baby.

# Journeying as Sage Femme

There was a sign on the door which had the protocol for fetal distress. It read:

## For 1st Stage Of Labour
- Lie patient on left lateral position
- Secure IV line of D/W 5% or DNS to run fast
- Give oxygen by face mask (instruct patient to open mouth and deep breath)
- If no improvement in 30 minutes, knee chest position
- If cervix not fully dilated and fetal head more than 1/5 above sypmhasis pubis and fetal head is about 0 station, deliver by C/S

## For 2nd Stage Of Labour
- If cervix fully dilated and fetal head in not more than 1/5 above the symphasis pubis or fetal head is at 0 station
- Do episiotomy to hasten delivery
- Do instrumental delivery (vacuum extraction/forceps)
- Be ready for neonatal resus

Once your baby was born, you were moved to the postnatal ward, which was a large room, with no curtains/dividers, that was full of beds. It smelled terrible, like sour grapes and it was hot and there was no cooling. To me, it seemed so shocking to see people invading the space of others. Strangers going up to women they don't know to touch and look at their babies, but to them it was a non-issue. The women were happy that they were alive. That their babies were alive. That they were being fed food and water. And that their babies were given clothes.

Women often didn't attend the hospital until it was too late, that is, that the baby had already died. Most women labour at home in their villages with their traditional birth attendants and will transfer only if labour is taking a long time or if something visibly wrong is happening

## The Wild Rainbow

to the mother (haemorrhaging or having seizures generally). Deciding to transfer to hospital isn't always an easy task. It often involves a long walk (or being carried by a team of people within their village) and can take 1-2 days walk. You can imagine the outcome of being a poverty stricken, malnourished woman, who has been in labour for 3 days, becoming obstructed, and knowing that your baby has died, to then begin a full day journey whilst still having contracting, to the closest hospital to have your baby surgically removed from your body.

On the $2^{nd}$ day I was at the hospital, a woman came in after being carried by 4 people for almost a whole day walk, contracting every 5 minutes the whole time she was being transferred. Before the transfer, she had already been in labour for around 20 hours. Her baby had her shoulder presenting, so was unable to naturally come out. This baby died, but the woman lived. There was a bittersweet moment of saving a life, but mourning another. I went to bed not knowing whether to be happy or sad, so I just let myself be both.

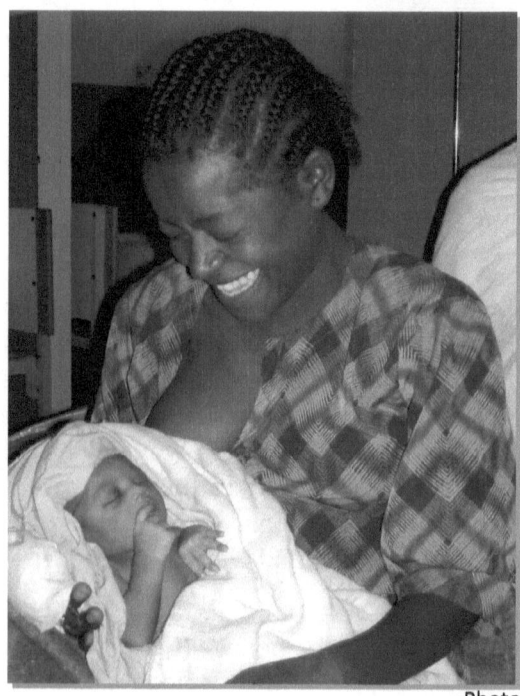

Photo: Sheree Stewart

### Womens' Income Generating Program

*Empowering and enabling women to take a more prominent role in their communities is central to the work of Maternity Worldwide. Their idea and implementation of the Women's Income Generating Scheme is that it helps to raise the status of women and enables them to increase their income. This allows women to make more choices about how their money should be spent for example on maternal or child health, improved food for the family or to save for future health or education needs. Through their work, weaving businesses were started and the women slowly started to save money from their sales. After some time, these women who were once in poverty are now starting to improve their lives. Some of them have even been able to send their children to school.*

### Community Health Programs

*A central part of Maternity Worldwide's Programme is to provide women and communities with the information they need to be able to make informed decisions about their health care, including family planning. In West Wollega they found a huge unmet need for this sort of information and many women and families walk over two hours to attend the sessions. Both men and women come to learn about making and saving money, family planning and health information. Many men have walked away with new knowledge of family planning and that pregnancy and birth take a lot of work from the woman and that having too many babies whilst living in poverty can be very dangerous to the woman and her unborn child.*

### Training Skilled Birth Attendants

*Being able to access regular care from a Skilled Birth Attendant (that is a trained midwife, doctor or nurse) is recognised as being one of the key ways of increasing the quality of maternal health services and preventing women dying in pregnancy and childbirth.*

### *Gimbie Adventist Hospital*

*Gimbie Adventist Hospital (GAH) is located in Gimbie Town, West Wollega Zone in the Oromia Region of Ethiopia, approximately 450km west of Addis Ababa.*

*In Ethiopia, one in fourteen women will die as a result of problems during pregnancy or childbirth. Beginning last January, health professionals from Gimbie Adventist Hospital in West Wollega, Ethiopia, have been working to fight those odds.*

*To help solve these problems staff and volunteers at Gimbie Adventist Hospital, a member of Adventist Health International, have started a program of community education, focusing on women's health and pregnancy problems.*

*The main emphasis of the education is "Be prepared!"*

*"The communities have been very receptive to the education and every meeting has been followed by lengthy discussion, with lots of questions asked," says Ruth Lawson, MBChB, MSc, MRCOG, MFPH, administrator, Gimbie Adventist Hospital.*

*Separate meetings have also been held with the leaders of the villages to encourage them to mobilize their communities and address maternal health problems.*

*There are many reasons for the high rate of difficulties during pregnancy in Ethiopia, including difficulties in accessing medical treatment and poor understanding of pregnancy and childbirth and the types of problems that require medical care.*

*Often women will wait two or three days in labor before they make the decision to come to the hospital, and by then it will often be too late.*

*Even travelling to the hospital is very difficult. Normally women have to be carried on an improvised stretcher for many miles—across rivers and mountains, which can be extremely difficult during the rainy season.*

*Sometimes a team of up to 20 people are needed to transport the woman on a journey which can be up to one day's walk.*

*One of the main causes of maternal death is bleeding in pregnancy or during childbirth. Unfortunately, there is a lot of fear in the community about blood transfusions and people are very unwilling to donate blood even in the event of an emergency. As a result, even after women arrive at Gimbie Adventist Hospital, they still may die because they cannot be treated adequately with blood transfusion.*

*Community reception to the programs have been very positive. In fact, in one instance, Ayantu, a senior nurse, and Moya, volunteer midwife, were returning from giving a health education class in another village nearby. They drove past a group of women walking along the side of the road and the women beckoned them to stop. Ayantu and Moya gave an ad hoc health education session right then and there to the women on the side of the road.*

*The message for these education meetings is very simple: As soon as you know you are pregnant, start to save a little money every month; Prepare a stretcher, and find a group of people who will carry you to hospital if needed; Make an arrangement with someone who is willing to look after your children, animals, crops, etc., in case you need to go to hospital; Find some friends or relatives who are willing to donate blood if needed; and "Don't let the sun set twice on a woman in labor." In other words, if a woman has been in labor for 24 hours she should come to hospital.*

*The government health department is also enthusiastic about this education and has been very helpful in facilitating meetings and helping staff at Gimbie Adventist Hospital to make contact with villages and village leaders.*

*"We intend to continue this education program and will also develop it further to cover other areas related to maternal and child health such as family planning, HIV/AIDs, and women's rights," adds Dr. Lawson.*

*05/16/06*

http://www.adventisthealthinternational.org/globalpartners/ethiopia/ethiopianews/051606ethiopia.html[1]

### *Days in a daze*

I spent my days in the hospital ground helping out other volunteers and staff members and walking around Gimbie with the locals. I will always remember the smell of that country. It smelled like mud and wet forest. I was always surprised at the laughter that always seemed to be lingering in the air. In the mornings I would walk around the postnatal ward and talk to the patients that were there. The conversations were simple and often we didn't understand what the other was saying, but we smiled and pointed at the babies together. I learned how to ask how many children they have, and was mostly answered with 'lots but some died'. It was such a contrast to the answers I would receive on the postnatal back home in Melbourne where I worked. The babies were all so beautiful with their huge mops of black curly hair. Their eyes always looked so magnificent against the darkness of their skin. They all looked so chubby and healthy as they would thrive on their mumma's milk. In the afternoons I would wonder through the town. I remember walking to a little store with 3 of the bike riders with me and we ordered a papaya smoothie. The woman was so excited as she made them for us, and then when we ordered a second round, she was sad to tell us that we had eaten everything in her whole shop! We just smiled at the thought of her going home that night with money to feed her family.

The children of Gimbie followed us everywhere. They would hold on to my hands and at one point I remember I had 9 children holding on to my hands, with many more trying to find space where they could hold. Some of the children who spoke English would tell us stories of their families, where they work and what they want to be when they grow up. It was wonderful. We were all fascinated with each other and most of them didn't understand the idea of where I lived. Most had never seen the ocean or knew what it was, so trying to explain that I came on something with wings across big water must had made me seem like I as from an old make believe story that the grandmothers tell.

I had such a wonderful time there. I loved just being with people, learning from them, as they did from me. Understanding a way of life that was so completely different to my own was a great learning to me. It shifted my perspective; it gave me new ideas, new insights into who we are as people. I guess one of the main things that I have learned while there is that we are all ultimately the same. We, as people, all have hopes, fears, beliefs, dreams. We all want love. We all want to feel safe. We all want to be happy.

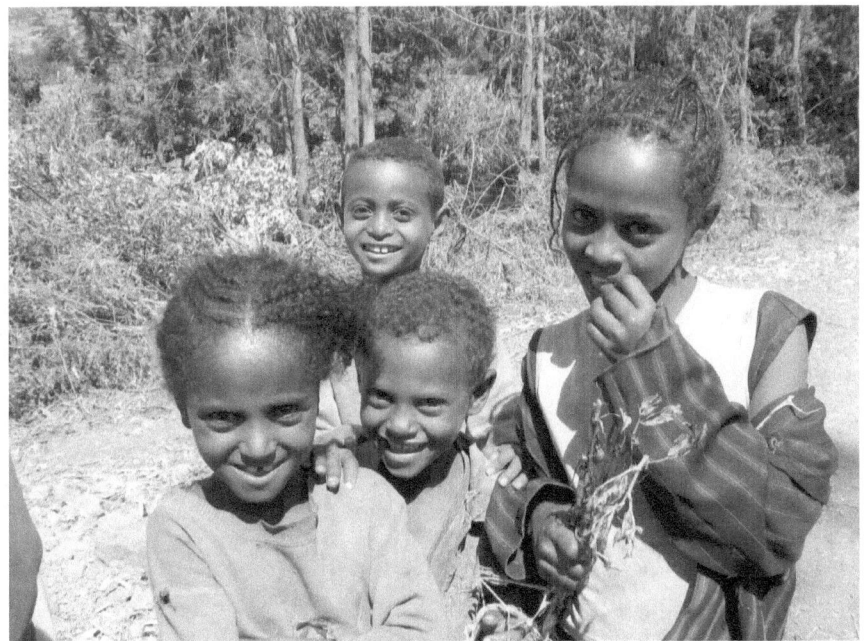

Photo: Sheree Stewart

## *There's no place like home – leaving Africa*

Leaving the hospital, I was met by a young man who was standing out the front of the hospital. I had seen him many times before, but never spoke to him. I did sometimes wonder what he was doing. Was he waiting for someone?

We caught eyes and both smiled. He quickly came up to me.

# The Wild Rainbow

"I am Birak" he said

I introduced myself and told him what I had been doing and that I was now going back home.

"I always stand out here every day" he said

"I'm just waiting. I can wait" he continued.

"Why?" I asked

"Because I want to help my people. This hospital saved my mother. I want to save lives. I want to be a nurse" he smiled and looked at the ground and then continued talking

"One day I want to work here. I am just saving my money so I can do this. For now, I stand here and wait."

I could see the potential in him. He had patience and compassion. I believed he could do this.

I told him my thoughts.

"It's time for me to leave now" I said and waved to him as I hopped in the back of the jeep.

He came up to the window and tapped on it.

"Don't forget us" he said "when you get home"

"I won't" I promised

"We will still be here living like this when you go back to your home. Please don't forget we are here"

I nodded my head and then turned my head so he didn't see the tear from my eye.

Of course I won't forget. That is impossible. I could never erase this place from my memory no matter how hard I tried.

~*~*~*~

The bumpy 7 hour ride home in the back of the Isuzu and then the 17 hour flight through the skies took me far away from Africa, back to my home, to my husband and my children. Walking through the doors at the airport to the safe, warm arms of my husband, my overexcited children and my ever so relieved mother was comforting to my heart.

They all asked in excitement about my journey. How was Africa? What was it like? How was the bike ride? What was my best part? What was my worst part? What was the weather like? What did you eat? Would I go back?

The questions seemed so simple, yet I found I couldn't answer them. I just couldn't explain what it was like. I was sitting at the table sipping whiskey and nibbling chocolate covered macadamia's in my beautiful house in my beautiful country. It really was a moment when I realised how lucky I am.

I had the realisation that I was able to go to bed at night, knowing that in the morning, I would be able to feed my children. Even the knowing that I had a bed to sleep in made me feel teary. I had a roof over my head and I could keep my family warm if it was cold outside and cool if it was hot outside. I didn't have to find a shady tree to take my children to if the weather was hot or to shelter them from torrential rain. We are able to watch a blazing hot sun or torrential rain from looking outside the window in the comfort of our home. I don't need to force my 4 and 6 year olds to go and work in fields for long hours every day so that we can have the simple basics of life. I know that if my legs were to be amputated from illness or accident that I would have access to medical care and a wheelchair and I wouldn't be left to work it out on my own, having to get around the place by using my hands as my feet. I knew that if Steven and I died, that my children would go to loving family and friends and the eldest would never be forced to go and work to send money back to his siblings.

After everyone went to bed that first night I came home, I stayed up in the dark, sipping my whiskey and I cried and cried at what I had seen in this world.

My heart has never been the same since being there, since witnessing that harsh place and I always thought that one day I would go back. But as the years pass, I don't actually think that I will. I can do other things that can help that ageless and broken country, such as encourage others to work there or help train a midwife or nurse to go

## The Wild Rainbow

over. I can speak about my experience in the hope that someone else hears the call of those rugged highlands. But no matter what happens, I will always hold on to that promise that I made to that young man with hope in his heart, standing there in his wild, raw country. I will not forget.

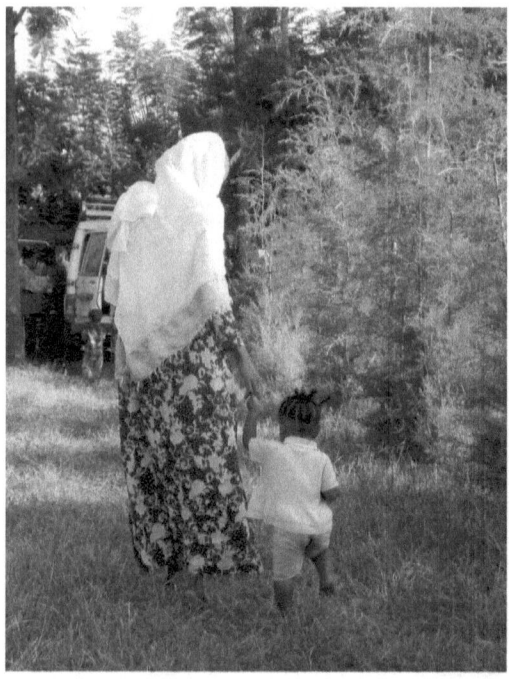

Photo: Sheree Stewart

*"To love. To be loved. To never forget your own insignificance. To never get used to the unspeakable violence and the vulgar disparity of life around you. To seek joy in the saddest places. To pursue beauty to its lair. To never simplify what is complicated or complicate what is simple. To respect strength, never power. Above all, to watch. To try and understand. To never look away. And never, never, to forget."*

*- Arundhati Roy*

# Cambodia

*This chapter was first published as a Blog, can still be found online at http://teamsmartmummas.blogspot.com.au*

*To find out more about the work of Denise Love and LifeOptionsAsia, or to make a donation, please visit http://www.lifeoptions.asia*

## The end is the beginning is the end

Monday, May 2, 2011

The year 2011 has been a strange one. One of ups and down, ups and downs and ups and downs again. Ecstatic highs, desperate lows and everything in-between. The decision to go to Cambodia with my baby was not an easy one to make. It took a lot of thinking about – it was a big decision! The woman who I was planning to stay and work with was Denise Love and she is the creatrix of Life Options. She has so much experience, knowledge and kindness and has taken this with her as a doula from Australia, to the remote villages of Cambodia.

Once I made the decision to actually do it, it made my heart sing. It felt perfect. I sent Denise a short and sweet email that went something like 'Hi Denise, I want to come to Cambodia very soon. Can my baby come? She has attended births and usually lives in a sling on me anyway'. And I pressed send. And waited. She replied half an hour later with an 'oh yes, yes, yes' and I knew that was it. Screw the logistics. It will all work. My heart was on fire, it was so bright and full. Myah and I are going to Cambodia for a month, in about a month!

As a Mumma to 5 awesome, wild, free-spirited children, it means I can't go on such big adventures without the support of my man. My husband, Steven, will be staying at home with 4 of them. He is a loving, capable father and husband and is very excited about his adventures as stay at home Dad (He has been the stay at home Dad for longer than I have been the stay at home Mum). My baby who is 6 months will be travelling with me on the plane across the water to live and learn amongst the gentle peoples of Cambodia.

I let the people closest to me know of my sudden decision and although some of them reacted very differently to how I was hoping, the majority of people have been so loving, supportive and generous. So loving, supportive and generous in fact, that one of my closest sister women, Courtney wanted to come along with me.

I first met Denise one week after I had just done an amazing bike ride across Ethiopia to raise money for a hospital and women's clinic in the Ethiopian Highlands. I was attending a Hypnochildbirth course which Denise was teaching and I fell in love with her straight away. She was very down to earth, passionate and had the belief that we all have the right to live our lives as we choose, with love, happiness and respect. I knew in my heart that we would journey together one day – and now we will be! Denise is the one who has set up LifeOptions Inc. and has initiated some amazing work and healthcare for the people in Cambodia.

When I go there, we are going to live and work in villages in developing countries to share skills, learn new ones, and develop an environment for a healthy sustainable life style. I am a registered midwife and doula so there is plenty for me to share and do there. There are birth centers, schools, orphanages and many families that will benefit from me going, and for me – I am hoping that it will bring a whole new perspective on life as I spend and share my life with them. I am hoping my life will be changed forever.

### *Give us your undies!*

Sunday, May 8, 2011

After the absolutely horrific genocide in the late 1970's – 1980's, the gentle people of Cambodia are striving to regain their community, peace, health and education. Many of the skilled birth attendants were killed in the genocide and I am not exactly sure what sort of care a women now receives who is pregnant or birthing.

Poverty is also a massive issue in Cambodia. Living on next to nothing per day is the pits, and seeing humans' living in such conditions is heartbreaking and soul shattering. If you are female, it seems to isolate and restrict you even further in the world you live in.

From what I know, many of the girls stop attending school during the time they menstruate, simply because when they bleed they don't have sanitary items, so choose to stay home for this time. This of course makes them fall behind in their studies, with a high possibility of them dropping out of education –thus continuing the cycle of poverty.

A very simple and life altering donation suggestion from Life Options Inc. has been that we donate underwear! New, cotton undies, from sizes 8 – 12 in adults and all kids sizes. Giving underwear seems almost silly in our western culture of abundance and over-consumerism, but for many women, giving them a new, clean pair of underwear can make a difference on whether or not they get an education and break the cycle of poverty.

Cloth pads are also massively useful. If you are able to donate some cloth pads, whether you sew or buy them, we promise you that the women of Cambodia will enormously appreciate it! It is amazing that what we take for granted and what we think is 'just the basics' is something that many women around the world don't have. To be honest, I have NEVER linked underwear and education together until a couple weeks ago. To realise that young women won't go to get an education if they don't have underwear to wear when they menstruate and thus continuing the cycle of poverty breaks my heart. We can do something about this. And we can do it right now.

## *Week of Wonder*

Sunday, May 22, 2011

There has been wonderful generosity shown in the last week towards my volunteering adventures in Cambodia. I have a box of stationary – pens, paper, pencils, textas, amongst other goodies that was donated by a friend who is off on an adventure of her own to an orphanage in

Bali. She got more boxes of stationary donated than she could take over, so she passed one on to me to take.

I've had undies in the postbox from people I know and people I don't know, both from Victoria and from interstate. Zip lock bags, gloves, bandages. 2$^{nd}$ hand kids clothes. It is piling up and looking fantastic!

Donations of money have been put into an account with the hope of reaching $2000 so that we can fund a Tuk Tuk Ambulance for the women and babies in desperate need of medical assistance. I love receiving emails which say 'I want to donate!'. It makes my heart sing. Every dollar helps and changes lives of women, families, villages, communities.

Courtney has made jars of delicious tomato relish and nectarine & ginger jam and has donated them to me to sell with all money going straight towards the ambulance. Steven bought the first jar, as he is a bit of a relish fan, and I am guessing he will buy one or two more too. He may end up funding half the Tuk Tuk if he keeps eating all the relish! Books have been donated and chillies have been picked from my garden and bunched up to sell. As I have already said, every little bit helps.

On Saturday, two really awesome events were held in honour of the the peoples of Takeo. Firstly, we screened a documentary called Babies, which was a gorgeous little film that followed four babies from birth across the first year of their lives. There weren't many attendees, there were around ten of us, but those who came loved the film, loved the atmosphere, loved the cause and we raised $120. Thank you to those who came – your support fills my heart and I am sure the hearts of women in Cambodia!

Secondly, a group of gorgeous women (and one spunky man I believe, plus a tribe of children) who hold the same passionate heart as my own, created a day of sewing and made many, many menstrual cloth pads for me to take over.

## I've got your bum covered

Sunday, May 29, 2011

Cambodia is poverty stricken. Bare minimum, and a lot of the time it seems that there is not even that. Denise said something to me which reminded me just how much I take for granted. How fortunate I am!. She said *Yesterday when I sent a new mum and her brand newborn baby home on the back on the motorbike, I wished for her that she had a pair of undies on and a pad between her legs."*

With that information, which touched me to my core as a woman, mother and a decent human being, I have been on a bit of a mission to get some undies and pads for these women. I have been blessed to be acquainted with some pretty spirited people whose hearts are as passionate as my own: The beautiful Jo has really gone above and beyond and 343pecializ a get together with some other wonderful women and had a craft day sewing cloth menstrual pads. In my mind, I was thinking they may do 40. Maybe 50. Definitely not much more than that! Imagine my surprise and complete excitement when it was announced that they reached the 100 mark!! A few days later, the number kept climbing even further! Once they were done, I I this little message from Jo:

> "I'm so proud and ecstatic to announce on behalf of fabric, PUL, snap and cloth donations from Emily of Happy Nappy, Esther from Ferny Hills, Sarah MaClean, Sarah Leslie, Natalie McQueen AND the time and skill donations of seamstresses Loz Woods, Veronica Ingram, Kintara Phillips, Victoria, Leah Timms, Ben Dechrau and Myself (Jo Dechrau) – we created together 155 cloth menstrual pads."

The Wild Rainbow

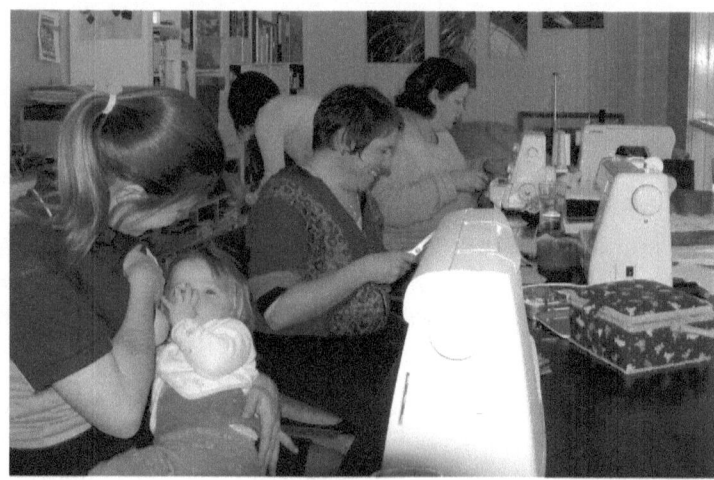

*"The Sewing Crew"*

So many cloth pads were created with the hands of hearts of these beautiful people! Hours and hours of crafting these beautiful bits of material for the women of Cambodia. I feel like I am bursting with pride!

Thank you to those who are generous. Thank you to those who responded to the call

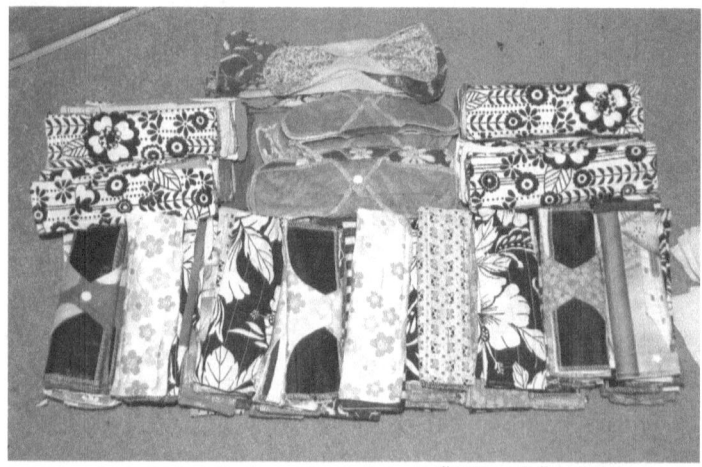

*"155 pads"* – Photos: India Dechrai

So, women of Cambodia, it's not long now. I've got your bum covered!

## *Target 2000 and beyond!*

Thursday, June 2, 2011

It is with extreme ecstasy, delight, gratitude and love, I announce that all money donated and pledged so far has not only reached the $2000 target, but has *exceeded* it!!!

When all monies are in, we are able to purchase a Maternity Tuk Tuk Ambulance for the work of LifeOptions Direct Empowerment, Cambodia & Nepal.

All extra money will be used for petrol, midwives wages, building toilets, and many, many other things! Money donations are still encouraged. These people need as much as we can give.

For instance:
- $1 will buy a litre of petrol
- $45 is what it costs in petrol to transfer a woman to the big hospital in Phnom Penh
- $25 will put in a village toilet
- $2000 is a Tuk Tuk transfer vehicle
- $5 will feed a poor family for a week

I'm not sure what was happening in the stars, but it seems almost unbelievable how the funds came in. For 6 weeks I tried my hardest and struggled to reach the target. I had donations of $320 which slowly came over 1 and a half months. I was feeling a little disappointed and a little lonely in this adventure. Then one evening, a few nights ago, I received an email from a beautiful family whose birth I attended, and they told me they wanted to donate a big chunk of money towards the ambulance. I was ecstatic, reeling in delight, wrapped in gratitude. How generous!

Around this same evening, one of my friends asked how much I had raised so far, and once I told her, she spread the word across Facebook that I need more funds. And then others posted it. And then others posted it. And then others posted it. The following morning I had over 20 emails asking me for details of where they would deposit money. I was so amazed, I almost didn't believe it. I was sitting at the computer screen blurry eyed from many tears being shed. My faith in the human spirit was restored.

To date, money donated and pledged so far is $2226. And there is more to come! Please know that although I have reached the target for the Tuk Tuk, the peoples in Cambodia have so very little. And as I said earlier, the additional money can go to many, many different things, including paying the local midwives, buying petrol for the Tuk Tuk so it can actually transfer women to emergency care, supplies for the birth centre and school, building toilets in the village, and the list goes on and on and on and on!

Thank you so much to those who donated money – You all rock, and will have a place in my heart forever and ever and ever. Thank you for sharing the same dream as me.

### *Here I am! The beginning of it all!*

Friday, June 24, 2011

Where do I start!?!

I travelled from Melbourne to Cambodia with a 7 month old, all on my own! And for someone who is such a cowardly lion about most things, I think I have done ok! I was picked up at the airport after a long overnight flight with Myah. After leaving the wintery 9 degrees weather in Melbourne, Myah and I still are working out how to deal with this 32 degrees sticky hot heat! Sleeping right next to a fan helps!

I've been introduced to the staff, they are all gorgeous and friendly, particularly the elder midwife Chong Nai Hy, who lived through the devastating Pol Pot times. She is also willing to learn new ways of being with women, with treating women with different remedies and is fascinated in what us *'birang'* (westerners) do in birth. Denise is wanting to bring the idea of water birth and delayed cord clamping here, but it is one step at a time, as birth in such a way here is unknown.

Generally, what happens is that a woman will come to hospital when she is labouring and will be examined. If she is in early labour, which basically means until her waters break or she starts pushing, then she will just wait in the waiting area with the other women who are in the same boat as her. Once she is called into the other room, she is on the small half bed with stirrups and directed to push until the baby is out. Cord clamped and cut immediately and then generally a quick cuddle with mum and then baby is on a bed next to mum. It is so hot here, there is not much skin to skin! It is very rare for women here to have breastfeeding problems. They just do it.

What makes the places Denise and Life Options Asia are involved in so special, is that women are given privacy, respect and kindness. This doesn't happen in any other hospital or health clinic here. The women that come here always leave saying that they felt listened to and it makes them feel happy.

So, since I've been here, I've been to two hospitals – the big one in Phnom Penh and one out here in Takeo Province- , as well as the places I am volunteering with Life Options with – the Women's Health Clinic (which is where I live, well just across the road) and to the new Birth Centre which officially opens on Saturday!

On quiet days I am hoping to do education sessions with the midwives here. Rachael has already done a few, one was about using garlic vaginally to treat different infections. The women here are poor and we are offering a free service and want to be able to give them remedies to use that is affordable to them. I had a short chat yesterday about lotus birth, but would like to talk about it more if they are open to it. There were lots of giggles and a few questions. One of them was worried about the salt I talked about to salt the placenta with, would travel up the umbilical cord and enter the baby. Another asked how many days it takes for the cord to fall off and what happens with the smell. They are all willing to learn and listen. It is just one small step at a time. And as I am often reminded by my 9 year old, *"how do you eat an elephant? One bite at a time!"*

Tomorrow I will be going to the village which I believe is 1 and a half hour by car and is very, very remote. There is another health and birth centre there and a school.

Oh, there is so much to say, I am probably just rambling. Before I go though, I wanted to say that all the undies and pads were sorted out by Rachael and I into little packs. Each woman will get three pairs of undies and eight pads after she gives birth. We will distribute these out to the three birth centres I am volunteering at. The women are ecstatic and so grateful for what we sisters in Australia have given them

I feel at the moment that I need to say some space to say THANKYOU to all those who have supported me in my adventure. I especially need to thank my 5 little humans in my life who have given me their blessings to come here. Caelan, Rhiannon, Aaliyah, Sage and Myah, I love you all, my little inspirations who drive me crazy but have shown me an amazing world.

And to Steven, for suggesting this adventure in the first place, and re-igniting my heart song once again. And a last one to my Mum who said "I will worry my ass off until you get home, but I know you need to do this, so go"

## *The Poor Family*

Saturday, June 25, 2011

I went out to a village in remote Takeo and met a family who is known as The Poor Family. When asked if they had names, we were answered 'No, we don't think so, everyone just calls them The Poor Family'.

The Poor Family were not always poor. The husband used to work, but hurt his back at work. He had a motorbike accident and needed an operation. To pay for this they sold their rice field. After the operation, he became an alcoholic. So, they began the downward spiral into poverty.

They have quite a few children, at least 5. Their fifth baby was born with a harelip so of course there was difficulty in feeding. In Cambodia, if you have a harelip, you don't have the operation until the baby is at least 6 month old. Until then, you need to somehow work out how to feed a baby that has deformities around the mouth. The midwives involved with LifeOptions went to visit them every week to see how they could help. Unfortunately, the baby had a bout of diarrheoa and died, returning to Mother Spirit.

From this baby's death, LifeOptions have decided to continue to help this family. They have help rebuilt their small 1 room shack, which was once falling down on one side, and also plant a small vegie garden. Whenever one of the midwives goes out to near that particular village, they stop at the market and get some rice and some bananas for them.

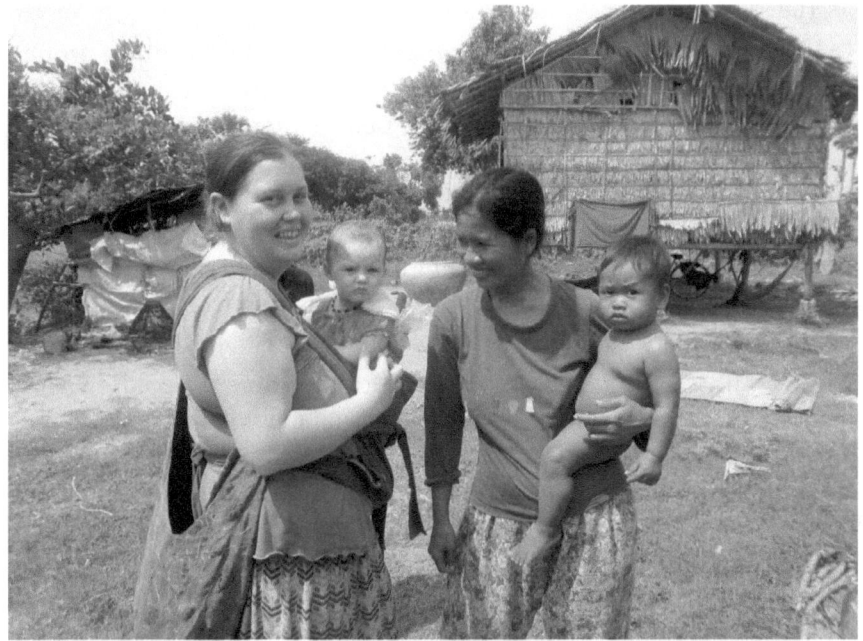

*"The Poor Family"* – Photo: Sheree Stewart

I talked to them while I was there – I don't speak Khmer and they don't speak English, but it doesn't seem to matter – communication is communication, and I felt we had some sort of understanding. We smiled at each other, our babies played whilst in our arms, and we got to paint a picture in each-others minds about who we are and what we are doing.

It's such a different world over here, one that you can see images of and read about, but can't really understand unless your feet are on the same soil and you look in each other's eyes.

### Tuk Tuk!

Wednesday, June 29, 2011

Thank you beautiful people who have donated to raise money for the Tuk Tuk! Because of your generosity and spirited hearts, we had enough money and went and purchased the Tuk Tuk in Phnom Penh on Tuesday and it is now in Takeo!

There are several Birth Centres / Women's Health Centres around Takeo that LifeOptions is involved with. It was decided that this Tuk Tuk would go to a Women's Health Centre that has recently lost a woman during birth. This women came into the centre during labour, bleeding. It was the middle of the night, and the hospital she was transferred to debated whether she could pay for care or not. So the decision was for her to wait until morning and catch a bus, to urgent medical care in Phnom Penh which she didn't have to pay upfront for. Unfortunately, she died on the bus on the way to help.

The Tuk Tuk is going to stay at that particular Womens Health Clinic so that if a scenario like that ever happens again, it will hopefully have a different, much happier ending. Also, there will be no charge to the woman if she needs to be transferred; it is funded by LifeOptions and the donations given by people like you.

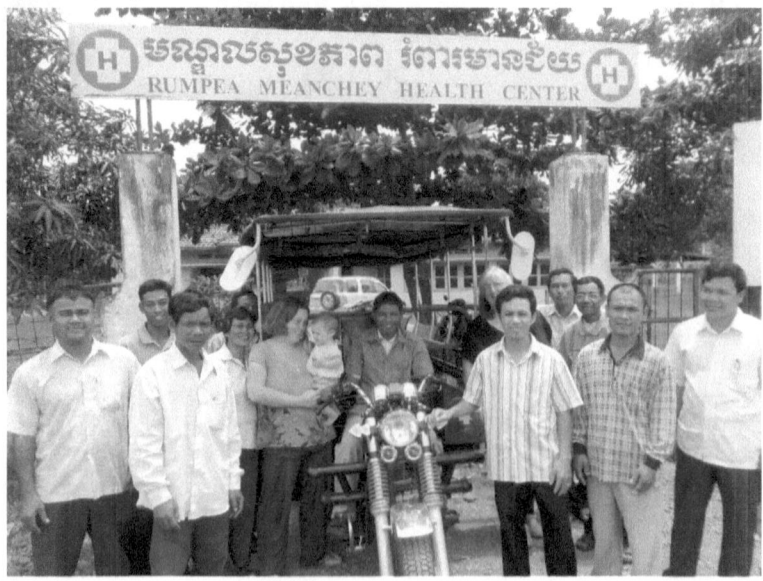

*"Rumpea Meanchey Health Center"* – Photo: Rachael Findlay

So, there you go. All those donations I was given where you said 'Its not much, but I hope it helps', definitely has! Please know that it was all your donations of $10 and $20 that ultimately got us to the $2000 and look at what we have achieved together. A little red motorbike Tuk Tuk that is going to save lives of women, and therefore children, families, villages and communities.

## *Revisiting The Poor Family*

Friday, July 1, 2011

As humans, we need to keep in mind the way we speak and act, and it must always be done with integrity and authenticity. I am finding myself experiencing this daily here.

Last week, when I met the Poor Family for the first time, we gave them some soap powder so that they could wash their clothes.

Yesterday we went back down to the village and stopped by The Poor Family. When the husband saw us pull up, he scurried along, and started looking very busy all of a sudden. It wasn't until we got over to their little house that we realised the husband was pulling all the clothes of the line and putting them in a pile, setting them on fire! I was absolutely gobsmacked as to why he was doing that. When asked what he was doing, he said that he is burning them because the clothes are too old. We realised that he had set them on fire because they hadn't been washed since we saw them last, and he felt ashamed. How sad.

Their 3 year old also looked hot and floppy; apparently she has been that way for 3 days. The Mumma didn't want to take her to the nearby health clinic, even though if they say they are poor they don't have to pay. It is so shameful for her to have to admit that they don't have any money. If that young girl gets diarrheoa, then she is probably going to die.

## The Wild Rainbow

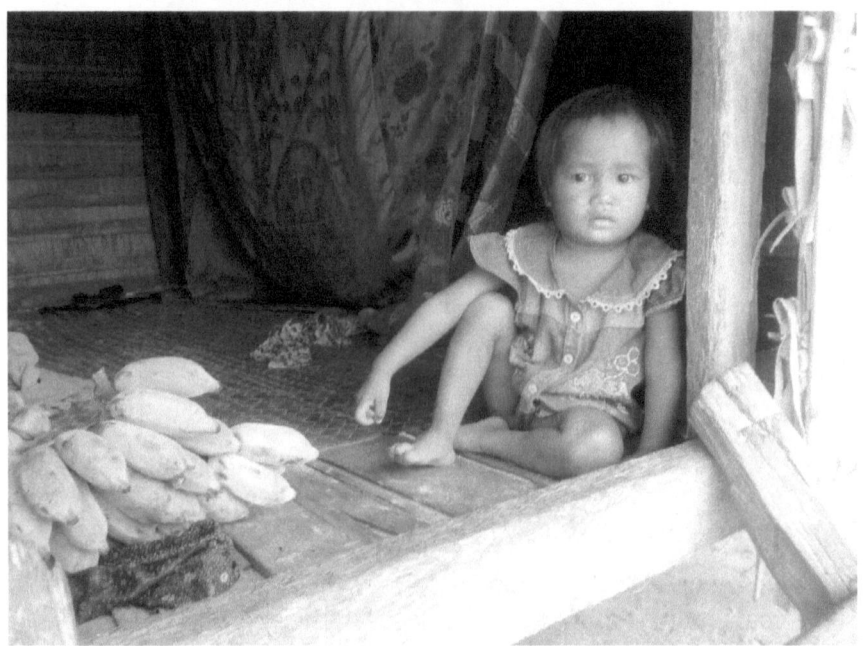

*"The Poor Family"* – Photo: Sheree Stewart

We all left that place feeling overwhelmed. There have been many attempts to help, some of the plans in place are still being done by LifeOptions, such as bringing them rice, but what else can we do? What can we do to help them that isn't rescuing them, but is helping them to find their own feet on the ground so that their children have a chance to survive and grow into healthy adults? The phrase 'give a man a fish and you feed his family for a day or teach a man to fish and you feed his family for a lifetime' feels like what needs to work here.

There are ideas of a school for that particular village so the children get a chance to be educated, clean up days each fortnight, drunk groups for the husbands.

The main thing that stays with me is not giving up hope. This family is on the brink of hopelessness. If you have nothing, at least you have hope. If you lose hope, I believe you die. So, as overwhelming as it is, we can't give up hope for The Poor Family, because it may be our hope for their futures that ultimately keeps them alive.

## *In my eyes*

Sunday, July 3, 2011

In the car, travelling around Takeo: My heart and eyes are open, and out the window is a world I have never experienced.

There are people in the rice fields, harvesting. They wear the traditional Khmer scarf, soaked in water, wrapped around their heads to keep cool. They see us and wave and smile. They have hope in their faces.

Up the road is full of brothels. The young women stand out the front with a face full of makeup and big, high shoes. They laugh when they see us and I can't help but wonder what is behind the laugh. It is nearly always the Mummies, Daddies and Aunties of these young women that actually put them there in this work to help pay off debt. A motorbike with 2 adult men and 1 small boy child pull up near one of the sex workers and starts talking. I feel sad when when I see it. These girls are forced into a life they didn't choose.

Passing by each village is a huge archway entrance. It is full of intricate designs and patterns. Huge statues of elephants, tigers, or heads are on each side of the archway. They look magnificent, lined up along the main road. I almost want to drive up each village, to see these little worlds within worlds.

There are children with big bellies. They don't have enough protein. How does that affect brain function? My heart feels so open. These children have nothing.

The weather here is so hot and sticky, so not much baby wearing happens! The baby is usually sitting on the hip of mum, dad, grandma, sister or cousin. And they often have hammocks under their homes (which are on stilts) and the baby lays in there while the elders swing, swing, swing them. I see children surrounding a hammock out the window, and one is swinging it back and forth. They are all smiling.

It's such a world of contrast here. And it makes me think of the power of the human spirit. It was only 30 years ago that Pol Pot and the horrific, unspeakable acts of the Khmer Rouge took over and destroyed everything. Cambodia truly is a place that is building everything from scratch again. They have had everything taken from them, but their human spirits, and it is that that is helping to slowly recover and rebuild this ancient Kingdom.

Out the window of the car, my heart skips a beat. The beauty and ugliness of this place is quite overwhelming.

## *Birth around the world*

Wednesday, July 6, 2011

After days of our neighbour, Noon, telling me she wants her baby born and out, her baby's birthday finally came.

Women in Cambodia often birth their babies easily and with no fuss. They walk around all during first stage, often with their mothers, stopping and holding onto something when a contraction comes, then continue on walking when the contraction passes. The majorities come in to centres during advanced labour and push their babies out. These women have incredible inner strength and resilience. They get on with what needs to be done, without being in their heads.

No one has breastfeeding problems. No one has 'not enough milk', 'too much milk' or 'my mum couldn't breastfeed so I can't' voices playing in their mind. Their babies attach to the breast sometime after birth, it doesn't have to be within the first hour and it normally isn't after time of skin to skin. It's so hot here that baby usually just lays next to Mumma, and then when baby makes a noise, Mumma picks it up and gives it breastmilk. There are not many families here that formula feed. It is simply a very dangerous choice in this country to do so, either because the water or the bottle is not clean enough and has deadly germs. I saw a sign once which said: 'Breastfed babies look like this' and there was a picture of a healthy plump child. Next to it it said 'Formula fed babies look like this': and there was a picture of a gravestone with a little flower on it.

Anyway, I'm going off track. Noon came into the centre after a restless night and morning at home. She lay on her bed on her back and we encouraged her to try a new position. She moved around freely, from her side, to the squatting, to kneeling, hardly making a sound. It was only about 2 hours of her being there that her black eyed, black haired

Khmer daughter was born. The placenta was born easily and fuss free physiologically and the cord was cut once it had stopped pulsating. Baby went to Mumma's chest and she looked relieved that her baby was here. It was beautiful.

This birth has bought up so many questions about birth around the world. Why is that it seems some cultures can just 'do birth'? These women in Cambodia all just get on with birth. They don't seem to need or want childbirth preparation classes, meditation for birth, spiritual guidance or hypnosis. It was the same in Ethiopia. No one asked for hypnosis and no one asked for epidurals or pain relief during birth. At home in the west, it seems that birth is a huge market and we all pay (me included) large amounts of money to be empowered, pain free, hypnotised, processed, zen and spiritual for our birth, and we still have an incredibly high caesarean rate and and even higher percentage of traumatised Mummas and Bubbas. Is it because in the west we are all in our heads that we physically can't get on with birth and we really do need all these other tools to help us out? Is it because in $3^{rd}$ world countries, they don't really have an option, so they just 'get on with it'? And it's not that one is right and one is wrong, it's just an observation and a thought.

One thing I have noticed from being both here and Ethiopia is that women all sit together and spend their days in each other's company. They have that village support and understanding without judgment. Is that the secret?

I don't know.

I don't have the answer.

But it has certainly got me thinking about the world and birth and the way we live within it.

## *Kindness and sharing knowledge*

Denise was approached by a midwife and asked if she can come to Cambodia to teach the midwives kindness.

This moved my heart.

# The Wild Rainbow

I feel as though it is an obvious statement to make that women deserve to be treated with kindness and respect during their pregnancy, birth and mothering days. My own experience of having my first born child in a hospital was that the staff were too busy, uncaring and had no compassion to who I was or what my experience was like. This is a huge contrast to the unassisted homebirth of my last two daughters where I had support and kindness from friends and doula's for a month post birth.

The idea of bringing kindness to birthing women reminds me of how it is easy to get caught up in our own world, in our own beliefs, in our own judgments of what a birthing mother should be, act, think, do or say. I sometimes think we are so caught up in our own beliefs that we forget to honour the woman.

The other night we watched some dvd's together. We watched women birthing while in a deep squat, women birthing in the ocean, women birthing with doulas, midwives, at home, hospital, birth centre, lotus birth, twins, women birthing with no one touching her perineum when her baby is coming earthside. It was beautiful. And after watching those dvd's it gave us a quiet sharing space of what we thought, and how we would be, or not be in some of those situations. I loved it, and felt it was so important to have that space with kindness and no judgment so that we could actually share our thoughts and question what we saw without fear of being judged.

The kindness and the sharing that took place made me feel that this is possibly the best way to start to assist these midwives. If we come in with our 'save the world' attitude, we will get nowhere. We don't actually know how these people work, and what works for them. I think when we come in to their country, into their space; we need to start with kindness and with sharing knowledge. Sharing our stories gives us perspective and may give us some common ground in which to work with. When we have this sharing of knowledge, we get mutual respect. And maybe then we can work alongside each other as we will have a better understanding of where the other is coming from.

A quick story, before I go, relating to this: when I was speaking to a midwife about lotus birth, sharing the reasons why I chose lotus birth for two of my children, and one of the reasons was because of the space it holds in the first few days. Visitors respect the space more and there is a certain quiet and observing energy around the baby. We talked about how in western culture, it's the norm for babies to be passed to everyone in the room except mum and that the mumma baby space is often interrupted and intruded. She was very interested and said she sees how people would choose lotus birth. She shared with me that they wouldn't need lotus birth here because everyone always respects the mumma baby space and no one picks up the baby unless it is grandma passing the baby from the hammock to the mothers breast. In the first month the mumma does nothing but recover and restore with her baby and her food is cooked and delivered to her. That space is just naturally honoured. Our conversation feels like a beautiful example of kindness and sharing, without judgment or blame, and it give us perspective and mutual respect.

## *Birthing and postpartum practices in Cambodia*

Monday, July 11, 2011

After a baby is born, there is a big knife placed near their head for the first month. This is so that Mother Spirit doesn't take them back home. As they get older the babies and kids have a colored string tied around their wrist or waist for the same reason. It is a protective amulet. I had to look twice when I first saw a huge meat cleaver sitting above the head of a newborn baby.

The girls all have earrings before they are one year old. Everyone thinks Myah is a beautiful boy because her ears aren't pierced.

Babies have a herb mixture that is made fresh and placed on the fontanelle with the belief that it will heal over, and perhaps protect their brain.

In the first month, the Mummas lie in bed. The food is bought to her. Her other children are around but their needs are met by other family members. It is never questioned. This is just what they do. Makes perfect sense to me!

Some women have a ritual called "roasting" post birth. Women live in elevated houses and a fire is lite under the house and extreme smoking and heat for the woman helps her regain her strength. Many mothers and babies experience burns to their bodies! They also admitted, it helps to keep the men away from them sexually for 7 days.

## Midwife Extraordinaire

Wednesday, July 13, 2011

Pec is an amazing midwife who works solo at a village birth centre. She is responsible for the health of the village which has around 10,000 people. On her own, she is the midwife for approximately 30 – 40 births per month and around 5 abortions.

She does everything relating to health of women and babies that needs to be done, whether that is STD checks, breast checks, antenatal, postpartum and birth care, discussions about birth spacing, sex and caring for a newborn. She has incredible skill and an incredible commitment and passion to help the people in her village. She is at the centre pretty much 24/7 and rarely comes out of the village.

She transports women who need emergency care to a hospital when they need it. She deals with hemorrhaging post abortion and birth, babies not breathing, women with eclampsia all on her own in a village health centre with barely any resources. She is midwife extraordinaire.

## Orphanage

Friday, July 15, 2011

Not far passed the Birth Centre is an orphanage that LifeOptions donates clothes and books to. We went for a visit there today.

Many curious, shy faces peered from behind the walls. Many smiled, many waved, and some simply stared.

I always feel such a dark heaviness to see children who have no love.

But it seems that as well as no love, these children will soon have no food.

Journeying as Sage Femme

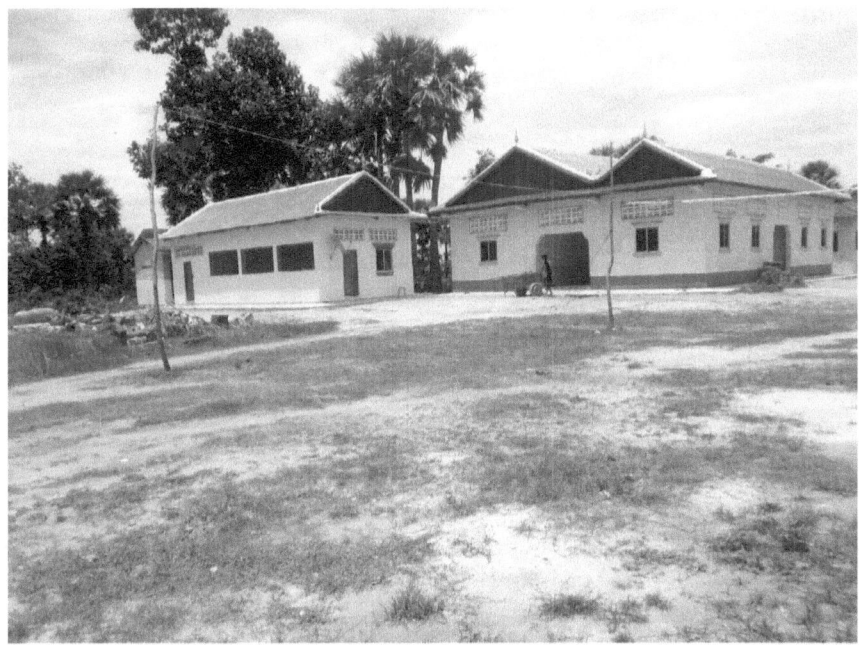

*"The Orphanage"* – Photo: Sheree Stewart

UNICEF has done an amazing thing by making a promise to pay for the food of these children for three years. At the end of this month, the 3 years is up. There is going to be no food.

I find this extremely distressing, especially when I think of families back home who spend $600 per week on food shopping alone with families of only 4! It costs $500 per month to feed the orphans a nutritious diet.

And the distressing thing is that it isn't just this Orphanage. There are many Orphanages around Cambodia that in the same position.

It's so hard. This Earth is a place of such extremes.

## *Thankyou Cambodia*

Saturday, July 16, 2011

My time in Cambodia is almost up! Tomorrow afternoon Myah and I start the long journey home.

It's been a month. One whole amazing month to observe, learn and experience the way of life for the Khmer people.

I've been thinking of my highlights, what things have touched me the most, and what things gave me the most joy. I'd like to share with you some of these amazing moments in my life.

The biggest one is that I actually managed to get me and my baby to Cambodia all by myself! That was a huge step to freedom to me, a huge step to independence, of being a strong woman, a capable woman, a woman who follows her heart. It reminded me of my own potential and capabilities as a human being. I can step out of the box and allow myself to experience the bigger world that is out there.

Other amazing moments involve mostly just hanging out with the Khmer people. I learned so much from their behavior, their way of life by being present with them. Myah and I would hang out with the kids next door, all the mumma's gathered at the little stall, the teenage orphan who lived in the next room to me (who was a part of LifeOptions 'Spread Your Wings And Fly Program'), and the midwives all working downstairs. We would chat, not speaking much of each-others language, but we would laugh and sign and have fun. I'm sure Myah was speaking Khmer with them! She would say something, and they would all giggle and say 'khmer, khmer!'

I got to be a part of our neighbour's birth. It was beautiful and simple. Women in Cambodia are strong. They have so much courage.

Sharing information and having education sessions with the midwives was lovely. We shared our customs and our ideas around birth. I talked to them about some practices in the West, such as lotus birth, water birth, doula support and physiological $3^{rd}$ stage.

Being able to help set up a new Birth Centre was fun! Organising the antenatal room, the postnatal ward, the STD clinic and the postpartum ward was just so exciting, I really love organising and setting up spaces, so having the opportunity to help set up a whole Birth Centre was a dream!

Being a part of the Blessing for the Birth Centre! The monks came and began and ended with chanting, and after each segment of chanting, the circle of people present would move forward an inch and the monks would continue to chant and bless the people and space with chant, water and flower petals. It was really special to be a part of and to be so welcomed into ancient ceremony. The ceremony finished and we drank iced tea and cold lychee drinks.

Meeting amazing people! I have never known resilience until I came to Cambodia. I have talked to some extraordinary human beings. The Traditional Birth Attendants are full of knowledge of a different kind, and I admire them greatly. I've met midwives who were trained in the Border Camps during Pol Pot times. They have incredible skill, more than any western midwife I have ever met. I have heard stories of resilience and the power of the human spirit. The beautiful midwife here at the Centre shared stories of when she was a little girl in Pol Pot times, who walked for a month with no food through the mountains. I've met several people, including one of the 7 only survivors of the prison camp of the Khmer Rouge. He is an old man, with sad eyes, who saw the most atrocious acts of human evil. I've met with poor families out in the remote villages, who don't have names, orphanages that are about to run out of food, 100's of women who come in to centre for STDs who choose us over the other centres because we are kind. I've met the kids at the school, their faces so happy with minds enthusiastic and eager to learn.

It's been life changing being here. My eyes are open, my heart is full. It's been such a privilege to be here. I'll come back one day, when my kids are older, and the time is right. But now it's time for me to come home.

Thank you Cambodia. You are a country of resilient, courageous and strong human beings. I honour you.

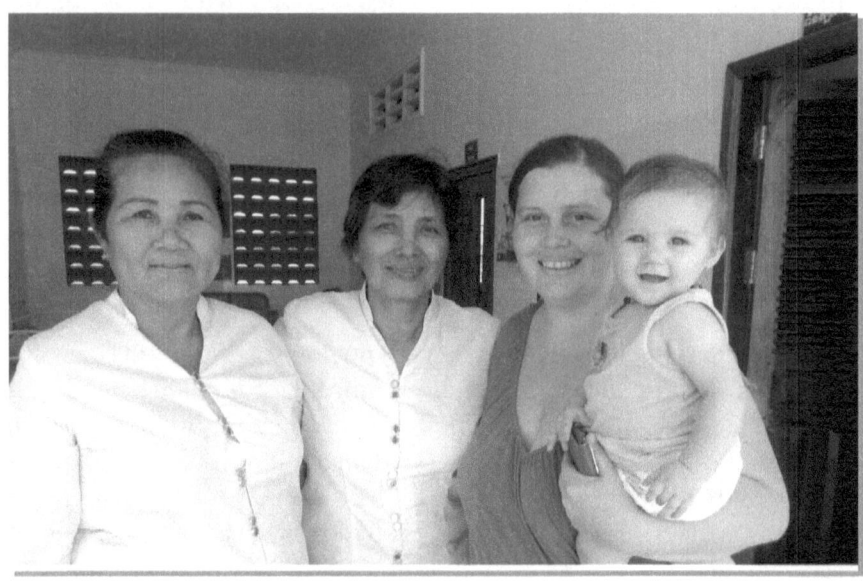

*"Women's Health Cambodia"* – Photo: Denise Love

*The world is not separate from you and me. There is a common thread of relationship weaving us all together. Deep down we are all totally connected...*

Satish Kumar

## *Earth Midwife*

There she goes, with her long coloured hair, happy in her heart, singing her own song.

She plants her herbs, watches them grow and makes them into medicines, salves and tinctures.

She waters her plants and lets the sun shine down on them.

She waters her spirit and lets the sun shine down on her.

She knows the ancient ways, the secrets of the earth, because she listens to the earth.

She follows the cycles of the moon, and acts accordingly.

She follows her intuition and is guided by her heart knowledge as well as her head knowledge. She is not easily fooled and she has her wits about her.

She hears the call of women with their birthsongs', and she hears the call of the earth, as it pulses deep and long, waiting to be tended to.

She heals herself first so that she can be healer.

She is present to her journey, she is courageous, she is lion fireheart.

She goes to bed at night knowing that she may be woken by the call of birth, by the call of earth, by the essence of spirit.

She is the witness to all things sacred. She is constantly alive and part of the magic.

She is the one who witnesses the babies first cry and the flowers first bloom.

She is the one who is courageous and willing, humble and kind, soft and strong. She is the tree does not break, but bends as she needs to.

She is the one who remembers.

> *You are a divine being. You matter, you count. You come from realms of unimaginable power and light, and you will return to those realms.*
>
> - TERENCE MCKENNA

## *Afterword*

> *And the day came when the risk to remain tight in a bud was more painful than the risk it took to blossom.*
>
> - ANAIS NIN

So, here I am. What started off as journals, as stories I shared with my friends, as fears that lurked like shadowy monsters in my head in the night, as poetry I wrote that I thought no one would ever see, has now become my book of love.

Although I always dreamed as a little barefoot, blonde haired girl in the Mallee of writing stories that others would read, to me it seemed like a world far away, a world I thought may never exist or be possible to visit.

I was always, and still am, so shy and never felt worthy enough to have people listen to my stories. But over the years, my fascination of listening to the lives of others – of listening to their heartaches, their triumphs and their own impossible dreams, made me realise how important sharing stories is to healing the soul.

Sharing stories really does heal us. It is medicine. Word medicine. It unsticks us from ourselves; it takes us out of the mud and places us on a spiral. It connects us. It unites us. Sharing stories changes us and inspires us, making us cry and laugh and give us new directions and perspectives on the world we live in.

Having had all this written down, my life until now, I am feeling so free. It feels as though my life from this point now is a new adventure. It is as though these past 30 years, I have been the flower in its bud gestating. Growing strong enough, nourished enough until I was at a point where I could feel the world that was holding me move and quiver. The pain of that quivering was so intense that even with living an already busy life with then 5 children (pregnant and birthed my 6$^{th}$ baby in the making of this book) plus relationships, work and life in general, I had to write this book.

It was a burning urge, a writing passion overflow, an explosion that consumed me so much that I could do nothing about it, but ride with it. The more I tried to fight it and resist it, the more it hurt.

At times it was challenging. There were many times when my children needed my attention right when I was in the midst of a creative wave and I had to put that creative wave on hold, which was incredibly frustrating. But knowing that I couldn't put my parenting on hold, I mostly learned to hold in the words, as frustrating as it was, until the rare times when I could write them out uninterrupted.

And now it is finished and I feel like I am at the beginning of something new. Of something so beautiful that I cannot even see it yet. I can feel it in my bones that my life can be more beautiful than what I could ever imagine it to be in my wildest dreams. And this writing down of myself has been what has set me free. This has been a birthing of myself. Even though it was painful; it has been what has bought me home.

I welcome my new world now. And I welcome all of it with courage, authenticity, humbleness, clarity and love.

Thank you for journeying with me. May your life be blessed with bliss, love and magic and be full of joy and big, jolly, uncontrollable belly laughs.

## *Contributors*

### *Julie Bell*

Julie Bell is a mother of three daughters and a son, all born at home – in Ireland, New Zealand and Australia. Julie and her American husband lived in Asia for nearly 20 years and moved to Australia in 2004. She completed her doula training here and is the WAHM of Blissful Herbs, which provides therapeutic herbal teas and topical herbs, specialising in women's health. Motivated by justice for all, Julie is a passionate activist for human rights, reconciliation, the environment, women's rights & gender equality, the welfare of refugees and immigrants, and of course, birth rights.

http://blissfulherbs.blogspot.com.au

### *Simone Surgeoner*

Simone Surgeoner is mother to four divine creatures of the female form, ranging from 1yo to 15yo. The first two were born in water – in a birth centre, the third in water – unassisted at home and the fourth, very lucky child, was born on the banks of a creek in the Daintree Rainforest. Simone is a Journey Practitioner (Brandon Bays) and Doula. Her passion is human potential and living as purely as possible, whether that be eating a high raw food diet, clearing stuck emotional energy and limiting beliefs, or giving birth in nature.

www.birthinnature.com.au

### *Jessica Pritchard*

Jess is mumma to four amazing souls, following her passion of supporting women through all major life changes. Dedicated hypnotherapist, doula and childbirth educator, she currently spends her time between Sydney and rural Victoria.

## Contributors

*Avalon Darnesh*

Avalon facilitates heart connection & authentic self-expression through coaching, workshops and creative arts. She inspires women to embrace their feminine essence for more flow, joy and fulfilment in their lives. Avalon honours motherhood as a sacred path and intimacy as a doorway to transformation and runs various programs for women, including 'The Sacred Journey of Pregnancy', 'Mama Nurture' for healing birth and motherhood, and 'Full Bloom' Coaching Packages. See more on her website:

http://www.blossomingwoman.com.au


*Charlie Young*

Charlie Young is a writer and movement meditations facilitator. Her debut novel will be out later this year; Ora's Gold is a story for young adults about birth, death the imagination and love.
When Charlie isn't busy mothering or writing she offers workshops to women and girls where she encourages them to connect with their bodies through movement and the imagination.
Charlie lives close to Melbourne and the Yarra River with her life partner, three children, dog and cat.
www.charlieyoung.com.au


*Denise Love*

Denise is an internationally recognised educator in sound antenatal, safe birthing, neonatal care, breastfeeding and family planning practices that are congruent with the cultural needs of the client demographic. Established in 1988, LifeOptions today delivers training across Australia, Thailand, Cambodia and consults to agencies and individuals in India and Nepal.
"I believe everybody has the right to choose how and where they live, how and where they give birth. I believe all people are good, but can be driven by life experiences to behave differently."
"I know that the way we are born, influences the way we live our lives"
Peace on earth begins at birth

http://www.lifeoptions.asia

### Jane Hardwicke Collings

Jane is a homebirth mother, midwife and grandmother.

She is a Priestess of the Goddess and serves with a mission to help women reclaim feminine power through reconnection with the women's mysteries. She facilitates workshops, presents at conferences and is author of several books: Ten Moons - the Inner Journey of Pregnancy, Thirteen Moons - the how to chart your menstrual cycle handbook and journal, Spinning Wheels - a guide to the cycles, Becoming a Woman - a guide for girls approaching menarche. Jane founded and teaches at The School of Shamanic Midwifery - a Women's Mystery School in NSW, Australia:

http://www.moonsong.com.au/
http://www.schoolofshamanicmidwifery.com/
http://www.placentalremedy.com/
http://schoolofshamanicmidwifery.blogspot.com/
http://janehardwickecollings-moonsong.blogspot.com/

### Janet Fraser

Janet Fraser is the National Convener of the Australian Homebirth Network, Joyous Birth. She lives in Sydney and divides her time between community birth education, birth activism, supporting women and families in healing from birth trauma. She has been writing since she was seven. She writes because she has to and reads because not to do so would thus appear churlish. She prefers cake. She is on a lifelong odyssey to locate the best coffee. She is clearly over run with bourgeois notions and pastimes and therefore with sufficient time to advocate revolutions of various kinds in the best white, middle class tradition. She is intimidated by poetry and startled when it emerges from her keyboard but persists nonetheless. She hopes to live a very long time and see social change unfold worldwide. Sometimes things she writes end up on t-shirts which is an unusual form of publishing but better than the alternative.

http://www.joyousbirth.info/
http://janetfraser.id.au

# Contributors

*Shivam Rachana*

Shivam Rachana is the founding principal of the International College of Spiritual Midwifery and was co-director of the Centre for Human Transformation, a residential spiritual community, for 28 years. Rachana's teaching career spans 40 years. A pioneer of conscious birthing practices since the 1970's and specialising in Water Birth and Lotus Birth, she brings insight to the significance of the pre- and perinatal experience and teaches the healing of birth trauma. Her 'Women's Mysteries' 5 day retreat program, attended by thousands of women during the past 25 years, connects women to the source of their feminine power and wisdom. She trains Doula's and Rebirther's. Her book, Lotus Birth, now in its second edition and translated into Italian, Polish and Czech, is a world-first publication. She is the executive director of the acclaimed DVD The Water birth Of The Malcolm Twins and co-author of The Tantric Path. For further information on Rachana's work, please visit:

http://www.womenofspirit.asn.au

*Dr Sarah Buckley*

Sarah is a NZ-trained GP, mother of four homeborn children and currently a full-time writer on pregnancy, birth and parenting. She is author of the bestselling book Gentle Birth, Gentle Mothering, with a new edition published in 2009. Sarah's work critiques current practices in pregnancy, birth and parenting from the widest possible perspectives, including scientific, evolutionary, psychological and personal.

For more about Sarah and her work, including her new membership website see www.sarahbuckley.com and www.gentlenaturalbirth.com

*Mikailah Rachael Gooda*

Mikailah is a Shamanee Medicine Woman and her deep passion is healing the Songlines within Mother Earth.

In her intuitive work, Mikailah celebrates the cycles of nature, the moon & the stars. She creates a place of truth & beauty to support people in remembering their natural state of Being through ceremony, creative therapies and instinctual body wisdom.

Mikailah embraces all Relations and connects to the Earth energies and Star Consciousness. This is the language spoken from her heart. She is a dancer between the Worlds ~ mystical, yet very earthy.

Mikailah offers private consultations for both men & women, combining her unique style of soul astrology, along with spirit messages and ceremonial smudging.

Her eclectic and unorthodox journey has honed her skills of intuition. She shares in a down to earth, compassionate way, offering spiritual guidance, wisdom and understanding.

She also presents 'Medicine Woman' private sessions, where women deepen their understanding of their connection to the Cosmic Earth Mother & the Shamanee.

http://www.mikailah.com

### *Kerry Baulch*

Kerry is a mother of 3 amazingly lovely children that brighten up her day the min the wake up and give her cuddles. She has a wonderful husband that loves and supports her no matter what her dreams are and where they lead them. She welcomes all into her life with no judgment and will run the min they drop a line asking for help. Kerry has just recently decided to open up more to her spiritual side and go where life takes her enjoying every moment that comes along and the friends and loved ones that take that journey with her.

### *Sarah Langford*

Sarah Langford is a mother of two freebirthed/lotus born girls (expecting a third baby at the time of writing). She is a birth servant or doula, who trained at the International College of Spiritual Midwifery in 2008. Sarah is a fierce advocate for homebirth and breastfeeding. More of Sarah's writing can be found on her website

http://ilithyiainspired.com

## Contributors

*Bree Downes*

Bree is a mother of 3 beautiful children and she lives in the luscious Dandenong Ranges. Her first son being born in 2006 via caesarean after 'failure to progress' through the hospital system. In 2009 her second son was born, a repeat caesarean, after an attempted home birth did not progress. She became a doula in 2009, completing her training with Rhea Dempsey, and achieved a beautiful vaginal birth at home with her daughter in 2010. She is very passionate about informed, empowered and 'present' birth, in whatever form it takes for that mothers' journey. Her own birthing journey has opened her heart to being a woman, mother and sister, and she deeply holds that light for every woman and friend she supports.

Facebook Page: Bree Downes Birth Support


*Lauren Gibbins*

Lauren is a young single mama who lives in the mountains with her 2 wild daughters.
They can usually be found adventuring with their community of wayward parents and kids or drinking tea in their garden.
She is passionate about human rights and empowering women and is currently at university putting into reality her dream of becoming a travelling midwife.
She spends all of her spare time spinning on a Spanish web at the women's circus because it makes her happy.


*Tamara Travaglia*

Tamara is a single mum to 3 amazing young children. Aside from being a full time mama and a milk making machine for her two youngest, she likes to get out in the sunshine as much as possible, check out local cafes and drink lots of good coffee with her friends. She is passionate about all things pregnancy, birth and breastfeeding and hopes to one day further her lactation knowledge and help and support women and their babies to breastfeed successfully.

### Steven Booth

Steven is Sheree's husband, and dedicated father of their six children. Steven is teacher of Qigong, Meditation, and the internal martial arts of Taijiquan and Baguazhang. Steven is also a deeply empathetic and intuitive healer, and a practitioner of Oriental Medicine. He is passionate about helping others reach their potential and live a full, heart driven, and meaningful life.

Primarily using Shiatsu therapy as the basis for his treatments, Steven deals with Transpersonal and Esoteric elements in his work. Steven is particularly interested in working with people that are experiencing shifts on the emotional and psycho-spiritual levels, and who are transitioning through various kinds personal or spiritual transformations.

http://www.melbournetaiji.com
http://www.sevenstarshiatsu.com.au

### Star Davis

Cornflakes. Cornflakes, cornflakes, cornflakes. Cornflakes, cornflakes. Cornflakes. Cornflakes. Cornflakes. Cornflakes. That is all. Oh, and she is also the Mother of 2 superhero babies, Seven Blaez and Raven Starr.

### Lucy Johnston

Lucy is a daughter, granddaughter, sister, doula and midwife. As life has unfolded so has her fascination with birth, pregnancy, sisterhood and all domains of the feminine. She feels honoured to be a birth worker and blessed to know the women she knows, or has met, through this line of work (or rather, line of passion). This is her calling in life – an urge even – to support and preserve the sacred art of giving birth, in any small way she can. To empower women in their womanhood, their bodies - to normalise birth. She believe that women are amazing- they are strong – and she is so deeply blessed to know birth the way that she does.

# Contributors

### *Annette Joy*

Annie was born in Altona 1961 and is the fifth child out of seven children. Her mother is Australian Aboriginal and father Australian/English. Her life journey so far is from the sea to the Mallee, and she has mothered 3 amazing Mallee born children, Adam, Sheree and Kyana.

Her love and life are her children and grandchildren, art and nature. She creates art and crafts from her heart and from life. Her animal totems are the Black Cockatoo/Pelican and Earth totem is Thunder. She is a descendant of the Gourmjanyuk and Wergaiia tribes.

### *Melanie Rees (Daisy Mabel)*

Melanie's art is inspired by the many special, magical, moments that come from being a mother. She is also deeply spiritual and inspired by the wonders of the natural world. Melanie is mother to five children and she has been creating art for over 24 years. She is a passionate natural birth advocate and is a certified doula. Mel is well on her way to becoming a certified childbirth educator.

http://daisymabel.weebly.com

### *Melissa Shemanna - Visionary Artist*

Living in the beautiful Yarra Valley in Victoria, Australia. On a Sustainable Co-op Community called Moora Moora, which is situated on the apex of Mt Toolebewong. Melissa and her two children; Jasper and Liwanu live in a beautiful octagonal, solar powered, spring water fed home of natural organic abundance and creativity.

http://www.honeybeetemple.com.au

### Brooke Patel

Brooke Patel is a daughter, granddaughter, wife, lover and mother to 3 beautiful, spirited, lively boys who make her heart burst with love and her eardrums burst with noise!

Besides having her arms full being loved by so many little men, she enjoys having a coffee (or wine!) with friends, listening to good tunes, banging on a djembe and the occasional sleep-in.

She is passionate about conscious, loving, present birth and parenting. Her calling in life has taken her to become a professional photographer where she has the great honour of capturing blossoming bellies, birth in all its glory, beautiful, squishy newborns and other magical moments. This gives her great joy!

http://www.brookepatel.com.au

### Courtney Gale

Courtney Gale is a passionate mother, lover and healer. In touch with her calling to be the mother of many, she loves to nourish, nurture and support. She believes women should feel supported through their childhood, menarche, pregnancies, birth and motherhood, so that they can love and give to their calling and creativity, whether this is in the form of a baby or projects.

Courtney is currently gathering the tools to support people grow through their experiences, so that they can find their strength within. Some of these tools have been learned through doula work, Birth into Being traineeship, holistic counselling, energetic work and now excitingly and passionately, kinesiology.

http://www.nourishinggrowth.com.au

## *About the Author*

Sheree is a woman, a mother and a midwife. She is the mother of 6 wild hearted, freespirited children and the wife of a very patient and loving man. Raised under the hot sun of the Mallee, she moved to Melbourne when she was 16 with her sweetheart, who is now her husband. Following her heart, she became a midwife, and continues to journey this path, answering the call of being with women. As well as being with women in birth, in her independent business, BirthSong, she runs women's circles, antenatal classes, mother and baby groups, infant massage sessions and a range of workshops all with the focus on women's health and wellbeing. She has travelled far with her work, ranging from working independently to large inner city private hospitals, tertiary level public hospitals, small rural hospitals and birth centres in Ethiopia and Cambodia. She believes that birth matters. That women matter. That we all matter.

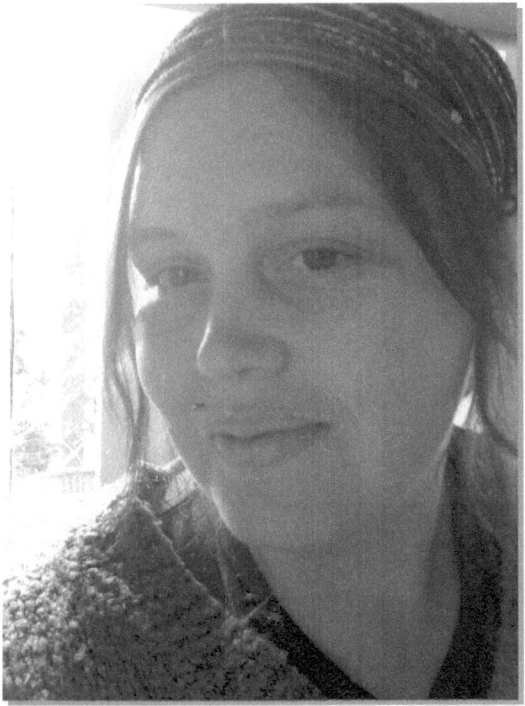

She likes to spend her days in the sunshine drinking tea, chatting about nothing and everything with those closest to her. Her life is full of messy faced children, a rainbow tribe of women whose hearts sing the same as her own and a wonderful man to continuously reminds her who she is. Besides the obvious love of writing and creating, she also loves big belly laughs and drinking wine, gazing at the moon, singing (especially when no one else can hear her) and being snuggled by the arms of those that love her.

## The Wild Rainbow

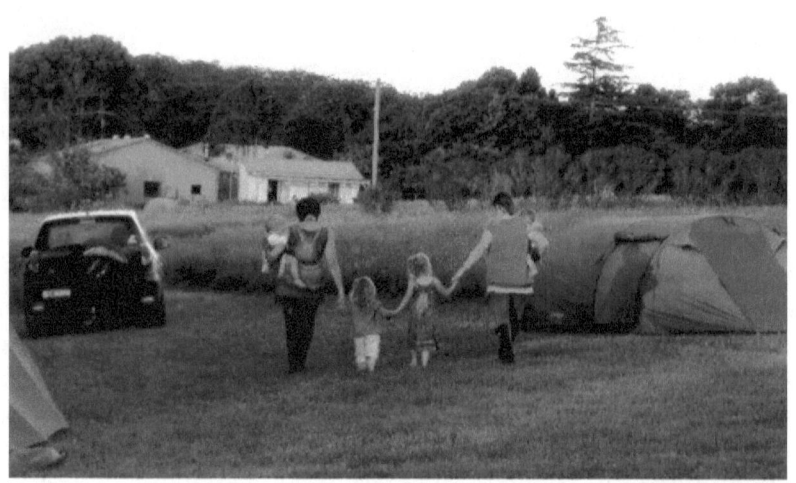

*"A school of mermaids"* – Photo: Jane Hardwicke Collings

I promised all the Rainbowbabies that their names will be in my book. So, my big love to the next generation of children who will one day soon be the ones in the forefront, making the change. Love you all:

Caelan, Rhiannon, Aaliyah, Sage, Myah, Eli, Kyana, Lusimba, Taioma, Jasper, Seven, Raven, Zakiyya, Milan, Taj, Lilith, Indigo, Jack Jack, Aliyah, Klarysa, Trystan, Ollie, Wil, Archie, Malachai, Jasper, Tuesday, Skye, Max, Marnie, Nyah, Amelia, Blake, Imogen, Woodley

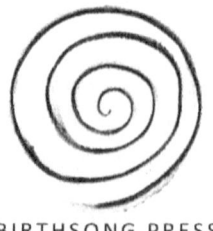

BIRTHSONG PRESS

www.ingramcontent.com/pod-product-compliance
Lightning Source LLC
Chambersburg PA
CBHW030238170426
**43202CB00007B/44**